Psychiatric Genetics

Guest Editor

JAMES B. POTASH, MD, MPH

PSYCHIATRIC CLINICS OF NORTH AMERICA

www.psych.theclinics.com

March 2010 • Volume 33 • Number 1

SAUNDERS an imprint of ELSEVIER, Inc.

W.B. SAUNDERS COMPANY
A Division of Elsevier Inc.

1600 John F. Kennedy Boulevard ● Suite 1800 ● Philadelphia, PA 19103-2899

http://www.theclinics.com

PSYCHIATRIC CLINICS OF NORTH AMERICA Volume 33, Number 1
March 2010 ISSN 0193-953X, ISBN-13: 978-1-4377-1867-6

Editor: Sarah E. Barth
Developmental Editor: Donald Mumford

Psychiatric Clinics of North America (ISSN 0193-953X) is published quarterly by Elsevier Inc., 360 Park Avenue South, New York, NY 10010-1710. Months of issue are March, June, September, and December. Business and Editorial Offices: 1600 John F. Kennedy Blvd., Suite 1800, Philadelphia, PA 19103-2899. Periodicals postage paid at New York, NY and additional mailing offices. Subscription prices are $248.00 per year (US individuals), $430.00 per year (US institutions), $125.00 per year (US students/residents), $297.00 per year (Canadian individuals), $535.00 per year (Canadian Institutions), $369.00 per year (foreign individuals), $535.00 per year (foreign institutions), and $185.00 per year (international & Canadian students/residents). Foreign air speed delivery is included in all *Clinics'* subscription prices. All prices are subject to change without notice. **POSTMASTER:** Send address changes to *Psychiatric Clinics of North America*, Elsevier Health Sciences Division, Subscription Customer Service, 3251 Riverport Lane, Maryland Heights, MO 63043. Customer Service: 1-800-654-2452 (US). From outside the United States, call 1-314-447-8871. Fax: 1-314-447-8029. E-mail: journalscustomerservice-usa@elsevier.com (for print support) and journalsonlinesupport-usa@elsevier.com (for online support).

Reprints. For copies of 100 or more, of articles in this publication, please contact the Commercial Reprints Department, Elsevier Inc., 360 Park Avenue South, New York, New York 10010-1710. Tel.: (212) 633-3813, Fax: (212) 462-1935, E-mail: reprints@elsevier.com.

Psychiatric Clinics of North America is covered in *MEDLINE/PubMed (Index Medicus)*, *Current Contents/Social and Behavioral Sciences*, *Social Science Citation Index*, *Embase/Excerpta Medica*, and PsycINFO.

Printed and bound by CPI Group (UK) Ltd, Croydon, CR0 4YY

Transferred to Digital Print 2011

Contributors

GUEST EDITOR

JAMES B. POTASH, MD, MPH
Arlene and Robert Kogod Associate Professor of Psychiatry and Medicine, Johns Hopkins
School of Medicine, Baltimore, Maryland

AUTHORS

DIMITRIOS AVRAMOPOULOS, MD, PhD
Associate Professor, Department of Psychiatry, McKusick Nathans Institute of Genetic
Medicine, Johns Hopkins School of Medicine, Baltimore, Maryland

KELLY S. BENKE, PhD
Department of Epidemiology, Johns Hopkins Bloomberg School of Public Health,
Baltimore, Maryland

LAURA J. BIERUT, MD
Professor, Department of Psychiatry, Washington University School of Medicine,
St. Louis, Missouri

JENNIFER DONALD, BA, PhD
Associate Professor, Department of Biological Sciences, Macquarie University,
Sydney, New South Wales, Australia

JUBAO DUAN, PhD
Department of Psychiatry and Behavioral Sciences; and Research Institute, Center
for Psychiatric Genetics, NorthShore University HealthSystem Research Institute,
Evanston, Illinois

PAUL EL-FISHAWY, MD, JD
Post-Doctoral Fellow, Child Study Center; Department of Genetics, Yale University School
of Medicine, New Haven, Connecticut

M. DANIELE FALLIN, PhD
Associate Professor, Department of Epidemiology, Johns Hopkins Bloomberg School
of Public Health, Baltimore, Maryland

STEPHEN V. FARAONE, PhD
Professor, Department of Psychiatry and Behavioral Sciences; Department of
Neuroscience & Physiology, SUNY Upstate Medical University, Syracuse, New York

JANICE FULLERTON, BSc, PhD
Senior Research Officer, Prince of Wales Medical Research Centre, Prince of Wales
Medical Research Institute, Randwick, Sydney, New South Wales, Australia

PABLO V. GEJMAN, MD
Department of Psychiatry and Behavioral Sciences; and Research Institute, Center
for Psychiatric Genetics, NorthShore University HealthSystem Research Institute,
Evanston, Illinois

MARCO GRADOS, MD, MSc
Assistant Professor, Department of Psychiatry and Behavioral Sciences, Johns Hopkins
School of Medicine, Johns Hopkins Hospital, Baltimore, Maryland

STEVEN P. HAMILTON, MD, PhD
Associate Professor, Carol Cochran Schaffner Endowed Chair, Department of Psychiatry,
Langley Porter Psychiatric Institute, University of California, San Francisco,
San Francisco, California

SARAH M. HARTZ, MD, PhD
Instructor, Department of Psychiatry, Washington University School of Medicine,
St. Louis, Missouri

JENNIFER T. JUDY, MS
Department of Mental Health, Johns Hopkins Bloomberg School of Public Health,
Baltimore, Maryland

BETTINA MEISER, PhD
Head of Psychosocial Research Group, Department of Medical Oncology, Prince
of Wales Clinical School, Prince of Wales Hospital, University of New South Wales,
Randwick, Sydney, New South Wales, Australia

ERIC MICK, ScD
Assistant Professor, Department of Psychiatry, Massachusetts General Hospital and
Harvard Medical School, Boston, Massachusetts

PHILIP B. MITCHELL, MBBS, MD, FRANZCP, FRCPsych
Scientia Professor and Head, School of Psychiatry, Prince of Wales Hospital,
Randwick; Director, Bipolar Disorders Clinic, Black Dog Institute; Convenor,
Brain Sciences UNSW, University of New South Wales, Sydney,
New South Wales, Australia

GERALD NESTADT, MD, MPH
Professor, Department of Psychiatry and Behavioral Sciences, Johns Hopkins
School of Medicine, Johns Hopkins Hospital, Baltimore, Maryland

JACK F. SAMUELS, PhD
Assistant Professor, Department of Psychiatry and Behavioral Sciences, Johns Hopkins
School of Medicine, Johns Hopkins Hospital, Baltimore, Maryland

ALAN R. SANDERS, MD
Department of Psychiatry and Behavioral Sciences; and Research Institute, Center
for Psychiatric Genetics, NorthShore University HealthSystem Research Institute,
Evanston, Illinois

PETER R. SCHOFIELD, PhD, DSc
Executive Director and CEO, Prince of Wales Medical Research Institute, Randwick;
School of Medical Sciences; Brain Sciences UNSW, University of New South Wales,
Sydney, New South Wales, Australia

THOMAS G. SCHULZE, MD
Assistant Director of Clinical Research, Unit on the Genetic Basis of Mood and Anxiety
Disorders, National Institute of Mental Health (NIMH), National Institutes of Health (NIH),
Bethesda; Department of Psychiatry and Behavioral Sciences, Johns Hopkins University,
Baltimore, Maryland; Department of Genetic Epidemiology in Psychiatry, Central Institute
of Mental Health, Mannheim, Germany

STANLEY I. SHYN, MD, PhD
Research Fellow, Department of Psychiatry, Langley Porter Psychiatric Institute, University of California, San Francisco, San Francisco, California

MATTHEW W. STATE, MD, PhD
Donald J. Cohen Associate Professor of Child Psychiatry, Child Study Center; Associate Professor, Department of Genetics; Deputy Chairman for Research, Department of Psychiatry; Co-Director Program on Neurogenetics, Yale University School of Medicine, New Haven, Connecticut

ALEX WILDE, BSc, MA
PhD Student, School of Psychiatry, University of New South Wales, Prince of Wales Hospital, Randwick, Sydney, New South Wales, Australia

KAY WILHELM, MBBS, MD, FRANZCP
Conjoint Professor, School of Psychiatry, Consultation Liaison Psychiatry, University of New South Wales, Sydney, New South Wales, Australia

PETER P. ZANDI, PhD
Associate Professor, Department of Mental Health, Johns Hopkins Bloomberg School of Public Health, Baltimore, Maryland

Contents

The practice of psychiatry has long suffered from the limited information available on the biological basis of mental disorders. This limitation is now coming to an end. Advances in DNA analysis technologies and in our understanding of the human genome, together with our new knowledge of the properties of the genome and significant efforts toward generating large patient and control sample collections, have paved the way for successful genome-wide association studies. As a result, reports now appear in the literature every week identifying new genes for complex disorders. Next-generation sequencing methods, combined with the results of association and perhaps linkage studies, will help us uncover missing heritability factors, achieve a better understanding of the genetic aspects of psychiatric disease, and devise the best strategies for incorporating genetics in the service of patients.

Given the potential benefits of gene identification in psychiatry, genetic epidemiology has become a mainstream discipline within the field. This article discusses the main tools for gene discovery. The focus is on the designs and analytic approaches for each of these methods. Because most gene discovery has now moved to genetic association studies, and most recently to genome-wide association studies, the focus is on methods for this design. Also highlighted are the current challenges of genetic epidemiology as a prelude to future approaches that may be applied to psychiatric disorders in the coming years.

Schizophrenia is a complex genetic disorder manifesting combined environmental and genetic causation. Recently, genome-wide association experiments yielded remarkable new experimental evidence that is leading to a better understanding of the genetic models and the biological risk factors involved in schizophrenia. These studies have discovered uncommon copy number variations (mainly deletions) and common single nucleotide polymorphisms with alleles associated with schizophrenia. The aggregate data provide support for polygenic inheritance and for genetic overlap of schizophrenia with autism and with bipolar disorder. It is anticipated that the application of a myriad of tools from systems biology, in combination with biological functional experiments, will lead to a delineation of biological pathways involved in the pathophysiology of schizophrenia, and eventually to new therapies.

Genetic Research into Bipolar Disorder: The Need for a Research Framework that Integrates Sophisticated Molecular Biology and Clinically Informed Phenotype Characterization

Thomas G. Schulze

Research into the genetic basis of bipolar disorder (BD) has reached a turning point. Genome-wide association studies (GWAS), encompassing several thousand samples, have produced replicated evidence for some novel susceptibility genes; however, the genetic variants implicated so far account for only a fraction of disease liability, a phenomenon not limited to psychiatric phenotypes but characteristic of all complex genetic traits studied to date. It appears that pure genomic approaches, such as GWAS alone, will not suffice to unravel the genetic basis of a complex illness like BD. Genomic approaches will need to be complemented by a variety of strategies, including phenomics, epigenomics, pharmacogenomics, and neurobiology, as well as the study of environmental factors. This review highlights the most promising findings from recent GWAS and candidate gene studies in BD. It furthermore sketches out a potential research framework integrating various lines of research into the molecular biological basis of BD.

The Genetics of Autism: Key Issues, Recent Findings, and Clinical Implications

Paul El-Fishawy and Matthew W. State

Autism spectrum disorders (ASDs) are highly heritable. Gene discovery promises to help illuminate the pathophysiology of these syndromes, yielding opportunities for the development of novel treatments and understanding of their natural history. Although the underlying genetic architecture of ASDs is not yet known, the literature demonstrates that it is not a monogenic disorder with mendelian inheritance, rather a group of complex genetic syndromes with risk deriving from genetic variations in multiple genes. This article reviews the origins of the common versus rare variant debate, highlights recent findings in the field, and addresses the clinical implications of common and rare variant discoveries.

Genetics of Addictions

Sarah M. Hartz and Laura J. Bierut

Addictions include a group of common, heritable psychiatric illnesses that have multiple psychiatric and medical comorbidities. Robust genetic associations have been found for alcohol dependence, nicotine dependence, and cocaine dependence. Common genetic associations have been found between alcohol dependence and aerodigestive cancers and between nicotine dependence and lung disease. These associations highlight the importance of understanding the genetics of substance dependence in the context of its multiple medical and psychiatric comorbidities.

Efforts to unlock the biology of major depressive disorder (MDD) are proceeding on multiple fronts. In this article, the authors review the current understanding of epidemiological evidence for a heritable component to MDD risk, as well as recent advances in linkage, candidate gene, and genome-wide association analyses of MDD and related disease subtypes and endophenotypes. While monoamine signaling has preoccupied the bulk of scientific investigation to date, nontraditional gene candidates such as PCLO and GRM7 are now emerging and beginning to change the landscape for future human and animal research on depression.

Obsessive-compulsive disorder is a common debilitating condition affecting individuals from childhood through adult life. There is good evidence of genetic contribution to its etiology, but environmental risk factors also are likely to be involved. The condition probably has a complex pattern of inheritance. Molecular studies have identified several potentially relevant genes, but much additional research is needed to establish definitive causes of the condition.

Although twin studies demonstrate that ADHD is a highly heritable condition, molecular genetic studies suggest that the genetic architecture of ADHD is complex. The handful of genome-wide linkage and association scans that have been conducted thus far show divergent findings and are, therefore, not conclusive. Similarly, many of the candidate genes reviewed here (ie, DBH, MAOA, SLC6A2, TPH-2, SLC6A4, CHRNA4, GRIN2A) are theoretically compelling from neurobiological systems perspective but available data are sparse and inconsistent. However, candidate gene studies of ADHD have produced substantial evidence implicating several genes in the etiology of the disorder, with meta-analyses supportive of a role of the genes coding for DRD4, DRD5, SLC6A3, SNAP-25, and HTR1B in the etiology of ADHD.

Existing psychotropic medications for the treatment of mental illnesses, including antidepressants, mood stabilizers, and antipsychotics, are clinically suboptimal. They are effective in only a subset of patients or produce partial responses, and they are often associated with debilitating side effects that discourage adherence. There is growing enthusiasm in the promise of pharmacogenetics to personalize the use of these treatments to maximize their efficacy and tolerability; however, there is still a long way to go before this promise becomes a reality. This article reviews the progress that has been made in research toward understanding how genetic factors influence psychotropic drug responses and the challenges that lie ahead in translating the research findings into clinical practices that yield tangible benefits for patients with mental illnesses.

Philip B. Mitchell, Bettina Meiser, Alex Wilde, Janice Fullerton, Jennifer Donald, Kay Wilhelm, and Peter R. Schofield

The recent advent of commercially available genetic tests for the diagnosis of several mental illnesses has led to intense controversy amongst the psychiatric research community. In this article the authors review these developments, and contrast these with the growing evidence from genome-wide association studies that highly heritable psychiatric conditions such as schizophrenia are due to the contributions and interaction of multiple allelic variants, each of small effect size. There is also evidence for the contribution of some highly penetrant rare de novo copy number variants, though the lack of disease specificity for these is of concern. This article outlines the prerequisites for predictive and diagnostic genetic tests, such as clinical validity and utility, and reviews the opportunity that genetic tests for mental illnesses present. As the scientific discourse on genetic tests for complex disorders is not limited to psychiatry, the authors outline current thoughts on the significance of genome-wide association studies across health, and the phenomenon of direct-to-consumer tests in medicine. The attitudes and understanding of patients, families, and clinicians about the future (currently hypothetical) scenario of psychiatric genetic tests are discussed, as is the potential for such testing to increase, rather than diminish stigma. Finally, recommendations on the future development and availability of genetic tests in psychiatry are provided.

THE CLINICS ARE NOW AVAILABLE ONLINE!

Access your subscription at:
www.theclinics.com

Preface

Promises Kept: Robust Discovery in Psychiatric Genetics

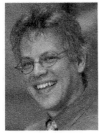

James B. Potash, MD, MPH
Guest Editor

The end of the last decade marked the beginning of a new phase in psychiatric genetics. It was a time when the previously uncharted territory of the genome came into much sharper focus and our tools for probing this territory became far more sophisticated. In his recent book, *The Age of Wonder: How the Romantic Generation Discovered the Beauty and Terror of Science*, Richard Holmes[1] describes the excitement in the 1780s when William Herschel, using a telescope more powerful than any that had come before, discovered Uranus, the first new planet identified since ancient times. While our field spent 20 years in search of genetic variants contributing to psychiatric illness, only in the past few years have our instruments become powerful enough that we can effectively scan the universe of DNA inside ourselves at a resolution sufficient to unlock its secrets.

We have remarkable new tools that can screen the whole genome for two types of genetic variations: single nucleotide polymorphisms (SNPs) and copy number variants (CNVs). The former refers to places where a single nucleotide commonly varies across individuals; there are some 10 million of these in the genome. CNVs are places where whole chunks of chromosomes can be deleted, leaving just one copy, or duplicated, resulting in three copies. These are rarer, but can be highly functionally significant because they can involve many genes at a time. In this issue, Dimitri Avramopoulos explains these tools, and Kelly Benke and Daniele Fallin describe the statistical approaches required to make sense of the resulting data.

There have been great successes in the research on genetics of common diseases over the last 2 years, with robust discoveries implicating over 400 SNPs in disease.

Psychiatr Clin N Am 33 (2010) xiii–xvi
doi:10.1016/j.psc.2009.12.008
0193-953X/10/$ – see front matter

Some of these robust genetic findings have been in psychiatry, which is very satisfying because for a long time molecular genetic studies in psychiatry and behavioral disorders found nothing definitive, with the exceptions of an *ALDH2* variant as a protective factor in alcohol dependence[2] and *APOE* ϵ4 as a risk factor in Alzheimer's disease.[3] There have been more than 20 papers reporting robust psychiatric genetic findings in *Nature*, *Science*, and *Nature Genetics* over the last 2 years, with most using genome-wide platforms to screen for SNPs and CNVs. In particular, exciting results have come in the fields of autism (described in this issue by Paul El-Fishawy and Matthew State), schizophrenia (Pablo Gejman and colleagues), bipolar disorder (Thomas Schulze), and nicotine dependence (described in an article on the genetics of addictions by Sarah Hartz and Laura Bierut). We also review developments in major depression (Stanley Shyn and Steve Hamilton), obsessive-compulsive disorder (Gerald Nestadt and colleagues), and attention deficit hyperactivity disorder (Stephen Faraone and Eric Mick).

Of course, the goal of psychiatric genetics is not merely knowledge of cause for its own sake, intellectually satisfying as that may be. Rather, it is to make use of that knowledge in the service of improved patient care. This might mean improved ability to determine which patients will respond to particular medications and which will not. This area, often referred to as personalized medicine, has been much discussed recently, though there are surprisingly few examples of success to date. Two examples that do exist are Herceptin in breast cancer and KRAS in colorectal cancer. The discovery that 25% to 30% of patients with early-stage breast cancer overexpress *HER2* led to the development of a recombinant monoclonal antibody, trastuzumab (Herceptin). Trastuzumab is indicated for patients with tumors that overexpress *HER2*, and it improves the efficacy of available therapies in all stages of breast cancer. Patients are tested for *HER2* overexpression first with immunohistochemistry, which measures *HER2* protein levels on the cell surface and, if that is unclear, then with fluorescence in situ hybridization (FISH), which measures the number of copies of the *HER2* gene.[4] In colorectal cancer, *EGFR* is frequently overexpressed in human malignancies and transmits signals instructing cancer cells to grow and metastasize. Anti-EGFR drugs interrupt the cancer-triggering signaling cascade. But if the *KRAS* gene, which encodes a downstream signaling molecule, is mutated, as is the case in 35% of patients, then the *KRAS* protein is locked into an active conformation regardless of whether *EGFR* is therapeutically blocked by the monoclonal antibody drugs cetuximab and panitumumab.[5] Therefore, these drugs are only indicated in patients who test negative for the mutations. In this issue, Peter Zandi and Jennifer Judy describe the work that has been done in pharmacogenetics of psychiatry to date, cautioning that our field has not yet produced any genetic variants that can robustly predict response to medications or side effects from them.

Another way in which we hope that patient care will benefit from genetic studies is through the development of DNA-based diagnostic testing. There is a history of the successful use of genetic tests for several neuropsychiatric disorders, including developmental disorders such as phenylketonuria (PKU)[6] and forms of dementia such as Huntington's disease (HD).[7] Such tests can be used to screen for the disorder before symptoms develop (PKU) or to establish the diagnosis in someone with symptoms (HD). In this issue, Philip Mitchell and colleagues outline the prerequisites for predictive and diagnostic genetic tests, and review the opportunity that genetic tests for mental illnesses present, along with the attitudes and understanding of patients, families, and clinicians towards these potential tests. They emphasize that the genetic variations uncovered so far in major mental illnesses explain only a minor fraction of the inherited risk. What that means for patients is that what we have uncovered so far can tell us relatively little about their diagnosis. Whereas some tests are being marketed that claim to provide information along these lines, they are premature and should be avoided, as there are real risks to their use such as having people act on results by taking unnecessary treatments, not taking necessary treatments, and changing life plans, including making decisions about whether or not to have children.

Perhaps the most momentous developments that could come from psychiatric genetics discoveries would be the identification of novel pathophysiologic mechanisms underlying the illnesses we study and treat. These would pave the way for rational drug development and, potentially, medications that work faster, more effectively, and with fewer side effects. An example of this process comes from the discovery that the gene DISC1 is disrupted in a very large family with schizophrenia and mood disorders. The strong evidence implicating this gene in disease has spawned a major pharmaceutical effort to develop novel drug targets for psychiatric disorders based on pathways related to the DISC1 protein.[8] A more definitive success story from outside of psychiatry is the way in which discovery of the genetic basis of familial hypercholesterolemia[9] helped stimulate a drug development program that led to the isolation of lovastatin, the first of the HMG-CoA reductase inhibitors, which reduce cholesterol levels and death from heart disease.[10]

After 20 years spent wandering in the desert in search of the causes of psychiatric disorders, it now feels as if we have crossed the Jordan River and entered the Promised Land flowing with the milk and honey of scientific discovery. We now, wondrously, have some highly robust genes for major mental illnesses. In addition to the powerful new tools mentioned above, another one of the keys to this success is that many in the field, 111 scientists from 48 institutions and 11 countries, have banded together against the common enemy of disease, forming a Psychiatric Genome-Wide Association Consortium (PGC), led by Patrick Sullivan.[11] The PGC has been able to pool more than 60,000 samples to date, and the preliminary results suggest the power of these very large sample sets to identify new genetic variants involved in disease. In spite of unprecedented progress, though, there remains much to be accomplished in the realm of genetics and in the challenge of connecting genetics to neurobiology and to pharmacology. Personalized medicine in psychiatry has not arrived yet, though it may not be very far off.

James B. Potash, MD, MPH
Johns Hopkins Hospital
600 North Wolfe Street
Meyer 4-119
Baltimore, MD 21287, USA

E-mail address:
jpotash@jhmi.edu

REFERENCES

1. Holmes R. The age of wonder: how the romantic generation discovered the beauty and terror of science. New York: Pantheon Books; 2009.
2. Harada S, Agarwal DP, Goedde HW, et al. Possible protective role against alcoholism for aldehyde dehydrogenase isozyme deficiency in Japan. Lancet 1982; 2(8302):827.
3. Strittmatter WJ, Saunders AM, Schmechel D, et al. Apolipoprotein E: high-avidity binding to beta-amyloid and increased frequency of type 4 allele in late-onset familial Alzheimer disease. Proc Natl Acad Sci U S A 1993;90(5):1977–81.

4. Pietras RJ, Fendly BM, Chazin VR, et al. Antibody to HER-2/neu receptor blocks DNA repair after cisplatin in human breast and ovarian cancer cells. Oncogene 1994;9(7):1829–38.
5. Lievre A, Bachet JB, Le Corre D, et al. KRAS mutation status is predictive of response to cetuximab therapy in colorectal cancer. Cancer Res 2006;66(8): 3992–5.
6. Guthrie R, Susi A. A simple phenylalanine method for detecting phenylketonuria in large populations of newborn infants. Pediatrics 1963;32:338–43.
7. Brandt J, Quaid KA, Folstein SE, et al. Presymptomatic diagnosis of delayed-onset disease with linked DNA markers. The experience in Huntington's disease. JAMA 1989;261(21):3108–14.
8. Wang Q, Jaaro-Peled H, Sawa A, et al. How has DISC1 enabled drug discovery? Mol Cell Neurosci 2008;37(2):187–95.
9. Brown MS, Goldstein JL. Expression of the familial hypercholesterolemia gene in heterozygotes: mechanism for a dominant disorder in man. Science 1974; 185(4145):61–3.
10. Stossel TP. The discovery of statins. Cell 2008;134(6):903–5.
11. Psychiatric GWAS Consortium Steering Committee. A framework for interpreting genome-wide association studies of psychiatric disorders. Mol Psychiatry 2009; 14(1):10–7.

Erratum

A typographical error appeared in the author affiliation information for article, "Management of Schizophrenia with Obsessive-Compulsive Features" by Drs Michael Y. Hwang, MD, Sung-Wan Kim, MD, PhD, Sun Young Yum, MD, and Lewis A. Opler, MD, PhD, published in the December 2009 issue of *Psychiatric Clinics of North America* (Vol. 32, No. 4, p. 835). Only Dr Hwang is affiliated with Mental Health Service, Franklin Delano Roosevelt Hospital, Veterans Affairs Hudson Valley Health-care System. The other authors are not affiliated with this institution. All other affiliation information is correct.

doi:10.1016/j.psc.2009.12.007
0193-953X/10/$ – see front matter. Published by Elsevier Inc.
psych.theclinics.com

Erratum

Genetics of Psychiatric Disorders Methods: Molecular Approaches

Dimitrios Avramopoulos, MD, PhD

KEYWORDS

- Human Genome Project
- Next-generation sequencing methods • Linkage analysis
- Genetic association studies • Epigenetics

Today, the genes responsible for the majority of Mendelian disorders are known. The Online Mendelian Inheritance in Man (http://www.ncbi.nlm.nih.gov/omim/) database lists 2517 Mendelian phenotypes with a known molecular basis and 1741 with an unknown molecular basis. This knowledge stems mainly from the power of linkage analysis, which enabled the genetic mapping of diseases to narrow genomic intervals so that, even before the availability of the genome sequence, they could be readily investigated for the presence of genes and mutations responsible for each disease. This valuable tool, however, proved much less effective for more common and genetically more complex disorders, including psychiatric disorders. The need for more powerful tools for molecular genetic analysis became obvious and the importance of developing such tools was clear given the public health impact of these disorders. The Human Genome Project was the first big step toward the development of technologies and tools that today enable the successful genetic investigation of complex phenotypes. In the postgenomic era, the need to understand such phenotypes has driven the development of new technologies. There have been many scientific breakthroughs in genetics in the last century. However, when it comes to technological breakthroughs, this is undoubtedly one of the most significant times in the history of genetics.

THE GENOME AND GENETIC VARIATION

In 1990, the National Institutes of Health, the Department of Energy, and international partners launched the Human Genome Project, which reached its first major milestone with the publication of a first working draft of the human genome in 2001.[1] The

The author is supported by funding from the National Institute of Aging (grant R01AG022099) and an award from the Neurosciences Education and Research Foundation.
Department of Psychiatry, McKusick Nathans Institute of Genetic Medicine, Johns Hopkins School of Medicine, BRB-509, 733 North Broadway, Baltimore, MD 21205, USA
E-mail address: adimitr1@jhmi.edu

Psychiatr Clin N Am 33 (2010) 1–13
doi:10.1016/j.psc.2009.12.006
0193-953X/10/$ – see front matter © 2010 Elsevier Inc. All rights reserved.

simultaneous publication of a genome draft from a parallel genome project outside the public sector[2] highlighted the tremendous technological advances that made possible ahead of schedule the achievement of what originally seemed to many an overambitious undertaking. The availability of the human and other genomes subsequently led to renewed interest and further advances in the field of population genetics and provided new tools and information for the study of polymorphism, recombination, linkage disequilibrium, and genetic association, leading to knowledge instrumental for the study of complex disorders.

In the study of complex disorders, it became quickly apparent that the practice of testing one or a few polymorphisms within a gene for association with a disease was insufficient. The number of known genetic variants increased exponentially, making it clear that a gene can contain dozens or hundreds of single nucleotide polymorphisms (SNPs) that could influence its function. Although information on coding sequence and phylogenetic conservation information from the newly emerged field of comparative genomics could provide a means to assess the likelihood of function for any given SNP and reduce the number of tested SNPs, an approach that tests just one or a few polymorphisms within a gene clearly could miss important variants.

Fortunately, the first studies that performed high-throughput genotyping showed that, to survey all common variations, it is not necessary to determine the genotypes of all common SNPs.[3–5] This shortcut in surveying is made possible because of linkage disequilibrium, an old genetic concept that came to enjoy renewed popularity. As shown in **Fig. 1**, when a mutation arises in the population, it generates a new

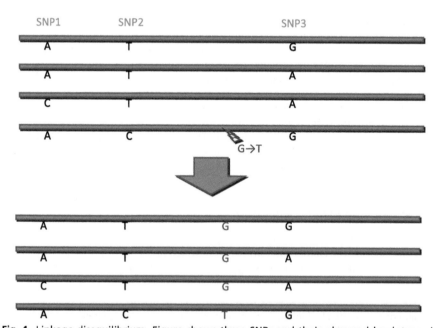

Fig. 1. Linkage disequilibrium. Figure shows three SNPs and their observed haplotypes in the population. A new mutation generates an additional variant on one of the haplotypes. In the simplistic example shown here, the mutation is in perfect linkage disequilibrium with SNP2 ($r^2 = 1$) and any disease association would also be observed with that SNP. The other SNPs are correlated with the mutation, but not perfectly ($r^2 < 1$). As long as recombination does not break this haplotype block, the variants remain in complete linkage disequilibrium ($D' = 1$) and certain combinations of alleles are never observed.

variable location. The newly generated allele resides on a preexisting haplotype, a DNA strand that carries a specific sequence of alleles on the other variable positions. The new allele will then be transmitted to the next generations always on this haplotype except where the haplotype continuity is broken by recombination. As a result, the genotype of every variant in the genome is correlated with the genotypes of neighboring variants, and this correlation is reduced with increasing distance and with increasing phylogenetic age of the variant. Furthermore, due to the nonuniform recombination rates in the genome and the existence of recombination "hot-spots,"[6] the correlation between genotypes, or linkage disequilibrium, has a patchy distribution with regions of higher linkage disequilibrium separated, often abruptly, by regions of lower linkage disequilibrium, a phenomenon that gave rise to the term *islands of linkage disequilibrium* (**Fig. 2**).[5] Regions of high linkage disequilibrium are often termed *haplotype blocks*, which refers to short haplotype fragments that contain only some of the possible combinations of alleles across their length. These blocks should not be confused with the traditional meaning of the word *haplotype*, which does not assume any correlation between alleles at the population level, but only their coexistence in the same strand in an individual.

Analysis of linkage disequilibrium in the genome has made it clear that the correlations of genotypes are often so strong that one variant can fully predict (or "tag") the genotype of another perfect linkage disequilibrium (see **Fig. 1**), making it possible to examine all common variations by genotyping only a fraction of common SNPs. The HapMap project, launched in 2002,[7] has genotyped millions of SNPs in multiple populations, achieving its goal to characterize linkage disequilibrium across the genome. These results, which have already been used to enhance the efficiency of current genotyping technologies, are valuable everyday tools for researchers studying the genetics of complex diseases.

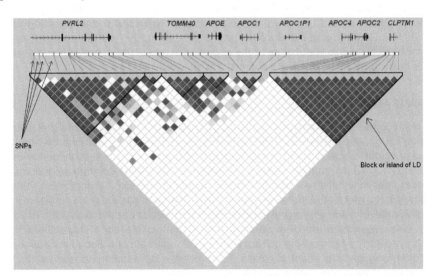

Fig. 2. Example of linkage disequilibrium islands. A 100-kb region around the APOE gene is shown using data from the HapMap project and the Haploview software (www.broadinstitute.org/mpg/haploview). Colored diamonds show the strength of linkage disequilibrium between the SNPs corresponding to the extension of their sides up to the SNP line-up at the top. Red is for strong linkage disequilibrium (high D') while purple signifies insufficient information to infer linkage disequilibrium. Islands of linkage disequilibrium are revealed as large red triangles. An island of strong linkage disequilibrium is labeled.

The sequencing of the human genome and the high-throughput technologies that emerged in part as a consequence of the Human Genome Project resulted in the identification of an additional source of genetic variation, the significance of which had previously remained unrecognized. Using highthroughput methods originally developed for the study of cancer, Sebat and colleagues[8] and Iafrate and colleagues[9] found that the genome of normal individuals (not affected by a specific disorder) contains multiple sites where DNA sequences are either deleted or present in multiple copies. These sites sometimes include one or more genes. Today we know that more than 10% of the human genome is subject to copy number variation and that these regions often include genes. Recent literature[10,11] has shown that these copy number variations often influence the transcription of genes, not only those included in the copy number variation, but also at some distance, enforcing their perceived importance and the necessity to examine them when exploring the genome for complex disease liability loci.

In 2003, the ENCODE project (Encyclopedia of DNA Elements) was launched (http://www.genome.gov/10005107) with the ambitious goal of identifying all functional elements in the human genome. Recently, the investigators completed and published[12] results of the pilot phase of the project (for a series of resulting articles see *Genome Research*, vol. 17, issue 6, at http://www.genome.org/content/vol17/issue6/). The National Human Genome Research Institute funded new awards to scale the project to the genome level and to perform additional pilot studies. The encode data are incorporated in the University of California Santa Cruz genome browser together with multiple other tracks of information, including the HapMap data track, providing researchers with an increasingly valuable tool for genome-wide or targeted genetic analyses.

Today, less than 10 years after from the completion of the Human Genome Project, technological advances have enabled the launch of the 1000 Genomes Project[13] (http://www.1000genomes.org), an international collaboration for sequencing the genomes of approximately 1200 people from around the world and for acquiring an unprecedented wealth of information on human polymorphism and diversity. Like the Human Genome and the HapMap projects before it, the 1000 Genomes Project promises to bring this information to the fingertips of researchers, providing a tremendous push for human genetics research.

LINKAGE ANALYSES

As mentioned, linkage analysis led to the identification of most genes that cause Mendelian genetic disorders. Such disorders stem from rare mutations that trigger disease under a specific model (eg, autosomal dominant) with a high penetrance (close to 100% of mutation carriers are affected) and with very rare phenocopies (almost everyone affected has the same genetic condition). Unfortunately these criteria are not met by the more common human disorders that, although usually milder than Mendelian disorders, represent overall a much bigger burden to society. Psychiatric diseases, which are both common and complex, are often characterized by a relatively early age of onset and the need for lifelong treatment. Because treatments are often only partially effective, these diseases have devastating consequences for the quality of life of the patients and their caregivers.

When linkage was first applied to complex disorders, it was performed using the established methods of the time, which required the determination, a priori, of an inheritance model. Many early efforts failed to find linkage and often declared exclusion of parts of the genome based on such analyses. It slowly became clear, however, that the common disorders were much more likely to involve more than a single gene and that the "mutations" involved were likely to cause disease in some but not all carriers. This finding was consistent with results of prior segregation analyses for schizophrenia.[14] Traditional linkage methods were not meant for the investigation of such diseases. Numerous efforts for the development of new approaches to linkage analysis were undertaken in the 1990s. Most of these approaches involved what eventually became the standard for linkage analysis of complex disorders: the analysis, in each genomic location, of allele sharing among affected relatives as compared with expected allele sharing. This sacrifices power, but avoids assumptions about inheritance, bypassing a significant problem of parametric linkage. At the same time, technologies were developed enabling genotyping of short tandem repeat markers without polyacrylamide gels or radioactivity and with extensive marker multiplexing. It became possible to survey the genome at a cost and time investment that was realistic. Whole genome linkage studies were soon being published monthly or weekly. The results, however, did not deliver on the expectations. Linkage signals were most often weak, not providing the strong evidence for disease loci everyone hoped for. In 1995, Lander and Kruglyak[15] formalized the criteria for declaring genome-wide significant linkage. Few studies met these criteria and the few loci that did were rarely replicated in other samples. Complex disease genetics and psychiatric genetics were going through a confidence crisis.

Just 1 year later, in a paper that strongly influenced the field of complex disease genetics, Risch and Merikangas[16] showed that, if complex disorders were due to common genetic variants with small effects, linkage studies would need to examine many thousands of families to identify such loci. They also showed that performing genetic association studies rather than linkage was far more powerful for discovering these loci. At that time, the genotyping technologies did not allow a genome-wide scan for association. Also, such studies were only performed on a small scale for individual candidate genes and were often reserved for following up linkage signals. Today, through the use of microarrays and other similar array-based technologies, genotyping a million SNPs across the genome has become both fast and affordable and genome-wide association studies (GWAS) have mostly replaced linkage in the exploration of complex disorders. The few linkage studies now performed use SNP markers genotyped in large numbers to match and exceed the high information content of microsatellites. The genetic effect sizes of common alleles uncovered by most GWAS are so small that one would need millions of families to detect them by linkage, which seems to be a justification for favoring GWAS. However, one needs to be careful when comparing linkage and association. As opposed to association studies, linkage would detect a disease locus with multiple rare disease risk alleles, provided their combined effect is substantial. In view of the most recent GWAS results, where the identified variants do not explain much of the heritability of the respective disorders,[17] linkage is starting to look attractive again as it could provide target regions for next-generation sequencing and enable the inference of mutation segregation across pedigrees, leading to the discovery of disease variants not visible by GWAS.

GENOME-WIDE ASSOCIATION STUDIES

The concept of GWAS was formed in the 1990s and supported by theoretical work, such as that of Risch and Merikangas.[16] However, at that time, genotyping the genome at an adequate density was not possible. Association studies were performed for 1, 10, or sometimes 100 SNPs, covering targeted genes or regions. Claims of "lack of association" were obviously exaggerated and, to everyone's frustration, positive findings could only rarely be replicated and almost never consistently. Genome-wide scans became possible around the turn of the millennium, initially at low marker densities and often with sample pooling to reduce cost. Today, before the end of the decade, studies testing 1 million SNPs across the genome on many thousands of subjects are published weekly. There have been many success stories that have confirmed the value of the GWAS approach. In just the last 3 years, GWAS have led to hundreds of associations of common DNA variants with over 80 diseases and traits,[18] including schizophrenia, bipolar disorder, major depression, autism, attention deficit disorder, neuroticism, alcohol dependence, smoking behavior, and other psychiatric or related disorders and traits (see http://www.genome.gov/gwastudies/). In addition to connecting genetic variation to disease, we have learned many lessons from these studies. The newly identified variants are common and have small effect sizes, typically allelic odds ratios not exceeding 1.5.[19] The implicated genes are usually not among those considered candidates, and they are often involved in multiple disorders previously thought to be unrelated.[19] Although the identified associations involve nonsynonymous coding variants and 5-kilobase gene promoter regions more often than expected by chance, 88% are in the intronic or intergenic space, and are only slightly more often than expected in conserved regions.[18] As has been shown, many of those trait-associated variants are involved in gene regulation.[20] However, in the majority of cases, the functional link between the DNA variant and disease biology remains unclear.

Despite the tremendous success of GWAS in the last few years, there remain skeptics who question the value of the approach. Some doubt the value of observing associations of DNA variants to disease in the absence of knowledge of the underlying biology. The response to such reservations is simple: GWAS should only be considered a first step toward the identification of causal relationships between gene biology and disease. Much work needs to be done after a GWAS to move the knowledge through basic research to translational research and into the clinic. Others argue that, since the identified genetic variants only explain a small fraction of the disease heritability, they are of limited value. The heritability explained by variants identified through GWAS is most often less than 2% to 3% of the disease heritability.[21] Questions about why this percentage is so low have triggered much discussion. Underlying reasons might include a great number of small-effect variants, gene-gene interactions, multiple individually rare variables not detectable by GWAS, copy number variations (a type of variation that remains incompletely examined although it represents a significant fraction of interindividual variation), and perhaps epigenetic variation.[17,22,23] Whichever the case, it is the author's view that the fact that these variants explain little of the phenotypic variance takes nothing away from the value of the identified associations. Knowing a gene is involved in a disease provides knowledge about the disease mechanisms and potential therapeutic targets, especially once the relationship between the DNA variants and the gene's function in the relevant pathways is determined. Although the normally occurring variation within a gene might influence the risk only a little, pharmacological intervention targeting that gene's function could have a significant impact. For example, although genetic associations between peroxisome proliferator-activated receptor (PPAR) gamma and diabetes mellitus are relatively weak, with odds ratios below 1.2,[24] PPAR gamma is the target of thiazolidinediones, a class of oral antidiabetic agents.[25] Another striking example is the low-density lipoprotein receptor. While mutations related to this receptor only account for a small fraction of hyperlipidemias, the discovery of these mutations has been instrumental to the development of statins and to our understanding of their mechanism of action, which has revolutionized hyperlipidemia treatment.[26]

The insights from GWAS specific to psychiatric disorders are similar, but they include some additional interesting observations, suggesting new ways to look at

GWAS data. One is the possible involvement of rare copy number variations in schizophrenia and autism, a possibility that has received substantial support.[27–38] Another is the possible involvement of thousands of genes with very small effects in schizophrenia, genes that overlap significantly with those involved in other psychiatric disorders, such as bipolar disorder.[39] As shown in the paper from the International Schizophrenia Consortium,[39] a risk score can be generated from multiple variants with weak associations with schizophrenia (certainly including many false positives), and such a score will differ when comparing controls to schizophrenic or bipolar patients, but not to patients with nonpsychiatric disorders. Although, once again, the explained variance from such a score was small, the approach provides a glimpse of the power that genetics will have when such groups of variants become free of false positives and of how dissecting such groups of variants/genes will help us understand how different disorders both overlap and differ.

GENOME-WIDE GENE EXPRESSION STUDIES

Microarray technologies provided a strong push forward for high-throughput genotyping. However, they were originally introduced for the high-throughput analysis of gene expression. They were a natural evolution of classic DNA and RNA hybridization methods, such as Southern and Northern blotting, through technological advances that made it possible to print thousands of features on a chip and hybridize them to the RNA (or complementary DNA) under investigation, enabling the quantification of gene transcripts across the genome and comparisons between healthy and diseased tissues. What could be considered the first expression array experiment was performed as early as 1987 by Kulesh and colleagues[40] while searching for genes responding to interferon. The first microarray experiment was reported by Schena and colleagues[41] in 1995, followed by thousands of other reports.

Genome-wide gene expression (GWGE) studies can be useful for the identification of genes involved in a disease by pointing to the genes whose expression differs between patients and controls, presumably as a cause or consequence of the disease process, or to genes that respond to disease-relevant medication. The value of such studies to our understanding of the disease biology is significant and the knowledge of disease expression profiles can have many applications. A gene found to have altered transcript levels in a disease is not necessarily a culprit in its pathogenesis. Although one can clearly claim a relationship between the gene and the disease process, this might be distant and mediated by indirect associations, so that the gene might bear no meaningful connection to the disease risk. When GWGE studies are seen in the context of their potential limitations, they are invaluable for our understanding of complex disorders.

More recently, GWGE studies have also been used to identify functional DNA variation in the genome, variation that influences the expression or splicing of genes. The data generated from such studies are expected to be useful for the study of complex disorders because they will enable the assessment of the functionality of variants identified through GWAS. In a recent review, Cookson and colleagues[20] calculated that 10% to 15% of GWAS signals involved a known regulatory variant, often called an *expression quantitative trait locus*. This number will likely increase as we identify more expression quantitative trait loci through new gene expression mapping studies. The National Institutes of Health has recognized the necessity of linking gene regulation to genetic variation and has recently launched the Genotype-Tissue Expression project (http://nihroadmap.nih.gov/GTEx/), a pilot project that will ultimately lead to a gene regulation database involving multiple tissues from 1000 donors with genome-wide variation information, a much anticipated resource.

Many limitations, potential pitfalls, and confounding factors must be considered when interpreting the information provided by GWGE studies. Unlike analyzing constitutional DNA, which is expected to be almost identical across cell types and tissues (with the notable exception of tumors), the source of RNA is a defining parameter in GWGE studies. Different tissues and different cell types have distinctly different expression profiles and likely involve different regulatory mechanisms. Solid tissues contain multiple cell types that are hard to separate and, although such techniques as laser capture microdissection[42] have been developed for this purpose, their use in large-scale gene expression studies is not always practical. As a result, the observed expression profile is often the summation from more than one cell type and, in certain cases (eg, in the brain in neurodegenerative disorders), the relative cell type abundance might differ between cases and controls. Furthermore, the acquisition of some types of tissues (eg, brain) is almost entirely limited to postmortem specimens, introducing additional confounding parameters, such as the cause of death and the delay in the dissection of the tissue, which could lead to RNA degradation. Many studies attempt to bypass such limitations by examining lymphocytes or immortalized cell lines that are often readily available or easy to acquire. This practice reduces significant sources of variation, but might be of limited value for the study of a psychiatric disease. Although it can be argued that some of the gene expression differences will be similar in brain and lymphocytes, only a fraction of genes will be expressed in both tissues and those are likely to be subject to different regulatory mechanisms in tissues that have different functions. Many other limitations, including alternative splicing, environmental factors (eg, diet and drugs), and platform-specific characteristics, introduce additional levels of complexity and highlight the importance of careful experimental design in GWGE studies.

In the more-than-20-year history of expression array analysis, we have learned a lot from GWGE studies and have developed tools to help us tackle their complexities and interpret their results. Those results, combined with the data from GWAS, will provide one more powerful tool for untangling the genetics of complex diseases.

EPIGENETICS

The term *epigenetics* refers to changes that involve the genetic material and lead to phenotypic changes but do not alter the DNA sequence. Epigenetic changes mainly include the methylation of DNA and modifications of chromatin, such as methylation and acetylation of the histones, the DNA's packaging material. Epigenetic changes are acquired during the life of an organism and they are important for gene regulation, with big differences observed in epigenetic marks across different tissues. Environmental factors can also influence epigenetic marks through life, before they are reprogrammed in gametogenesis and early embryogenesis.[43] Occasionally epigenetic changes can escape reprogramming and be vertically transmitted across generations and, as a result, an acquired epigenetic state can persist in the next generation. In other words, an acquired epigenetic state can be inherited. The involvement of epigenetic modifications in cancer is well known[44] and many have argued that such modifications have potentially important roles in complex diseases.[45–47] It has been suggested that such epigenetic changes could be a source of missing heritability.[23] Although this view has been challenged,[48] it is clear that epigenetic variation can be causally linked to complex diseases, including psychiatric disease, and recognizing the interplay between epigenetics and genetics will help us discover complex disease genes.

Multiple tools now available enable the assessment of epigenetic variation across the genome. These tools employ methods using modification of methylated DNA or chromatin immunoprecipitation and microarray hybridization (ChIP-chip), the latter now being replaced by modern high-throughput sequencing methods (ChIP-seq, **Fig. 3**).[49–51] These tools, when appropriately applied to complex disorders, will likely lead to significant new discoveries of the mechanisms of disease, as they have for cancer. Many of the same problems encountered in GWGE studies also need to be considered here, including the differences between tissues and cell types that could mask differences or confound results. Additional complexity is added by the many different types of histone modification one needs to examine to obtain a thorough epigenetic assessment. Yet, however many the complexities, the promise is great, especially as pharmacological agents that can affect epigenetic modifications are already available.[52]

NEXT-GENERATION SEQUENCING

For more than 3 decades, the leading method for DNA sequencing was that described by Sanger in 1977[53] based on oligonucleotide-primed DNA synthesis and dideoxy termination. This was the method used for sequencing the human genome. Sanger sequencing remains the tool of choice in the modern laboratory for small-scale DNA sequencing. However, new technologies that evolved over the last few years, collectively termed *next-generation sequencing*, have taken over in the field of high-throughput sequencing.[54] These new technologies, which include such platforms as Roche 454 (454 Life Sciences, Branford CT, USA), Genome Analyzer (Illumina Inc, San Diego, CA, USA), SOLiD (Applied Biosystems, Carlsbad,

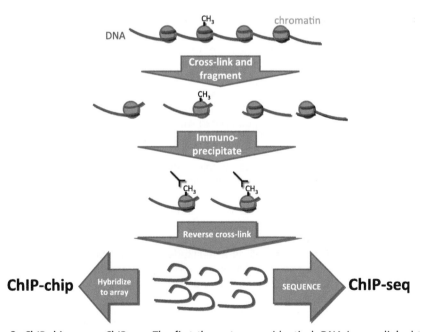

Fig. 3. ChIP-chip versus ChIP-seq. The first three steps are identical. DNA is cross-linked to chromatin and fragmented and then antibodies specific to modifications of interest are used for immunoprecipitation. Cross-links are reversed and the selected DNA is analyzed for content. This analysis was traditionally done through hybridization on a chip (hence ChIP-chip) and is now often done by next-generation sequencing (ChIP-seq).

CA, USA), Heliscope (Helicos Biosciences, Cambridge, MA, USA), and SMRT (Single Molecule Real Time; Pacific Biosciences, Menlo Park, CA, USA), each have specific advantages and one common feature that clearly set them apart from Sanger sequencing: They are highly parallel, generating 500 megabases to 40 gigabases of sequence in every run. These new technologies have reduced the price of sequencing a genome by many orders of magnitude (an estimate for the human genome today is under $100,000) and have made possible research projects that involve sequencing extensive genomic regions across multiple individuals. Beyond this revolution in sequencing capacity, they have opened up new approaches to genomics and epigenomics, including RNA-seq analysis for gene expression (see **Fig. 3**),[55] ChIP-seq analysis for DNA-protein interactions,[51] and metagenomics applications for the study of biodiversity by sampling specific environmental niches.[56] Each of these applications takes advantage of the new technologies' high throughput capabilities as well as the ability to generate sequence from DNA libraries without prior knowledge of the content.

With RNA-seq, next-generation sequencing is applied to survey the content of the transcriptome.[55] It is a step up from previously applied sequencing methods for gene expression, such as serial analysis of gene expression.[57] RNA-seq can provide a quantitative assessment of transcription, including sequence information across the transcriptome. That enables the identification and assessment of normal or disease-causing alternative splicing; the discovery of coding variation, including pathogenic mutations; and the assessment of allele-specific expression differences revealed by transcribed polymorphisms. It is clear that in the study of disease, this approach has significant advantages over hybridization-based microarray analysis.

ChIP-seq[58,59] is the sequencing of DNA that has been reversibly bound to protein and pulled down by immunoprecipitation, an evolution of ChIP-chip analysis, which used hybridization on tiled arrays instead of sequencing (see **Fig. 3**). Although the name implies that the proteins of interest are in the context of chromatin, any DNA associating protein can be analyzed. The method enables the identification of the DNA sequences at the location of interaction, and it has been used extensively in the study of epigenetic modifications, where the modified histones are used for immunoprecipitation, but also in the study of nucleosome positioning and transcription-factor binding. The additional information provided by ChIP-seq compared with ChIP-chip will enhance and accelerate our functional annotation of the genome sequence and bring us one step closer to linking DNA variation to function and to disease.

Next-generation sequencing also enables the complete sequencing of large genomic regions around association signals or linkage peaks for multiple individuals. The large number of DNA variants such studies identify, especially variants in intergenic space, makes it difficult to determine the roles of these variants in disease. However, many of the genomic approaches mentioned here (eg, gene regulation mapping, which can use RNA-seq, epigenomic, and other DNA-protein interaction analyses using ChIP-seq), as well as a multitude of other laboratory and *in silico* approaches outside the scope of this article, will help us sort through the identified sequence variants and identify those that underlie disease.

SUMMARY

Despite significant challenges in the genetics of psychiatric and other complex disorders, the sequencing of the human genome, together with a series of advances in biotechnology, is leading to new gene discoveries and the recognition of new disease mechanisms. As the pace of discovery accelerates, the geneticist's toolbox is also expanding and the future looks more promising than ever. The practice of psychiatry has long suffered from the limited information available on the biological basis of mental disorders, as compared with other conditions. This limitation is now coming to an end, and exciting new possibilities are on the horizon for psychiatry in the twenty-first century.

The launch of the Human Genome Project in 1990 triggered unprecedented technological advances in DNA analysis technologies. These were followed, after the completion of the first draft in 2001, by tremendous advances in our understanding of the human genome. Over this same period, interest shifted from the genetic causes of the Mendelian disorders, most of which were uncovered through linkage analyses and positional cloning, to the genetic causes of complex (including psychiatric) disorders that proved more of a challenge for linkage methods. The new technologies, together with our new knowledge of the properties of the genome, and significant efforts toward generating large patient and control sample collections, paved the way for successful GWAS. As a result, reports now appear in the literature every week identifying new genes for complex disorders. We still have along way to go to completely explain the heritable component of complex disorders, but we are certainly closer to being able to use the new information toward prevention and treatment of illness. Next-generation sequencing methods, combined with the results of association and perhaps linkage studies, will help us uncover the missing heritability factors, achieve a better understanding of the genetic aspects of psychiatric disease, and devise the best strategies for incorporating genetics in the service of patients.

ACKNOWLEDGMENTS

The author thanks Megan Szymanski for critical review of the manuscript.

REFERENCES

1. Lander ES, Linton LM, Birren B, et al. Initial sequencing and analysis of the human genome. Nature 2001;409:860–921.
2. Venter JC, Adams MD, Myers EW, et al. The sequence of the human genome. Science 2001;291:1304–51.
3. Daly MJ, Rioux JD, Schaffner SF, et al. High-resolution haplotype structure in the human genome. Nat Genet 2001;29:229–32.
4. Reich DE, Cargill M, Bolk S, et al. Linkage disequilibrium in the human genome. Nature 2001;411:199–204.
5. Goldstein DB. Islands of linkage disequilibrium. Nat Genet 2001;29:109–11.
6. Arnheim N, Calabrese P, Tiemann-Boege I. Mammalian meiotic recombination hot spots. Annu Rev Genet 2007;41:369–99.
7. International HapMap Consortium. The International HapMap Project. Nature 2003;426:789–96.
8. Sebat J, Lakshmi B, Troge J, et al. Large-scale copy number polymorphism in the human genome. Science 2004;305:525–8.
9. Iafrate AJ, Feuk L, Rivera MN, et al. Detection of large-scale variation in the human genome. Nat Genet 2004;36:949–51.
10. Cahan P, Li Y, Izumi M, et al. The impact of copy number variation on local gene expression in mouse hematopoietic stem and progenitor cells. Nat Genet 2009; 41:430–7.
11. Henrichsen CN, Vinckenbosch N, Zollner S, et al. Segmental copy number variation shapes tissue transcriptomes. Nat Genet 2009;41:424–9.

12. Birney E, Stamatoyannopoulos JA, Dutta A, et al. Identification and analysis of functional elements in 1% of the human genome by the ENCODE pilot project. Nature 2007;447:799–816.
13. Siva N. 1000 Genomes project. Nat Biotechnol 2008;26:256.
14. Risch N, Baron M. Segregation analysis of schizophrenia and related disorders. Am J Hum Genet 1984;36:1039–59.
15. Lander E, Kruglyak L. Genetic dissection of complex traits: guidelines for interpreting and reporting linkage results. Nat Genet 1995;11:241–7.
16. Risch N, Merikangas K. The future of genetic studies of complex human diseases. Science 1996;273:1516–7.
17. Manolio TA, Collins FS, Cox NJ, et al. Finding the missing heritability of complex diseases. Nature 2009;461:747–53.
18. Hindorff LA, Sethupathy P, Junkins HA, et al. Potential etiologic and functional implications of genome-wide association loci for human diseases and traits. Proc Natl Acad Sci U S A 2009;106:9362–7.
19. Manolio TA, Brooks LD, Collins FS. A HapMap harvest of insights into the genetics of common disease. J Clin Invest 2008;118:1590–605.
20. Cookson W, Liang L, Abecasis G, et al. Mapping complex disease traits with global gene expression. Nat Rev Genet 2009;10:184–94.
21. Goldstein DB. Common genetic variation and human traits. N Engl J Med 2009; 360:1696–8.
22. Maher B. Personal genomes: the case of the missing heritability. Nature 2008; 456:18–21.
23. McCarthy MI, Hirschhorn JN. Genome-wide association studies: potential next steps on a genetic journey. Hum Mol Genet 2008;17:R156–65.
24. Scott LJ, Mohlke KL, Bonnycastle LL, et al. A genome-wide association study of type 2 diabetes in Finns detects multiple susceptibility variants. Science 2007; 316:1341–5.
25. Day C. Thiazolidinediones: a new class of antidiabetic drugs. Diabet Med 1999; 16:179–92.
26. Goldstein JL, Brown MS. The LDL receptor. Arterioscler Thromb Vasc Biol 2009; 29:431–8.
27. International Schizophrenia Consortium. Rare chromosomal deletions and duplications increase risk of schizophrenia. Nature 2008;455:237–41.
28. Stefansson H, Rujescu D, Cichon S, et al. Large recurrent microdeletions associated with schizophrenia. Nature 2008;455:232–6.
29. Walsh T, McClellan JM, McCarthy SE, et al. Rare structural variants disrupt multiple genes in neurodevelopmental pathways in schizophrenia. Science 2008;320:539–43.
30. Xu B, Roos JL, Levy S, et al. Strong association of de novo copy number mutations with sporadic schizophrenia. Nat Genet 2008;40:880–5.
31. Kirov G, Gumus D, Chen W, et al. Comparative genome hybridization suggests a role for NRXN1 and APBA2 in schizophrenia. Hum Mol Genet 2008;17: 458–65.
32. Vrijenhoek T, Buizer-Voskamp JE, van der Stelt I, et al. Recurrent CNVs disrupt three candidate genes in schizophrenia patients. Am J Hum Genet 2008;83: 504–10.
33. Sebat J, Lakshmi B, Malhotra D, et al. Strong association of de novo copy number mutations with autism. Science 2007;316:445–9.
34. Christian SL, Brune CW, Sudi J, et al. Novel submicroscopic chromosomal abnormalities detected in autism spectrum disorder. Biol Psychiatry 2008;63:1111–7.

35. Kumar RA, KaraMohamed S, Sudi J, et al. Recurrent 16p11.2 microdeletions in autism. Hum Mol Genet 2008;17:628–38.
36. Weiss LA, Shen Y, Korn JM, et al. Association between microdeletion and micro-duplication at 16p11.2 and autism. N Engl J Med 2008;358:667–75.
37. Cho SC, Yim SH, Yoo HK, et al. Copy number variations associated with idio-pathic autism identified by whole-genome microarray-based comparative genomic hybridization. Psychiatr Genet 2009;19:177–85.
38. Glessner JT, Wang K, Cai G, et al. Autism genome-wide copy number variation reveals ubiquitin and neuronal genes. Nature 2009;459:569–73.
39. Purcell SM, Wray NR, Stone JL, et al. Common polygenic variation contributes to risk of schizophrenia and bipolar disorder. Nature 2009;460:748–52.
40. Kulesh DA, Clive DR, Zarlenga DS, et al. Identification of interferon-modulated proliferation-related cDNA sequences. Proc Natl Acad Sci U S A 1987;84:8453–7.
41. Schena M, Shalon D, Davis RW, et al. Quantitative monitoring of gene expression patterns with a complementary DNA microarray. Science 1995;270:467–70.
42. Best CJ, Emmert-Buck MR. Molecular profiling of tissue samples using laser capture microdissection. Expert Rev Mol Diagn 2001;1:53–60.
43. Rakyan V, Whitelaw E. Transgenerational epigenetic inheritance. Curr Biol 2003; 13:R6.
44. Feinberg AP, Tycko B. The history of cancer epigenetics. Nat Rev Cancer 2004;4: 143–53.
45. Feinberg AP. Epigenetics at the epicenter of modern medicine. JAMA 2008;299: 1345–50.
46. Ptak C, Petronis A. Epigenetics and complex disease: from etiology to new ther-apeutics. Annu Rev Pharmacol Toxicol 2008;48:257–76.
47. Jiang Y, Langley B, Lubin FD, et al. Epigenetics in the nervous system. J Neurosci 2008;28:11753–9.
48. Slatkin M. Epigenetic inheritance and the missing heritability problem. Genetics 2009;182:845–50.
49. Shendure J. The beginning of the end for microarrays? Nat Methods 2008;5: 585–7.
50. Park PJ. Epigenetics meets next-generation sequencing. Epigenetics 2008;3: 318–21.
51. Park PJ. ChIP-seq: advantages and challenges of a maturing technology. Nat Rev Genet 2009;10:669–80.
52. Papait R, Monti E, Bonapace IM. Novel approaches on epigenetics. Curr Opin Drug Discov Devel 2009;12:264–75.
53. Sanger F, Nicklen S, Coulson AR. DNA sequencing with chain-terminating inhib-itors. Proc Natl Acad Sci U S A 1977;74:5463–7.
54. Mardis ER. Next-generation DNA sequencing methods. Annu Rev Genomics Hum Genet 2008;9:387–402.
55. Morozova O, Hirst M, Marra MA. Applications of new sequencing technologies for transcriptome analysis. Annu Rev Genomics Hum Genet 2009;10:135–51.
56. Blow N. Metagenomics: exploring unseen communities. Nature 2008;453: 687–90.
57. Velculescu VE, Zhang L, Vogelstein B, et al. Serial analysis of gene expression. Science 1995;270:484–7.
58. Robertson G, Hirst M, Bainbridge M, et al. Genome-wide profiles of STAT1 DNA association using chromatin immunoprecipitation and massively parallel sequencing. Nat Methods 2007;4:651–7.
59. Mardis ER. ChIP-seq: welcome to the new frontier. Nat Methods 2007;4:613–4.

Methods: Genetic Epidemiology

Kelly S. Benke, PhD[a], M. Daniele Fallin, PhD[b],*

KEYWORDS

- Genetic epidemiology • Genome-wide association studies
- Linkage studies • Polymorphisms

It is now commonly accepted that genes contribute to the etiology of many psychiatric disorders. Estimates of the heritability for schizophrenia have been as high as 81%,[1] for bipolar disorder as high as 93%,[2] and for autism over 90%.[3] Evidence for a genetic component has motivated intense efforts to identify particular genetic variation related to psychiatric phenotypes. The applications of such discoveries are several-fold. First, unlike other disciplines of human disease, the field of psychiatry is often lacking in definitive biomarkers of disease or progression. Understanding the biological under-pinnings of particular disorders can target processes that may be measurable in the periphery or through noninvasive techniques. An even more hopeful purpose of illumi-nating the underlying biology is the possibility for intervention on particular processes, to prevent or delay onset of disease or to minimize symptoms and improve function-ality. Finally, gene identification is not limited to searches for etiologically relevant vari-ants, but also spans discovery of genetic predisposition to response to interventions. Genes may contribute to whether an individual responds favorably to a pharmaceutical or behavioral intervention, or may predict who will encounter adverse events and should avoid particular therapies. Identification of such genetic variation helps target recipients appropriately to allow more treatment options broadly, but with tailored approaches to avoid side effects and to improve efficacy.

Given the potential benefits of gene identification in psychiatry, genetic epidemi-ology has become a mainstream discipline within the field. This article discusses the main tools for gene discovery. Most of the articles in this issue cover findings for particular disorders from either linkage or genetic association studies. This article focuses on the designs and analytic approaches for each of these methods. Because most gene discovery has now moved to genetic association studies, and most recently to genome-wide association studies (GWAS), the focus is on methods for

[a] Department of Epidemiology, Johns Hopkins Bloomberg School of Public Health, 615 North Wolfe Street, W6033, Baltimore, MD 21205, USA
[b] Department of Epidemiology, Johns Hopkins Bloomberg School of Public Health, 615 North Wolfe Street, W6519, Baltimore, MD 21205, USA
* Corresponding author.
E-mail address: dfallin@jhsph.edu (M.D. Fallin).

Psychiatr Clin N Am 33 (2010) 15–34
doi:10.1016/j.psc.2009.12.005
0193-953X/10/$ – see front matter © 2010 Elsevier Inc. All rights reserved.

this design. Also highlighted are the current challenges of genetic epidemiology as a prelude to future approaches that may be applied to psychiatric disorders in the coming years.

DNA VARIATION

Although each human being carries almost entirely identical sequences, there are some loci where the genetic sequence is considered polymorphic, because more than one form or sequence can occur at the same locus across individuals. Polymorphisms, also called "genetic variants" or "genetic markers," exist in several forms including single nucleotide polymorphisms (SNPs), insertion-deletions, and duplications. SNPs are common alterations of a single nucleotide that occur at a frequency of about 1 every 1000 bases. SNPs have been the workhorse of most modern genetic epidemiology studies given their frequency in the genome, their ease of assay with modern genotyping technology, and the available public catalog of SNP locations in the genome. Insertion-deletions are a type of chromosomal abnormality in which a DNA sequence, either one or multiple nucleotides, is either inserted into or deleted from a genetic sequence. Finally, duplications, often called "microsatellites," are short sequences of DNA (usually 1 to 1000 nucleotides) that are repeated multiple times. Microsatellites are widely distributed across the genome and are highly polymorphic, such that many different repeated lengths exist at the same location from person to person. Certain types of both insertion-deletion and duplication polymorphisms can be considered as "copy number variants" (CNV). These CNVs are also very common in the genome and can now be assayed by modern genotyping methods.

LINKAGE ANALYSIS

There are two distinct but related paradigms for identifying genes or regions that confer disease risk: linkage analysis and association analysis. Linkage analysis relies on the observation of the cosegregation of genetic marker alleles and presumed genetic traits (eg, case status) through families. This is evidence of genetic "linkage" between the observed marker locations and the unobserved trait gene location. The concept of linkage relates to the probability of recombination between two locations on a chromosome during meiosis. When a gamete is formed by a parent to be transmitted to a child, the two grandparental genomes align in parallel (**Fig. 1**), and information may be exchanged by crossover and recombination. If genetic locations are very far apart, this can occur with 50-50 probability. When locations are very close together, however, it is difficult physically for crossover events to occur and the probability of recombination is much lower. The concept of genetic linkage is simply

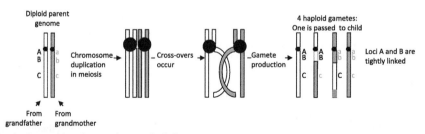

Fig. 1. Recombination and genetic linkage.

proximity between genetic loci such that this probability of recombination is less than 50%. When two loci are linked, they rarely recombine, and the particular alleles (eg, at locus A and at locus B in **Fig. 1**) are likely to be transmitted as a single unit from parent to child. If two loci are not close to each other, however, they should not cosegregate through families beyond chance.

The key concept for linkage analysis of disease is that one presumes the disease is caused by a genetic locus that is not directly genotyped in the families. Instead, case status (or a quantitative trait value) is used as a proxy for the presence of a disease allele. Linkage analysis looks for cosegregation of marker locus alleles and disease status through families. For example, in **Fig. 2**, family 1 shows an affected mother (shaded circle) who had three children (shaded circles and squares) who also developed disease. If one assumes all four cases were caused by a disease-risk allele, then it seems that marker alleles b, c, d, e, and f cosegregate with the disease allele in that family. In family 2, all cases share alleles c, d, E, and F, again suggesting no recombination between that region of the chromosome and a putative disease allele in that nuclear family.

Genetic markers used in linkage analysis are typically duplications or SNPs. Traditionally, a set of approximately 400 duplication polymorphisms (microsatellites) was used. These polymorphisms are highly informative, because there can be 10 to 20 different alleles at one locus. The resolution of these marker sets, however, was limited. More recently, SNPs have been used for linkage analyses. A standard set of

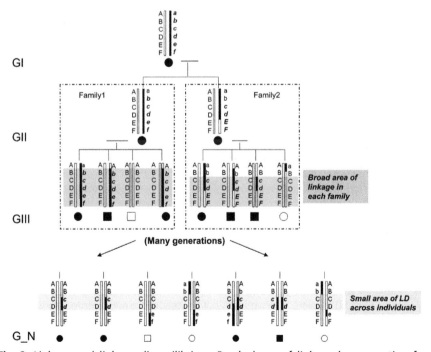

Fig. 2. Linkage and linkage disequilibrium. Break down of linkage by generation from a common ancestor. Black chromosomes reflect the ancestral chromosome on which a disease mutation occurred. Squares represent males, circles represent females. Shaded circles and squares indicate affected individuals. G_N is assumed to be many generations beyond GIII.

approximately 6000 SNPs for linkage analyses is available (www.illumina.com/pages.ilmn?ID=162), although any subset of independent SNPs from a genome-wide SNP panel can be used. Although individual SNPs are less informative (only two alleles per locus), the density of SNP panels allows greater resolution than previous microsatellite panels.

Parametric

Parametric linkage analysis specifically estimates a linkage parameter, θ, which is the probability of a recombination event between a particular marker and the disease locus, based on observed cosegregation in families.[4] Estimates of θ less than 0.5 indicate linkage. The actual θ estimate can be converted to a measure of genetic distance on a chromosome to help pinpoint the location of the putative disease locus. Estimates of θ are also used to perform a likelihood ratio test that compares the likelihood of the observed family data given the θ estimate and a particular inheritance model with the likelihood of the observed family data assuming no linkage (θ set to 0.5). The log10 of this ratio is referred to as a "LOD score," and is the most common metric of linkage reported in parametric linkage analyses. A LOD greater than or equal to three corresponds to a threefold log odds of linkage. A LOD of 3.3 is often taken as statistically significant evidence of linkage at a genome-wide P value of .05.[5] Because many believe diseases can result from multiple distinct genetic loci, a heterogeneity LOD score has been introduced that allows for some proportion of families to have linkage between a particular marker locus and a disease locus, and some proportion to be unlinked to that particular marker. Parametric linkage analysis is a powerful method for gene discovery if the correct genetic inheritance model and disease allele frequency can be specified. Model misspecification can lead to reduced power or spurious linkage findings, however, which has limited the use of parametric linkage methods for complex diseases.

Non-parametric

Because many psychiatric diseases are not thought to follow a simple mendelian form of inheritance, or because that model is not known, many linkage analyses in psychiatry have focused on a nonparametric approach that does not rely on specification of a particular inheritance model.[4] These nonparametric, or sometimes more appropriately called "model-free" approaches, rely simply on the expected genetic sharing for relatives of a particular type. For example, full siblings should on average share 50% of their genome, given that they share the same parents. If two siblings both have a genetic disease caused by a particular allele, however, at that locus they should share the same disease allele. If one samples many affected sibling pairs at the location of the disease gene, they share greater than 50% of their alleles. This design looks for sharing of alleles from a particular parent (such alleles are referred to as "identical by descent") among a collection of affected siblings and locations with greater than 50% allele sharing identical by descent are implicated as linked to the putative disease gene. Statistical evidence for model-free linkage is often reported in the form of a nonparametric linkage score, which can be converted to a nonparametric LOD score, with similar interpretation as the parametric LOD.[6] The advantage of this approach is the ability to pinpoint regions of the genome that may harbor a disease gene without having to specify an inheritance model. The disadvantage is a dramatic reduction in power compared with parametric methods if the inheritance model can be correctly specified.

ASSOCIATION STUDIES

Genetic linkage studies have been successful in mapping genes involved in mendelian disorders that have high relative risks in families.[7,8] These studies, however, have been less successful in mapping complex disorders. Genetic association studies, which are more similar to traditional epidemiologic studies that test for an association between an exposure and an outcome, offer an alternative to linkage studies,[9] although the two are conceptually related. A typical association study design compares the frequency of marker genotypes in cases with an appropriate control group. Although case-control designs among unrelated individuals are most common, association can be performed using family controls, or other types of epidemiological study designs. For example, data from a closed cohort population allow calculation of the rate, risk, or hazard of disease in those carrying risk genotypes compared with those unexposed to a risk variant. Likewise, differences in the trajectories of repeatedly measured traits between genetic groups can be evaluated.

The conceptual similarity between association and linkage is apparent when considering the ancestral population that gave rise to a current association study sample. Although linkage is performed in samples of closely related individuals from the same family, association is performed in a population that can be considered very distantly related.[10–12] For example, in **Fig. 2**, linkage studies may be performed among families like those depicted in generations II and III, whereas association studies typically sample seemingly unrelated people who are only very distantly connected to a common ancestor (as in generation N). **Fig. 2** assumes a disease mutation lies on a chromosomal background (in black) that is marked by the recessive alleles for six different loci: a, b, c, d, e, and f. By the third generation, recombination has resulted in a smaller region that harbors the disease locus, which is marked by cosegregation of disease with only five markers in family 1 and by four markers in family 2. After many generations, there have been so many meiotic events since the common ancestor that the genomic region still connected through linkage to the disease mutation (those with shaded circles or squares) is very small, marked only by alleles c and d across affected individuals. Both linkage and association studies exploit the concept of genetic linkage, but association studies, using only very distantly related individuals of a common genetic ancestry, can achieve greater resolution. This requires a much denser marker set. In generation N, information on markers B and E alone, for example, would not have distinguished those with and without disease, although they would have been informative for linkage within families.

Genetic Measurement for Association

SNPs are the most common source of genetic measurement in association studies. A SNP can have a direct functional role that is responsible for increasing risk of disease. For example, the APOE ε4 SNP variant, located in a nonsynonymous coding region that determines whether the resulting APOE protein is an e4 isoform versus another isoform, is directly associated with Alzheimer disease risk.[13] Functional SNPs in regulatory regions can also influence disease risk by altering the amount of expressed protein. Most SNPs in the genome, however, have no known function, and are used as indirect markers of surrounding genetic variation because of spatial correlation between alleles located very close together on a chromosome. This population genetic phenomenon, which was illustrated by the residual correlation among marker alleles in generation N of **Fig. 2**, is called "linkage disequilibrium" (LD). An indirect association can be detected for a marker SNP that is correlated with an unmeasured, functional variant. The linear sequence of marker alleles that travel together in the population because of linkage on the same chromosome is called a "haplotype." For a given region of LD, each individual has two haplotypes, one from each parent. Multi-locus haplotypes are analogous to single-locus alleles, and the pair of haplotypes, often termed a "diplotype," is analogous to a single-locus genotype. Haplotypes and diplotypes can be used as the measured genetic unit for association analyses much like genotypes.

Because an exhaustive set of functional variants in the genome is not currently known, and full sequencing is not yet technically feasible, most genetic epidemiology studies rely on this concept of indirect association using genetic markers at known locations throughout a gene (or throughout the genome) to act as proxies for any unmeasured variation. The location, prevalence, and correlation patterns among SNPs in several world populations have been genotyped and cataloged for over 3 million SNPs by the International HapMap Project.[14] A set of SNP markers for a gene or genomic region in a particular population can be chosen directly from this public catalog and used in a genetic association study. The optimal selection of markers depends on the structure of LD at a given location of the genome and in a given population. Highly correlated markers caused by LD in a region carry redundant information,[15–19] so that only a subset of all available markers is needed to achieve coverage of the known full variation in the region. One seeks a subset of markers that effectively "tag" the rest of the known genetic variation. Algorithms to identify the minimal set of efficient SNPs to genotype for a study are readily available.[17,18,20] The best set of tagSNPs depends on the location in the genome and on the population being studied; more tagSNPs are needed for populations with older genetic ancestry, such as Africans, because more generations have passed and more recombination events have occurred to break down linkage between loci.

Scope of Genetic Association Studies

Association studies range in scale from a particular candidate gene to the whole genome. There has been much debate about the strengths and limitations of targeted gene-based efforts versus studies of chromosomal regions or of the whole genome.[21–23] Candidate-gene studies begin with an a priori rationale for a gene's involvement in disease etiology, and selects markers to cover only particular genes. This approach has been lauded for following the traditional hypothesis-driven scientific method, and large-scale candidate gene studies focused on hundreds of genes relevant to a particular biological pathway are now commonly pursued.[24,25] Candidate-gene studies have been criticized, however, because most study findings have not been replicated,[26] and because the field lacks sufficient knowledge of all the genes or proteins that are involved in the etiology of a disorder.[27] To address this latter point other approaches, such as fine-mapping or GWAS, have been pursued. Fine-mapping studies target a chromosomal region, made up of several or hundreds of potentially unrelated genes, based on prior evidence from linkage or chromosomal abnormalities associated with a disease. These studies aim to narrow the focus of subsequent work to one or few genes. The most agnostic, hypothesis-generating approach, is to scan the entire genome for direct or indirect association through GWAS that genotype a set of LD tagging markers.[28] The particular issues related to this approach are discussed further later.

Analysis of Genetic Association Data

Once the genetic and phenotype data have been collected, statistical analyses correlating single marker information with phenotypes are performed. The type of statistical analyses depends on the study design. For case-control studies, odds ratios, their 95% confidence intervals, and P values from a logistic regression model are often estimated, although the Cochran-Armitage trend test is also commonly used.[29] For these analyses, the analyst must either create two dummy genotype variables, one for each genotype category compared with the most common homozygote (**Table 1**), or choose a genetic mode of inheritance that allows creation of a single genotype variable, such as recessive, additive (eg, on the log-odds scale), dominant, or multiplicative (see **Table 1**). The former requires a two-degree of freedom genetic test, whereas the rest contain only one risk parameter and allow a more efficient one-degree of freedom test. The additive model is often selected for this because it is viewed as a middle ground among the possible choices. Similar methods for using haplotypes or diplotypes as the unit of genetic measurement in analysis have been developed. These follow the same principles, but require additional estimation of haplotype phase.[30,31]

Statistical models for other study designs are also straightforward, using the same genotype variable coding. A cross-sectional study with a quantitative trait may use a linear regression or ANOVA model. Survival analyses may use Cox proportional hazards modeling or may parametrically model the distribution of event times. Finally, studies of quantitative, repeated measures allow modeling of the trajectory of change over time. In this case, marginal models, such as generalized estimating equations,[32] or mixed effects models that acknowledge heterogeneity in the population of trajectories can be used.[32]

These approaches for categorical and quantitative outcomes are also relevant to family-based association studies.[33] The key difference lies in the correlated genotypes among family members. This correlation is exploited in family-based association to protect against confounding caused by ancestry, which is discussed further in the section on biases. The most common design and analysis for family-based association is the case-parent trio design, where genotypes of parents are used as genetic controls for cases. The transmission disequilibrium test[34] is based on the null hypothesis of mendelian transmission, that parental alleles are transmitted to offspring with 50-50 chance. In a sample of cases who developed disease because of a particular disease allele, most cases carry the disease allele and it seems as though the parents transmitted that allele greater than 50% of the time among those trios, which are essentially an oversampling of the risk allele from the population. This test can be considered a matched analysis of transmitted alleles (contained in the case genotype) versus nontransmitted alleles (the other parental allele not given to that affected child), and odds ratios can be estimated by conditional logistic regression.[35,36] A suite of methods and accompanying software[37,38] has extended this thinking to accommodate both quantitative and qualitative phenotypes and larger family structures beyond a single affected child and his or her parents. These methods can also be extended to include covariates and interactions.[39,40]

GWAS

With the advent of marker panels that span the genome,[41] the criticism that candidate-gene studies are limited by lack of knowledge of all the genes that may be relevant to

Table 1
Coding choices for genotypes in association analysis

Single-Locus Genotype	I_{hom}	I_{het}	$I_{add/Mult}$	I_{dom}	I_{rec}
aa	1	0	2	1	1
Aa	0	1	1	1	0
AA	0	0	0	0	0

disease can be addressed. By covering the entire genome, all known and unknown functional variants can be covered simultaneously. The advantage gained by surveying the genome, however, does not come without a cost. Issues relating to coverage, quality, false-positive control, and design are challenges that must be addressed.

Coverage

Predefined, commercially available panels can measure between 300,000 and 1 million marker SNPs for a single study. The proportion of known genetic variation actually represented by this set of markers is termed "coverage" and is typically calculated with respect to the set of available SNPs in HapMap. For example, coverage is often characterized as the percent of all genotyped HapMap SNPs of a given frequency (eg, >5%) in a given ancestry group (eg, European white) that are correlated at a specified threshold (eg, pairwise correlation coefficient, r^2 >0.8) with markers available on the panel to be genotyped in a study. This is estimated to be between 70% and 92% of common variation in white populations.[14] GWAS panels leave a portion of the genome underrepresented, often omitting entire genes. An analysis comparing coverage for candidate genes obtained using a custom design panel with that of two different predefined GWAS panels illustrates that the coverage of predefined GWAS panels can be improved, at least for common SNPs (>5%) by targeted tagSNP selection for specific genes.[42] Coverage estimates are limited to those HapMap SNPs for which genotype information is available. To date, these represent only a fraction of the genetic variation in the population at large (**Fig. 3**), and true coverage of current GWAS panels may be much less than 70% to 92%. Further, coverage is lower for populations whose ethnicity is different from the population that served as the basis for SNP selection on the panel.

Strategies to improve coverage include imputing SNP genotypes that are not on a particular panel, based on outside data.[43–45] These methods work by imputing the untyped alleles for individuals based on their observed genotypes and the known LD (allelic correlation) structure for their relevant ethnicity from HapMap or other available data sets. This is limited by the available genotyped SNPs in outside data, such as HapMap. Another strategy to improve coverage is to type other markers in addition to SNPs that occur in the genome. Microscopic structural variations called "copy number variants" are of growing interest. A CNV can be defined as a stretch of

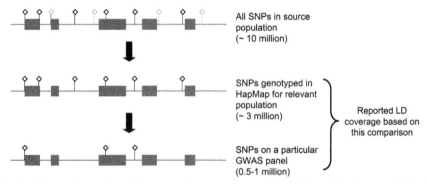

Fig. 3. SNPs used to calculate coverage for a genotyping panel. First row shows all SNPs in a given population, with those not cataloged in HapMap shaded in gray. Second row shows only those SNPs with genotype and LD information available in HapMap. Third row represents the subset of tagSNPs available on a GWAS panel.

DNA, 1000 base pairs or longer, that is present in a greater or smaller number of copies compared with a referent genome. CNVs can be several megabases in size and can contain many genes. They can be inherited or result from a de novo mutation, and may affect phenotypes by altered protein expression levels.[46] Examples of CNVs that are associated with autism and schizophrenia are discussed later.

Quality control
With so many markers, even a small percentage of measurement error can lead to incorrect inferences, making quality control efforts paramount for GWAS. Rigorous data checks are performed to filter poor-quality DNAs and SNPs before genetic association analyses.[47] Filters of individuals are often based on rates of missing or poor-quality genotype calls, identification of cryptically related or duplicate individuals, mendelian errors, and excess heterozygosity across all markers. Filters of SNPs are often based on rates of missing or poor-quality genotype across individuals, low minor allele frequencies, and departures from the expected ratio of heterozygous to homozygous genotypes under Hardy Weinberg equilibrium.[47] Without filtering, gross departures from the expected test statistic distributions can be seen on Q-Q plots of all SNP tests performed,[48] and this is typically corrected once filtering is applied. One other area of filtering is based on detection of outlier individuals who are from a different ancestry than most samples. This problem, and several solutions, is discussed further in the bias section as a potential source of confounding.

False-positive control
A major challenge for GWAS is the enormous number of statistical tests, between 300,000 and 1 million; even a small percentage of type I errors represent a large number of false signals that could frustrate efforts for replication and prove very costly. A number of statistical approaches can address this challenge. Statistical significance thresholds based on a Bonferroni correction for all SNPs are often used (α approximately 10^{-8}), which protects the probability of even one false-positive among all tests, assuming all SNPs are truly not associated with disease.[48,49] This is referred to as control of the "family-wise type 1 error rate." This approach is considered conservative because it controls the probability of any false-positive finding, which may be too stringent for an initial GWAS scan, and because the lack of independence among markers because of LD suggests that the effective number of tests is smaller. Methods to reduce the denominator of the Bonferroni correction to a more appropriate reflection of the LD structure are available.[50,51] Permutation approaches can also address this latter point, where the genetic LD structure is kept intact but phenotype status is shuffled many times so that empirical P values can be computed.[52] This is often prohibitively computationally intensive. Because the required sample size to detect a true association increases dramatically as the number of tests in either a Bonferroni or permutation approach increases, both have been criticized for their severe power penalty because of the attempt to control the family-wise type 1 error.

A potentially less stringent and more powerful approach, conceptually different from protection of the family-wise error rate, is to control the false discovery rate, defined as expected proportion of false-positive findings among the findings considered significant at a particular threshold.[53,54] Controlling the false discovery rate attempts to balance the opposing needs to limit the false-positive and false-negative rates. Whatever the statistical approach, sample sizes that provide adequate power for such a vast number of tests are on the order of thousands to tens of thousands.[14,28]

Design

Because it is often not feasible to recruit enough participants in a single study to achieve adequate power when correcting for the multiple tests inherent in GWAS, alternative design options have also been used. Many have pursued meta-analyses[55] where effect sizes are summarized across studies. Others have performed mega-analyses,[56] where individual genotype-phenotype data are pooled across studies and reanalyzed. Efforts to carry out both meta- and mega-analyses require careful consideration of the differences across studies in phenotype definitions, selection of study participants and ascertainment schemes, and genotyping platforms. The methods that are available for imputing untyped markers based on HapMap LD structures are particularly useful for this latter concern, and can minimize differences across panels.[57] Yet another option is to rely on replication in a separate sample, and guidelines for replication have been discussed.[48]

Genotyping a large number of markers in a large study sample is expensive. Although the cost of genotyping per SNP has decreased over time, the price of commercially available chips continues to be prohibitive for many research programs.[58] Staging designs have been suggested to lower the cost for this reason.[59–61] In a typical staged design, the full GWAS panel is typed for only a fraction of the original sample in stage one. Statistically significant regions are defined using liberal criteria, and only the markers that lie in these selected regions are typed in the second stage among remaining participants. Inferences are made using strict criteria for statistical significance in the second stage that accommodates the multiple testing across stages. Although the sample from the second stage can be considered an independent replication sample, it has been shown that joint analysis of both subsamples provides more statistical power, and the real advantage to this approach is budgetary.[62]

GWAS findings to date

At least 200 unique nonpsychiatric GWAS have found significant associations (www.genome.gov/26525384),[63] many of which have been replicated.[56] Psychiatric GWAS have also borne fruit, and some significant findings with replication exist for disorders including bipolar disorder,[64–66] schizophrenia,[67–69] and autism,[70,71] although results more generally have been conflicting. A large international mega-analysis project entitled the Psychiatric GWAS Consortium (http://pgc.unc.edu) is now underway to evaluate associations using GWAS methods for five disorders and also develop hypotheses for pleiotropic genetic signals that span two or more disorders[72]; the Psychiatric GWAS Consortium is sufficiently powered to find even modest-effect sizes for a single disorder.[63] Time will tell if the GWAS approach leads to meaningful findings with clinical applications in the area of psychiatric genetics. Major challenges in this pursuit are discussed next.

CHALLENGES
Biases

A common concern of most genetic epidemiological studies among unrelated participants is confounding bias caused by imbalanced genetic ancestry between cases and controls, even after adjustment or matching for self-reported race. Population substructure, or confounding by ethnicity, is of particular concern in association studies because both allele frequencies and disease frequencies may vary by race. Family based association studies handle this through matching on ancestry within families. Several methods have been developed to detect and adjust for substructure in unrelated samples. Three common strategies include (1) a genomic control method that corrects for inflated test-statistics resulting from population substructure,[73] (2) a "structured analysis" approach that estimates admixture proportions per individual and uses these empirical estimates as covariates for adjustment in regression-based association analyses,[74–76] and (3) a principal components method that estimates orthogonal ancestry variability and uses principal component ancestry scores as covariates for adjustment.[77,78] These methods have relative advantages and disadvantages. For example, genomic control may estimate the inflation factor imprecisely, whereas the structure analysis requires the assumption of the correct number of subpopulations. All of these require genotype data on at least 100 markers throughout the genome that are not related to the genetic variant under discovery.

In addition to race, age is also an important confounder if allele frequencies tend to change over the life course because of death or study drop-out. Other potential confounders in genetic studies, however, are likely to occur on the pathway to disease, and represent causal intermediates. Researchers must decide if an indirect pathway to disease is of interest, which determines whether or not to include these intermediates in the genetic association model.[79] If the genetic model includes important modification by environmental factors, consideration of other types of epidemiological biases is also important. For example, selection of controls in a case-control study that results in unequal prevalence of important modifying risk factors can affect results. This is especially important when considering a set of common controls, as was done in the Wellcome Trust Consortium GWAS.[64]

Common Disease Common Variant Versus Multiple Rare Variants Hypotheses

The ability to find signals in genetic association studies is heavily reliant on the validity of the common disease common variant (CDCV) hypothesis: that common disease susceptibility arises from a combination of common variants each with weak to moderate effects.[80–82] This rationale motivated the HapMap project, which was designed to have the power to characterize and catalog variants with allele frequencies greater than or equal to 5%. Because GWAS panels and selection of candidate genes typically borrow SNP information from HapMap, the success of GWAS will likely be determined by the validity of CDCV.

Although some data have provided support for CDCV, others argue that much of the genetic variation in complex disease is likely to be explained by multiple rare variants (MRVs). The MRV hypothesis, which posits that many rare, independent risk alleles with strong effects in different individuals account for observed disease,[14,83] implies that focus on the marginal effects of common variants is not fruitful. This problem is discussed later in this article. Support for the MRV hypothesis as the leading model for disease genetics is growing, given GWAS findings so far have been underwhelming, and that among those variants found, only a small percentage of the genetic variation in the trait can be explained.[84] Further, there is emerging evidence, especially in psychiatry, of rare variants, such as CNVs that seem to be causal in individual cases. Rare CNVs found in cases of schizophrenia and autism[85] motivate additional work under that assumption.[86–89] For most of these CNVs, the risks seem to be highly penetrant but exist in only a tiny percentage (<1%) of cases. An increase in the genome-wide number of CNVs in cases compared with controls has also been reported for schizophrenia[90,91] and autism.[92,93] This latter genome-wide approach provides a means for testing multiple rare CNVs simultaneously, but does not allow for the identification of specific variants or genes that may explain the underlying pathology. Future studies of CNVs need to evaluate the penetrance of CNVs using inheritance patterns in families or trios; standardize the criteria for calling a CNV in a given study (eg, location and frequency); and especially for psychiatric disorders, account for potential confounders, such as intelligence quotient.[85] Despite support for the MRV hypothesis, defenders of the GWAS approach highlight the successes of candidate gene and GWAS findings for common variants with small effects sizes,[84] and argue that that meta- and mega-analyses provide sufficient sample sizes to detect these very modest effects.[94] As a complement to the CDCV assumptions of HapMap, a better understanding of the rare variation in the genome may come from the 1000 genomes project (www.1000genome.org), which is now underway to provide a new genetic map with greater resolution for rare variation. Further, the advent of full genomic sequencing, likely available in the next 5 years, will provide data to explore both common and rare variation simultaneously, although many technical and analytic details must be sorted out.

Causal Heterogeneity

Regardless of the rare versus common nature of underlying causes, the ability to detect risk variants may still be low, given the complexity of causal models for most psychiatric diseases. Complexity arises from causal heterogeneity, which can be viewed from several perspectives. The sufficient-component cause model[95] in epidemiology describes a causal mechanism whose components represent a minimum set of factors that are sufficient to bring about the occurrence of an outcome. This minimum set of factors is referred to as a "sufficient cause" (SC). In a population, there can be several sufficient causes that bring about the occurrence of a psychiatric disorder. **Fig. 4**A depicts three different sufficient causes, each with separate components. The existence of more than one genetic variant that predisposes to disease is what geneticists refer to as "genetic heterogeneity." In **Fig. 4**A, there are three genetic mutations giving rise to three different sufficient causes. This type of heterogeneity can include situations where separate genes contain variation that can cause a disease (locus heterogeneity), or where separate mutations, or alleles, of the same gene can cause disease (allelic heterogeneity). For example, the APP, PS1, and PS2 genes each contain mutations that can cause Alzheimer disease in a small number of families, reflecting locus heterogeneity, and even within each gene, there are several different mutations that can cause Alzheimer disease (allelic heterogeneity).[7] Relating this idea back to the sufficient-component cause model, each mutation is a separate sufficient cause, and the number of sufficient causes in a population is at least as large as the number of unique mutations that predispose to disease. The challenge with multiple sufficient causes for disease is that if one were to look for association

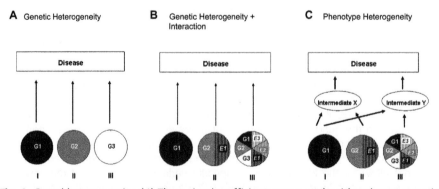

Fig. 4. Causal heterogeneity. (A) Three simple sufficient causes, each with only one genetic component. (B) Three sufficient causes, but with more complexity per sufficient cause: one with a single genetic component; one with two components (gene and environment); and one with six components of genes and environments. (C) Putative relationships between sufficient causes and intermediate phenotypes.

between any particular mutation and a psychiatric disorder, such as Alzheimer disease at the population level, they would likely not see a statistically significant association, because only a few of the cases in the study are caused by that particular sufficient cause. This problem of genetic heterogeneity potentially hinders the detection of any particular causal genetic variant.

Another perspective on causal heterogeneity is the potential for interaction, either between separate genes or between genes and environmental factors. For a particular sufficient cause, component causes interact to produce disease.[95] Often, genetic studies conceptualize a sufficient cause that contains only a single genetic variant, as depicted by SC I in **Fig. 4**. In reality, however, other genetic or environmental factors are likely to interact to make up a particular sufficient cause. SC II and III in **Fig. 4**B are examples of this, with SC II containing both a gene and an environment, and SC III containing a complex interaction of three genetic and three environmental factors. Where more than one component cause exists, analysis of "marginal" effects of a particular genetic variant, which considers only the average effect across all combinations of other risk factors, is only powerful in samples where those other component causes are quite common. In this case, the average effect is only detectable when a large proportion of the population with a particular variant also has the other risk factors in that component cause, because they are needed in concert with the genetic variant to cause disease. Genes that are part of sufficient causes with components that are rare in the population will likely be missed in marginal genetic analyses of single variants at a time. The complexity of disease etiology is described in part by the number of component causes in each sufficient cause model. When combined with the presence of genetic heterogeneity, the possible number of sufficient causes grows, as does the complexity of each sufficient cause. The detection of marginal gene effects in this situation becomes even less probable.

There is yet another perspective on causal heterogeneity that gives rise to complexity. One current theory is that distinct sufficient causes may give rise to subtly different phenotypic expressions of a clinical disorder. This is sometimes couched as "phenotypic heterogeneity." For example, one sufficient cause may result in schizophrenia with significant mood disorder, whereas another may result in psychosis without significant mood involvement. Separation of cases by this subphenotype may help to identify genes involved in each of these separate sufficient causes in a way not possible if they are considered together. This thinking can be extended to the concept of "endophenotypes," often defined as a set of intermediate phenotypes between the primary cause and the clinical classification, which may be measured quantitatively. Because endophenotypes are closer to a particular causal set, the strength of the relationship between a susceptibility allele and an intermediate phenotype should be stronger, and the causal etiology might involve fewer competing sufficient causes. **Fig. 4**C illustrates examples of sufficient causes that exert influence on intermediate phenotypes to ultimately affect a downstream clinical disorder. SC II only influences the disease by an intermediate X, whereas SC III only influences the disease by intermediate Y. SC I, however, has an indirect effect on disease through X and Y. Whereas SC I may be best detected using disease as the outcome for analysis, the most powerful way to identify genes in SC II is to focus on intermediate phenotype X rather than disease status, and for SC III to focus on intermediate Y. This endophenotype, or subphenotyping, strategy is now commonly used in most psychiatric genetics endeavors.[96–99]

Interaction methods

One solution to the causal heterogeneity challenge is to directly consider interaction models. The most standard approach is to incorporate a cross-product interaction term in the generalized linear modeling framework, which can accommodate most epidemiologic designs. This requires very large sample sizes to provide statistically significant evidence for interaction, however, and becomes intractable when many factors are studied. To overcome these limitations, population genetic isolates, such as the Amish or Ashkenazi Jews, have been studied to limit the number and complexity of sufficient causes in a study sample and reduce the problem of heterogeneity.[100] Beyond population isolates, specific design options include stratified or restricted studies where genetic analysis is performed only within groups defined by a potentially interacting factor (gene or environment). Case-only designs are also used, which can test for multiplicative statistical interaction as association between two interacting factors among cases.[101] This can be a more statistically efficient test of interaction than case-control studies.[102] Results from case-only studies are heavily biased when the two factors are not independent in the general population, however, and designs that exploit the power of case-only approaches while balancing this potential bias have been proposed[103,104] as especially useful for increasing power to detect gene × environment interaction in a GWAS setting.

Because the main goal of some research is to discover genes that are important risk factors at least in some portion of the population, the concept of interaction can be viewed as nuisance heterogeneity that is masking detection of a particular gene, as described earlier in this section. Only through accommodation of the heterogeneity can the genetic risk be powerfully discovered. For research of this sort, Kraft and colleagues[105] proposed a simple nested likelihood ratio test to identify important genetic factors by comparing the likelihood of observed data modeling the genetic factor, environmental factor, and possible interaction term, versus the likelihood of the data with gene or interaction terms. This "2 degree of freedom test" does not specifically test for interaction, but can provide greater power for detection of gene effects if G × E interactions exist (even if the interaction itself would not achieve significance).[105]

These approaches quickly become complicated with increasing numbers of genes or exposures. Full exploration of G × E combinations with multiplicity in both domains, such as SC III in **Fig. 4**C, is challenging. Methods to discover complex interaction models based on machine-learning and neural networks analysis have been explored, and model-building algorithms based on phenotype predictive ability, such as CART, logic regression, and multiple dimensionality reduction.[106–109] Each of these can be viewed as exploratory searching algorithms that can sample the huge space of potential interactions to find combinations of factors that must then be tested for importance in subsequent studies.

Other Genetic Mechanisms

Genetic involvement in psychiatry is not limited to inherited nuclear DNA. For example, mitochondrial DNA inherited from mothers, which codes for the critical energy production functions, may play a role. Also, epigenetic mechanisms, chemical modifications of DNA, such as DNA methylation, which do not involve the sequence itself but control tissue and time-specific expression, have been implicated in psychiatric disorders.[110,111] Interestingly, epigenetics may also be a way of connecting cumulative environmental damage with genetic mechanisms, because it may be the epigenetic chemistry that is modified by environments, providing a biological connection between genetic and exposure-focused epidemiology.[110,112] A role for epigenetics in psychiatric disorders has been suggested based on such factors as the lack of complete concordance in monozygotic twins, the overlap with known disorders associated with imprinting, the onset of illness in adolescence or adulthood rather than childhood, the demonstration of parent-of-origin effects for many linkage and association findings, the often episodic nature of the illnesses, and the apparent relationship to environmental factors that have known epigenetic vulnerability.[110,113,114] Although promising, findings to date likely represent only the tip of the iceberg,[115] given that few large-scale epigenetic studies have yet been performed for psychiatric disorders. Efforts are now in place to improve measurement and to catalog variably methylated sites in the genome in several human tissues[116] to provide the foundations for monitoring changes in the epigenome and connecting methylation to psychiatric phenotypes (discussed elsewhere in this issue).[110]

SUMMARY

Given the evidence for genetic contributions to the etiology of many psychiatric disorders, efforts to identify genes can have a great impact on prediction, prevention, and treatment of these diseases. This article highlights two common approaches to gene discovery: genetic linkage and genetic association studies. Although both exploit the concept of genetic linkage, association studies have recently gained popularity because of their increased resolution and feasibility with modern technology. In particular, the use of GWAS is now pushing discovery in this field, although several design, statistical, and technical hurdles remain. The current challenges include how to accommodate causal heterogeneity; how to incorporate seemingly competing hypotheses regarding whether genetic discovery should focus on common or rare variants; and how to integrate other types of information, such as epigenetic and mitochondrial data. Each is a topic of current debate, and the focus of intense technological and statistical development. In the near future, full genome sequencing will become available, potentially allowing for the convergence of several of these challenges by providing simultaneous data on both common and rare variation and on epigenetic marks on a single platform. There is much to be done toward this goal, but with careful consideration of the complexity of underlying causal models, attention to biases, clever designs, and larger samples, the field promises to continue to bring exciting new genetic information to light that may benefit both public health and clinical practice in psychiatry.

REFERENCES

1. Sullivan PF, Kendler KS, Neale MC. Schizophrenia as a complex trait: evidence from a meta-analysis of twin studies. Arch Gen Psychiatry 2003;60:1187.
2. Kieseppa T, Partonen T, Haukka J, et al. High concordance of bipolar I disorder in a nationwide sample of twins. Am J Psychiatry 1814;161:2004.
3. Freitag CM. The genetics of autistic disorders and its clinical relevance: a review of the literature. Mol Psychiatry 2007;12:2.
4. Dawn Teare M, Barrett JH. Genetic linkage studies. Lancet 2005;366:1036.
5. Lander E, Kruglyak L. Genetic dissection of complex traits: guidelines for interpreting and reporting linkage results. Nat Genet 1995;11:241.
6. Kong A, Cox NJ. Allele-sharing models: LOD scores and accurate linkage tests. Am J Hum Genet 1997;61:1179.
7. Goate AM. Molecular genetics of Alzheimer's disease. Geriatrics 1997;(52 Suppl 2):S9.
8. Mayeux R. Mapping the new frontier: complex genetic disorders. J Clin Invest 2005;115:1404.
9. Burton PR, Tobin MD, Hopper JL. Key concepts in genetic epidemiology. Lancet 2005;366:941.

10. Carlson CS, Eberle MA, Kruglyak L, et al. Mapping complex disease loci in whole-genome association studies. Nature 2004;429:446.
11. Collins A. Approaches to the identification of susceptibility genes. Parasite Immunol 2009;31:225.
12. Terwilliger JD, Haghighi F, Hiekkalinna TS, et al. A bias-ed assessment of the use of SNPs in human complex traits. Curr Opin Genet Dev 2002;12:726.
13. Corder EH, Saunders AM, Strittmatter WJ, et al. Gene dose of apolipoprotein E type 4 allele and the risk of Alzheimer's disease in late onset families. Science 1993;261:921.
14. Frazer KA, Ballinger DG, Cox DR, et al. A second generation human haplotype map of over 3.1 million SNPs. Nature 2007;449:851.
15. International HapMap Consortium, Donnelly P, Altshuler D. A haplotype map of the human genome. Nature 2005;437:1299.
16. Ardlie KG, Kruglyak L, Seielstad M. Patterns of linkage disequilibrium in the human genome. Nat Rev Genet 2002;3:299.
17. Carlson CS, Eberle MA, Rieder MJ, et al. Selecting a maximally informative set of single-nucleotide polymorphisms for association analyses using linkage disequilibrium. Am J Hum Genet 2004;74:106.
18. de Bakker PI, Yelensky R, Pe'er I, et al. Efficiency and power in genetic association studies. Nat Genet 2005;37:1217.
19. Reich DE, Cargill M, Bolk S, et al. Linkage disequilibrium in the human genome. Nature 2001;411:199.
20. Stram DO, Haiman CA, Hirschhorn JN, et al. Choosing haplotype-tagging SNPS based on unphased genotype data using a preliminary sample of unrelated subjects with an example from the Multiethnic Cohort Study. Hum Hered 2003;55:27.
21. Khoury MJ, Bertram L, Boffetta P, et al. Genome-wide association studies, field synopses, and the development of the knowledge base on genetic variation and human diseases. Am J Epidemiol 2009;170:269.
22. Pearson TA, Manolio TA. How to interpret a genome-wide association study. JAMA 2008;299:1335.
23. Sober S, Org E, Kepp K, et al. Targeting 160 candidate genes for blood pressure regulation with a genome-wide genotyping array. PLoS One 2009;4:e6034.
24. Anderson BM, Schnetz-Boutaud N, Bartlett J, et al. Examination of association to autism of common genetic variationin genes related to dopamine. Autism Res 2008;1:364.
25. Fallin MD, Lasseter VK, Avramopoulos D, et al. Bipolar I disorder and schizophrenia: a 440-single-nucleotide polymorphism screen of 64 candidate genes among Ashkenazi Jewish case-parent trios. Am J Hum Genet 2005;77:918.
26. Ioannidis JP, Ntzani EE, Trikalinos TA, et al. Replication validity of genetic association studies. Nat Genet 2001;29:306.
27. Tabor HK, Risch NJ, Myers RM. Candidate-gene approaches for studying complex genetic traits: practical considerations. Nat Rev Genet 2002;3:391.
28. Hirschhorn JN, Daly MJ. Genome-wide association studies for common diseases and complex traits. Nat Rev Genet 2005;6:95.
29. Slager SL, Schaid DJ. Case-control studies of genetic markers: power and sample size approximations for Armitage's test for trend. Hum Hered 2001;52:149.
30. Cordell HJ. Estimation and testing of genotype and haplotype effects in case-control studies: comparison of weighted regression and multiple imputation procedures. Genet Epidemiol 2006;30:259.

31. Kraft P, Cox DG, Paynter RA, et al. Accounting for haplotype uncertainty in matched association studies: a comparison of simple and flexible techniques. Genet Epidemiol 2005;28:261.
32. Fitzmaurice GM, Laird N, Ware JH. Applied longitudinal analysis. Hoboken (NJ): John Wiley and Sons; 2004.
33. Laird NM, Lange C. Family-based methods for linkage and association analysis. Adv Genet 2008;60:219.
34. Spielman RS, McGinnis RE, Ewens WJ. Transmission test for linkage disequilibrium: the insulin gene region and insulin-dependent diabetes mellitus (IDDM). Am J Hum Genet 1993;52:506.
35. Maestri NE, Beaty TH, Hetmanski J, et al. Application of transmission disequilibrium tests to nonsyndromic oral clefts: including candidate genes and environmental exposures in the models. Am J Med Genet 1997;73:337.
36. Schaid DJ. Likelihoods and TDT for the case-parents design. Genet Epidemiol 1999;16:250.
37. Horvath S, Xu X, Laird NM. The family based association test method: strategies for studying general genotype-phenotype associations. Eur J Hum Genet 2001; 9:301.
38. Lange C, DeMeo D, Silverman EK, et al. PBAT: tools for family-based association studies. Am J Hum Genet 2004;74:367.
39. Horvath S, Wei E, Xu X, et al. Family-based association test method: age of onset traits and covariates. Genet Epidemiol 2001;(21 Suppl 1):S403.
40. Lake SL, Laird NM. Tests of gene-environment interaction for case-parent triads with general environmental exposures. Ann Hum Genet 2004;68:55.
41. Barrett JC, Cardon LR. Evaluating coverage of genome-wide association studies. Nat Genet 2006;38:659.
42. Fallin MD, Matteini A. Genetic epidemiology in aging research. J Gerontol A Biol Sci Med Sci 2009;64:47.
43. Abecasis GR, Cherny SS, Cookson WO, et al. Merlin–rapid analysis of dense genetic maps using sparse gene flow trees. Nat Genet 2002;30:97.
44. Marchini J, Howie B, Myers S, et al. A new multipoint method for genome-wide association studies by imputation of genotypes. Nat Genet 2007;39:906.
45. Nicolae DL. Testing untyped alleles (TUNA): applications to genome-wide association studies. Genet Epidemiol 2006;30:718.
46. Henrichsen CN, Chaignat E, Reymond A. Copy number variants, diseases and gene expression. Hum Mol Genet 2009;18:R1.
47. Ziegler A, Konig IR, Thompson JR. Biostatistical aspects of genome-wide association studies. Biom J 2008;50:8.
48. McCarthy MI, Abecasis GR, Cardon LR, et al. Genome-wide association studies for complex traits: consensus, uncertainty and challenges. Nat Rev Genet 2008;9:356.
49. Risch N, Merikangas K. The future of genetic studies of complex human diseases. Science 1996;273:1516.
50. Duggal P, Gillanders EM, Holmes TN, et al. Establishing an adjusted p-value threshold to control the family-wide type 1 error in genome wide association studies. BMC Genomics 2008;9:516.
51. Nyholt DR. A simple correction for multiple testing for single-nucleotide polymorphisms in linkage disequilibrium with each other. Am J Hum Genet 2004;74:765.
52. Good P. Permutation tests. New York: Springer-Verlag; 1994.
53. Benjamini Y, Hochberg Y. Controlling the false discovery rate: a practical and powerful approach to multiple testing. J R Stat Soc Ser B Methodol 1995;57: 289.

54. Storey JD, Tibshirani R. Statistical significance for genomewide studies. Proc Natl Acad Sci U S A 2003;100:9440.
55. Zeggini E, Ioannidis JP. Meta-analysis in genome-wide association studies. Pharmacogenomics 2009;10:191.
56. The Psychiatric GWAS Consortium Steering Committee, Sullivan PF. A framework for interpreting genome-wide association studies of psychiatric disorders. Mol Psychiatry 2009;14:10.
57. Spencer CC, Su Z, Donnelly P, et al. Designing genome-wide association studies: sample size, power, imputation, and the choice of genotyping chip. PLoS Genet 2009;5:e1000477.
58. Kraft P, Cox DG. Study designs for genome-wide association studies. Adv Genet 2008;60:465.
59. Satagopan JM, Elston RC. Optimal two-stage genotyping in population-based association studies. Genet Epidemiol 2003;25:149.
60. Satagopan JM, Venkatraman ES, Begg CB. Two-stage designs for gene-disease association studies with sample size constraints. Biometrics 2004;60:589.
61. Skol AD, Scott LJ, Abecasis GR, et al. Optimal designs for two-stage genome-wide association studies. Genet Epidemiol 2007;31:776.
62. Skol AD, Scott LJ, Abecasis GR, et al. Joint analysis is more efficient than replication-based analysis for two-stage genome-wide association studies. Nat Genet 2006;38:209.
63. Cichon S, Craddock N, Daly M, et al. Genomewide association studies: history, rationale, and prospects for psychiatric disorders. Am J Psychiatry 2009;166:540.
64. Wellcome Trust Case Control Consortium, Donnelly P. Genome-wide association study of 14,000 cases of seven common diseases and 3,000 shared controls. Nature 2007;447:661.
65. Ferreira MA, O'Donovan MC, Meng YA, et al. Collaborative genome-wide association analysis supports a role for ANK3 and CACNA1C in bipolar disorder. Nat Genet 2008;40:1056.
66. Sklar P, Smoller JW, Fan J, et al. Whole-genome association study of bipolar disorder. Mol Psychiatry 2008;13:558.
67. Lencz T, Morgan TV, Athanasiou M, et al. Converging evidence for a pseudoautosomal cytokine receptor gene locus in schizophrenia. Mol Psychiatry 2007;12:572.
68. O'Donovan MC, Craddock N, Norton N, et al. Identification of loci associated with schizophrenia by genome-wide association and follow-up. Nat Genet 2008;40:1053.
69. Sullivan PF, Lin D, Tzeng JY, et al. Genomewide association for schizophrenia in the CATIE study: results of stage 1. Mol Psychiatry 2008;13:570.
70. Arking DE, Cutler DJ, Brune CW, et al. A common genetic variant in the neurexin superfamily member CNTNAP2 increases familial risk of autism. Am J Hum Genet 2008;82:160.
71. Wang K, Zhang H, Ma D, et al. Common genetic variants on 5p14.1 associate with autism spectrum disorders. Nature 2009;459:528.
72. Purcell SM, Wray NR, Stone JL, et al. Common polygenic variation contributes to risk of schizophrenia and bipolar disorder. Nature 2009;460:748.
73. Devlin B, Roeder K. Genomic control for association studies. Biometrics 1999;55:997.
74. Pritchard JK, Stephens M, Donnelly P. Inference of population structure using multilocus genotype data. Genetics 2000;155:945.
75. Pritchard JK, Stephens M, Rosenberg NA, et al. Association mapping in structured populations. Am J Hum Genet 2000;67:170.

76. Satten GA, Flanders WD, Yang Q. Accounting for unmeasured population substructure in case-control studies of genetic association using a novel latent-class model. Am J Hum Genet 2001;68:466.
77. Epstein MP, Allen AS, Satten GA. A simple and improved correction for population stratification in case-control studies. Am J Hum Genet 2007;80:921.
78. Price AL, Patterson NJ, Plenge RM, et al. Principal components analysis corrects for stratification in genome-wide association studies. Nat Genet 2006;38:904.
79. Vansteelandt S, Goetgeluk S, Lutz S, et al. On the adjustment for covariates in genetic association analysis: a novel, simple principle to infer direct causal effects. Genet Epidemiol 2009;33:394.
80. Pritchard JK, Cox NJ. The allelic architecture of human disease genes: common disease, common variant, or not? Hum Mol Genet 2002;11:2417.
81. Reich DE, Lander ES. On the allelic spectrum of human disease. Trends Genet 2001;17:502.
82. Wang WY, Barratt BJ, Clayton DG, et al. Genome-wide association studies: theoretical and practical concerns. Nat Rev Genet 2005;6:109.
83. Cohen JC, Kiss RS, Pertsemlidis A, et al. Multiple rare alleles contribute to low plasma levels of HDL cholesterol. Science 2004;305:869.
84. Goldstein DB. Common genetic variation and human traits. N Engl J Med 2009; 360:1696.
85. Joober R, Boksa P. A new wave in the genetics of psychiatric disorders: the copy number variant tsunami. J Psychiatry Neurosci 2009;34:55.
86. International Schizophrenia Consortium, Sklar P. Rare chromosomal deletions and duplications increase risk of schizophrenia. Nature 2008;455:237.
87. Kumar RA, KaraMohamed S, Sudi J, et al. Recurrent 16p11.2 microdeletions in autism. Hum Mol Genet 2008;17:628.
88. Stefansson H, Rujescu D, Cichon S, et al. Large recurrent microdeletions associated with schizophrenia. Nature 2008;455:232.
89. Weiss LA, Shen Y, Korn JM, et al. Association between microdeletion and microduplication at 16p11.2 and autism. N Engl J Med 2008;358:667.
90. Walsh T, McClellan JM, McCarthy SE, et al. Rare structural variants disrupt multiple genes in neurodevelopmental pathways in schizophrenia. Science 2008;320:539.
91. Xu B, Roos JL, Levy S, et al. Strong association of de novo copy number mutations with sporadic schizophrenia. Nat Genet 2008;40:880.
92. Marshall CR, Noor A, Vincent JB, et al. Structural variation of chromosomes in autism spectrum disorder. Am J Hum Genet 2008;82:477.
93. Sebat J, Lakshmi B, Malhotra D, et al. Strong association of de novo copy number mutations with autism. Science 2007;316:445.
94. Zeggini E, Scott LJ, Saxena R, et al. Meta-analysis of genome-wide association data and large-scale replication identifies additional susceptibility loci for type 2 diabetes. Nat Genet 2008;40:638.
95. Rothman K, Greenland S, Lash T. Modern epidemiology. 3rd edition. Philadelphia: Lippincott, Williams and Wilkins; 2008.
96. Chen PL, Avramopoulos D, Lasseter VK, et al. Fine mapping on chromosome 10q22-q23 implicates Neuregulin 3 in schizophrenia. Am J Hum Genet 2009;84:21.
97. Duvall JA, Lu A, Cantor RM, et al. A quantitative trait locus analysis of social responsiveness in multiplex autism families. Am J Psychiatry 2007;164:656.
98. Kebir O, Tabbane K, Sengupta S, et al. Candidate genes and neuropsychological phenotypes in children with ADHD: review of association studies. J Psychiatry Neurosci 2009;34:88.

99. Owen MJ, Craddock N, Jablensky A. The genetic deconstruction of psychosis. Schizophr Bull 2007;33:905.
100. Shifman S, Darvasi A. The value of isolated populations. Nat Genet 2001;28:309.
101. Umbach DM, Weinberg CR. Designing and analysing case-control studies to exploit independence of genotype and exposure. Stat Med 1997;16:1731.
102. Yang Q, Khoury MJ, Flanders WD. Sample size requirements in case-only designs to detect gene-environment interaction. Am J Epidemiol 1997;146:713.
103. Mukherjee B, Chatterjee N. Exploiting gene-environment independence for analysis of case-control studies: an empirical Bayes-type shrinkage estimator to trade-off between bias and efficiency. Biometrics 2008;64:685.
104. Murcray CE, Lewinger JP, Gauderman WJ. Gene-environment interaction in genome-wide association studies. Am J Epidemiol 2009;169:219.
105. Kraft P, Yen YC, Stram DO, et al. Exploiting gene-environment interaction to detect genetic associations. Hum Hered 2007;63:111.
106. Breiman L, Friedman JH, Stone CJ, et al. Classification and regression trees. Belmont (CA): Chapman and Hall; 1984.
107. Kooperberg C, Ruczinski I. Identifying interacting SNPs using Monte Carlo logic regression. Genet Epidemiol 2005;28:157.
108. Moore JH, Gilbert JC, Tsai CT, et al. A flexible computational framework for detecting, characterizing, and interpreting statistical patterns of epistasis in genetic studies of human disease susceptibility. J Theor Biol 2006;241:252.
109. Ritchie MD, Motsinger AA. Multifactor dimensionality reduction for detecting gene-gene and gene-environment interactions in pharmacogenomics studies. Pharmacogenomics 2005;6:823.
110. Bjornsson HT, Fallin MD, Feinberg AP. An integrated epigenetic and genetic approach to common human disease. Trends Genet 2004;20:350.
111. Petronis A. The origin of schizophrenia: genetic thesis, epigenetic antithesis, and resolving synthesis. Biol Psychiatry 2004;55:965.
112. Sutherland JE, Costa M. Epigenetics and the environment. Ann N Y Acad Sci 2003;983:151.
113. Petronis A, Gottesman II, Crow TJ, et al. Psychiatric epigenetics: a new focus for the new century. Mol Psychiatry 2000;5:342.
114. Petronis A, Paterson AD, Kennedy JL. Schizophrenia: an epigenetic puzzle? Schizophr Bull 1999;25:639.
115. Mill J, Tang T, Kaminsky Z, et al. Epigenomic profiling reveals DNA-methylation changes associated with major psychosis. Am J Hum Genet 2008;82:696.
116. Eckhardt F, Beck S, Gut IG, et al. Future potential of the human epigenome project. Expert Rev Mol Diagn 2004;4:609.

The Role of Genetics in the Etiology of Schizophrenia

Pablo V. Gejman, MD*, Alan R. Sanders, MD, Jubao Duan, PhD

KEYWORDS

• Evolution • SNP • CNV • Complex disorders
• Polygenic • GWAS

This article introduces the reader to the genetics of schizophrenia: its background; the status of a variety of genetic findings; new developments (which are many since the last review)[1]; and current and future challenges. Schizophrenia is a devastating psychiatric disorder with a median lifetime prevalence of 4 per 1000 and a morbid risk of 7.2 per 1000.[2] The age at onset is typically in adolescence or early adulthood,[3] with onset after the fifth decade of life and in childhood both being rare.[4,5] Although the prevalence for males and females is similar,[2] the course of schizophrenia is often more severe and with earlier onset for males.[3,6] The standardized mortality ratio (ratio of observed deaths to expected deaths) for all-cause mortality is 2.6 for patients with schizophrenia compared with the general population,[2] with excess deaths mainly from suicide during the early phase of the disorder, and later from cardiovascular complications.

Schizophrenia commonly has a chronic course albeit with fluctuating patterns, and cognitive disability. Its hallmark is psychosis, mainly characterized by positive symptoms, such as hallucinations and delusions, which are frequently accompanied by negative (deficit) symptoms, such as reduced emotions, speech, and interest, and by disorganization symptoms, such as disrupted syntax and behavior. Severe mood symptoms, up to and including manic and major depressive episodes, are present in many cases. There are no diagnostic laboratory tests for schizophrenia; instead, the diagnosis relies on clinical observation and self-report. It is then remarkable that ongoing epidemiological study over the last century using the clinical phenotype, but with variable ascertainment and assessment rules, has consistently shown the importance of genetic factors in schizophrenia.

This review was supported by funding from the NIH grant 5U01MOH79469-03 to Pablo V. Gejman, and by The Paul Michael Donovan Charitable Foundation.

Department of Psychiatry and Behavioral Sciences; and Research Institute, Center for Psychiatric Genetics, NorthShore University HealthSystem Research Institute, 1001 University Place, Evanston, IL 60201, USA
* Corresponding author.
E-mail address: pgejman@gmail.com

Psychiatr Clin N Am 33 (2010) 35–66
doi:10.1016/j.psc.2009.12.003
0193-953X/10/$ – see front matter © 2010 Elsevier Inc. All rights reserved.

THE PHENOTYPIC CONUNDRUM

The definition of caseness is fundamental to research design decisions. Bipolar disorder, schizoaffective disorder, and schizophrenia share some phenotypic aspects in common, both in terms of symptoms and also therapeutics, with all responding to antipsychotic drugs. Kraepelin[7] defined dementia praecox as a group of psychotic conditions with a tendency toward poor prognosis. He grouped under the term "manic-depressive psychoses" a set of conditions that included periodic and circular insanity, simple mania, and melancholia, which he thought did not result in deterioration. Kraepelin believed that dementia praecox and manic-depressive psychoses had specific and separate causes. Reality proved to be more complex, however, and in 1933 Kasanin[8] coined the term "schizoaffective psychosis" to refer to a disorder with mixed features of schizophrenia and affective disorder. Compared with the general population, family studies show that the clinically intermediate diagnosis of schizoaffective disorder is more common in families ascertained from probands with schizophrenia and in families ascertained from probands with bipolar disorder.[9–14] The diagnostic distinction between schizophrenia or bipolar disorder and schizoaffective disorder is not reliable.[15] The specific time criterion for affective symptoms relative to the schizophrenic symptoms is not well defined and varies in different modern classifications.[16,17]

COMPLEX GENETICS

Knowledge of the molecular mechanisms of schizophrenia pathophysiology remains very incomplete. False starts and research dead ends have taught the field the need for caution; the biological complexity of schizophrenia is much higher than was anticipated. This complexity also applies to simple Mendelian disorders, which although easily analyzed by studying pedigrees, can present unexpectedly intricate biology. Yet, the architecture of schizophrenia is incommensurably more difficult than simple genetic disorders. The idea that one or a few common major gene effects explain schizophrenia was empirically tested in genome-wide linkage scans but results mostly fell short of genome-wide significance.[18] That schizophrenia is very complex should not be surprising. First, the brain is more complicated than any other organ; the number of neuronal interconnections and permutations thereof in humans is enormous (approximately 2×10^{10} neocortical neurons and approximately 10^{14} synapses),[19,20] and knowledge of the physiological basis of higher brain functions is very incomplete. Second, the absence of well-defined, focal, and specific neuropathology has contributed to making schizophrenia particularly impervious to molecular progress, but this is starting to change (discussed later).

Schizophrenia belongs to a group of pathologies known as "complex genetic disorders." Understanding of complex genetic disorders is still evolving as new experiments uncover novel mechanisms of disease. It is commonly thought that many genes are involved in each disorder with each gene conferring only a small effect on the phenotype. The individual risk variants are without diagnostic predictive value, and any estimations of risk are probably going to change in the future as large epidemiological samples become available for analysis.[21] Epistatic interactions between these genes and among their products, and interactions with environmental risk factors are considered highly plausible. The study of genetic interactions using genome-wide data remains largely unexplored because of need to correct for an enormous number of statistical comparisons. Knowledge is shifting from oligogenic models to a polygenic model of schizophrenia, but its genetic architecture still remains largely unknown. The current evidence strongly suggests that the mutation frequency spectrum comprises a mix of many common and rare mutations. The idea that complex disorders do not result from abnormal function of individual genes but from dysfunction of entire molecular networks, the concept of system disorder, is making strong inroads in the literature.[22] Whether this applies to schizophrenia is still an empirical question that remains to be addressed.

It has traditionally been assumed that changes in DNA sequence are solely responsible for the transmission of schizophrenia. Twin studies show, however, that it is also conceivable that an epigenetic mechanism may contribute to the transmission of schizophrenia. The possibility of a role for epigenetics (ie, changes in phenotype not explained by DNA sequence) was raised first as an explanation of the incomplete concordance for schizophrenia in monozygotic twins,[23] but still remains little tested because of methodological difficulties.[24]

EVIDENCE FOR ENVIRONMENTAL FACTORS

The long-standing and influential belief that the incidence of schizophrenia is unaffected by place and time has been recently disproved, opening a remarkably productive period for the study of schizophrenia epidemiology. New epidemiological results show specific circumstances where risk for schizophrenia is increased, including various obstetric complications[25,26]; urban birth or residence; famines; migrant status; and seasonal effects (by prenatal infections [eg, influenza]).[2] Other epidemiological evidence strongly suggests that advanced paternal age[27,28] along with cerebral hypoxia and other severe pregnancy and perinatal complications[29,30] are also environmental risk factors. Overall, the landscape of environmental risks is fertile and growing rapidly, pointing to a myriad of risk factors acting early during development. Yet, the individual effects of environmental risks, even those that are biologically catastrophic, such as famines,[31,32] are relatively small. Although the specific pathophysiological connections between environmental risk factors and schizophrenia remain largely tentative, epidemiological findings can potentially provide strong guidance to molecular genetic experiments (eg, screening specific genes involved in prenatal nutrition and performing serologic assays from epidemiological samples).[33] Although the prevalence of some other complex disorders are rising, such as obesity[34] and diabetes,[35] there is no evidence for such a rapid change for schizophrenia (a registry analysis from Denmark has even detected a possible trend toward decreased incidence).[36] Finally, it is likely that additional environmental factors associated with increased risk for schizophrenia still remain to be discovered, and that an understanding of gene-environment interactions is necessary to unravel the biology of schizophrenia.

EVIDENCE FOR GENETIC FACTORS

The modern twin and adoption studies were instrumental in rejecting psychological hypotheses of schizophrenia causation[37] and became the main foundation for the search of molecular genetic risk factors.

Familial Clustering is a Characteristic of Schizophrenia

Ernst Rüdin, who was a disciple of Kraepelin, but later infamously became the main scientific leader of Nazi eugenics,[38] conducted the first systematic family study for a psychiatric disorder.[39] He realized that the data would not fit a model of simple monogenic Mendelian transmission, but missed the evidence for additional complexity. Many family studies of schizophrenia were conducted since then, with the available evidence showing that the child of a parent with schizophrenia has an elevated empirical risk about tenfold over the general population risk.[40] The risk of a disease in a type of relative compared with that in the general population is often called λ (if the risk is conferred by an allelic variant, it is further specified as an allele-specific λ). The relative risk to siblings resulting from having a proband with the illness is called λ_s.[41] Common disorders have a smaller λ_s than rare disorders, even with similar overall genetic effects. For example, the respective λ_s for the autosomal-dominant Huntington disease (assuming population prevalence 0.0001), the autosomal-recessive cystic fibrosis (assuming population prevalence 0.0004), and autism are 5000, 625, and 60 to 100,[42,43] although the λ_s for major psychiatric disorders of the adult typically are under 10 (λ_s is approximately 10 for schizophrenia). The risk for schizophrenia to a relative of an affected proband decays much more rapidly than the proportion of genes shared between them, which is also inconsistent with a simple Mendelian model.[40] Still, most cases of schizophrenia in the general population are sporadic,[44,45] which may seem surprising at first glance. Assuming polygenic inheritance (which explains the molecular findings of schizophrenia better than other models), for a disease with a prevalence of 1% and 90% heritability, more sporadic than familial cases are expected.[44]

Twin Studies

Differences between monozygotic (identical) twins are attributed to the environment, and differences between dizygotic (fraternal) twins to both hereditary and environmental factors in twin studies. The concordance rate, the probability that a second twin will develop a disorder if the proband (first examined) twin has the disorder, is commonly used. Heritability is the proportion of variance explained by genetic factors. The concordance rates of schizophrenia for monozygotic twins have been found to be about 40% to 50%, and heritability estimates are around 80%.[46,47] The reader should note that heritability per se is not an estimation of the cause of the disease, but rather of the cause of the variation of the disease in a particular population.[48] Studies from Denmark and Finland finding concordances consistent with older studies have used population registries,[49,50] which present two major advantages[46]: systematic ascertainment and an estimation of the population risk for the studied trait. Contemporary studies based on hospital registries from Germany, United Kingdom, and Japan also yielded similar results.[51,52] The risk of schizophrenia and schizophrenia-related disorders is similar for the offspring of both the unaffected and the affected monozygotic twins,[53,54] which suggests that the unaffected twins do carry a heritable genetic risk for schizophrenia without expressing the disease (supporting either or both, epigenetics and nonshared environments). It has recently been proposed that DNA methylation differences might be the cause of monozygotic twin discordance,[55] and also might provide a mechanism for a variety of environmental risk factors for schizophrenia.[33,56]

ADOPTION STUDIES

Such studies allow dissection of genetic from environmental contributions to a disorder in ways that twin studies cannot (see review,[57] which also explores methodological strengths and weaknesses of these approaches). The high-risk adoptees approach evaluates adopted away offspring of parents with schizophrenia to see if risk for schizophrenia (or often also schizophrenia spectrum disorders) is elevated. These studies have found an elevated risk for psychosis in such offspring, whether the parents had schizophrenia onset before or after adoption, and whether the rearing environment was foster parents or institutional.[58–64] Consistent with the risk traveling with the biological rather than the adoptive relationship, it was shown that the risk was similar for offspring of schizophrenia mothers, whether they were raised by the biological (schizophrenic) parent or an adoptive (nonschizophrenic) parent,[59] and that offspring of mothers without schizophrenia did not have an increased risk when raised by psychotic adoptive parents.[60] Furthermore, adoption studies can yield some insight into gene-environment interactions, for example by comparing communication deviance in adoptive parents of high-risk adoptees.[65] The adoptees' family approach starts with schizophrenic adoptees and matched control adoptees, and evaluates their adoptive and biological families for illness. These studies have shown elevated rates of schizophrenia and schizophrenia spectrum disorders in biological families of schizophrenic adoptees compared with biological families of control adoptees, coupled with low and equivalent such rates in adoptive families of both types of adoptees.[66–70]

DARWINIAN PARADOX

Schizophrenia has long been known to be associated with decreased fertility,[39,71] which is explained by the behavioral and social characteristics of schizophrenia. Fertility is substantially compromised in both genders,[72,73] although more markedly in males. Decreased fertility is anticipated to increase because of the delayed marriage patterns in Western societies, whereas age of onset for schizophrenia has not changed. It is expected that natural selection decreases the population frequencies of disorder genes that diminish fertility. The prevalence of schizophrenia remains high, however, much higher than for Mendelian disorders. How schizophrenia circumvents the effect of natural selection (sometimes called a "Darwinian paradox") remains an enigma and multiple hypotheses have been proposed.[74] Fananas and Bertranpetit[75] proposed that the relatives of schizophrenics might have a compensatory increase in fertility, but preliminary data did not replicate in larger samples.[72,73,76] Lack of evidence for increased fertility in relatives of schizophrenics weakens alternative explanations, such as heterozygote advantage (either homozygote shows reduced fitness compared with the heterozygote, such as with sickle cell anemia)[77] and antagonist pleiotropy (an allele might reduce fitness for one trait while increasing fitness of a related trait).[74]

Another proposed explanation is that the clinical phenotype might have poor correlation with the underlying genetic susceptibility (ie, genotype), and it has been suggested that endophenotypic variables (sometimes called "intermediate phenotypes"), such as structural and functional neuroimaging characteristics, constitute a better index of the underlying gene effects than the clinical phenotype.[78] There are two problems with this argument: a large body of genetic epidemiology is based on the clinical phenotype, and none of the proposed endophenotypes has been proved yet to be more heritable than the aggregate clinical phenotype.[79]

It is also conceivable that the alleles conferring susceptibility to schizophrenia might be maintained in the population against negative selection by a high mutation rate.[80] Advanced paternal age would then be a risk factor because spermatogonia replicate many more times over life than oocytes and the age of fathers is greater than expected for some autosomal-dominant diseases because of new mutations.[81] A study of an epidemiological sample of 87,907 individuals born in Jerusalem between 1964 and 1976 found that the relative risk of schizophrenia increased continuously with the age of the fathers to a maximum of 2.96 in offspring of fathers aged 50 and 54 years.[27] This finding has been replicated in larger samples from different populations, especially for older fathers,[28] and found to be a stronger effect in sporadic (family history negative) cases,[82] as is predicted for de novo mutations. As reviewed,[74] paternal age effects challenge neutral and balancing selection (such as heterozygote advantage and antagonist pleiotropy) explanations of schizophrenia's Darwinian paradox, but are expected under a mutation-selection model.[83] In addition, polygenic mutation-selection balance (where deleterious mutations have yet to go extinct: many older mutations of milder individual effect that are removed more slowly from the population, and rarer recent mutations of larger effect that have not had time to diminish over generations) is consistent other important aspects of schizophrenia (eg, its prevalence, reproductive fitness costs, and its expression by the body's most complex organ with an enormous "mutational target size"),[74] and also with recent findings detailed later from genome-wide association studies (GWAS), especially support for the importance of polygenic inheritance.

FIRST MODERN ASSOCIATION STUDIES

Before the availability of GWAS, most gene association studies consisted of tests of candidate gene involvement. Close to 800 genes have been tested for association (see www.schizophreniaforum.org/res/sczgene.[84] This makes schizophrenia one of the most studied disorders through a candidate gene approach. Unfortunately, none of them as of today can be considered fully established. Because samples frequently lacked sufficient statistical power, the problem of nonreplication has been far from trivial. In a comprehensive study of some of the most cited candidate genes (eg, *DISC1*, *DTNBP1*, *NRG1*, *DRD2*, *HTR2A* [*5-hydroxytryptamine (serotonin) receptor 2A*], and *COMT*), each of 14 genes were tested by genotyping a sample of 1870 cases and 2002 screened controls of European ancestry (EA).[85] A total of 789 single nucleotide polymorphisms (SNPs), including tags for common variation in each gene (tag SNPs are SNPs that are correlated with many other nearby SNPs, for which they are proxies), SNPs previously reported as associated, and SNPs located in functional domains of genes was genotyped, but no association was found (**Fig. 1**), which clearly contradicts odds ratios (ORs) predicted from the analysis of smaller samples (the effect size can be conceptualized as the strength of the association between a marker and the disorder, and it can be expressed as the OR, which is the odds for an event, here possessing a risk allele in the risk group [cases], divided by the odds in the nonrisk group [controls]). The dilemma for the field is interpreting the reasons for the abundance of positive and negative associations with candidate genes. It is likely that the use of small sample sizes and inadequate or loose statistical thresholds are behind many of the unreplicated observations. Other potential causes of false-positives are multiple analyses and selective reporting.[86] It is possible that genetic heterogeneity in some specific cases precludes a replication, but it seems unlikely that this is a robust general argument.[87] Multiplicative epistasis (where the individual gene effects might not be detectable but the product of the effects might become detectable) is another largely unexplored possibility that could in principle explain nonreplication, and environmental variation is another source of heterogeneity. Furthermore, very provocative work by Richter and colleagues[88] suggests that increased standardization (such as in experiments designed to decrease heterogeneity, which allows and frequently requires smaller sample sizes) can actually decrease reproducibility in animal behavioral experiments, challenging long-held ideas. Recent schizophrenia GWAS results (where each candidate gene is typically more comprehensively tested than in most candidate gene experiments) overall have not supported most associations to classical candidate genes (**Table 1**, also see supplementary data file 3 from),[89] a pattern consistent with the general results of GWAS in complex disorders (www.genome.gov/gwastudies).[90] Although some

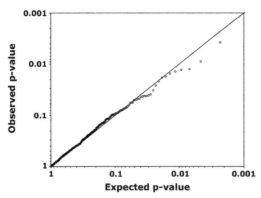

Fig. 1. Quantile-quantile plot of observed versus expected *P* values for tag SNPs for 14 schizophrenia candidate genes. Open circles represent the relationship between the expected (X axis) and observed (Y axis) *P* values for pointwise nominal Armitage trend tests for the 433 SNPs that represent tags (at *r²*>0.8) for common SNPs in each of 14 tested genes (*RGS4, DISC1, DTNBP1, STX7, TAAR6, PPP3CC, NRG1, DRD2, HTR2A, DAOA, AKT1, CHRNA7, COMT,* and *ARVCF*). The solid line represents the null expectation. The observed distribution is within the 95% confidence interval of the null expectation, consistent with a lack of evidence in the tested sample for association with schizophrenia in the tested candidate genes. The lowest *P* values are slightly below the line (less significant than expected), but still within the confidence interval. (*Reprinted from* Sanders AR, Duan J, Levinson DF, et al. No significant association of 14 candidate genes with schizophrenia in a large European ancestry sample: implications for psychiatric genetics. Am J Psychiatry 2008;165:497; with permission. Copyright 2008, American Psychiatric Association.)

candidate genes have been replicated (eg, *APOE4* in Alzheimer disease), most discovered associations from GWAS were either in genes that were not previously suspected to be involved in the disease or in regions of the genome with no obvious genes. Still, the evidence supporting some candidate genes is difficult to ignore (eg, *ERRB4*, the receptor for *NRG1*, has shown high significance in an African American [AA] GWAS sample).[89] Additional research and the analysis of cumulative data, with particular attention to both quality control and statistical rigor, are required for definitive conclusions. The interpretation of data can be treacherous. For example, the reader should be aware that gene pathway analyses do not specifically confirm individual gene associations. Although an association with *ERRB4* may suggest potential involvement of *NRG1* because both belong to the same biological pathway, it does not confirm, by itself, participation of *NRG1* in schizophrenia, which requires a genome-wide association signal between *NRG1* and schizophrenia.

GWAS

Genome-wide studies, in combination with system biology approaches, yield comprehensive information and have been demonstrated to be more useful to deal with complex phenotypes. In direct opposition to candidate gene studies, GWAS interrogate markers of common variation across the human genome one at a time, investigating all genes and most of the nongenic regions, whether or not they were previously implicated by pathophysiological hypotheses. The large number of tests in a GWAS makes the method highly susceptible to false-positive hits; the estimation of an appropriate genome-wide significance threshold is

Table 1
Top genes or genomic regions identified in recent schizophrenia GWAS

First Author and Year	Sample (Case/Control)	Gene or Region	Lowest P Values	OR	References
Lencz 2007	178/144 (EA)	CSF2RA, SHOX	3.7×10^{-7}	3.23	192
Sullivan 2008	738/733 (EA)	AGBL1	1.71×10^{-6}	6.01	193
O'Donovan 2008	Discovery: 479/2937 (EA) Follow-up: 6829/9897 (EA)	ZNF804A	1.61×10^{-7}	1.12	129
Need 2009	Discovery: 871/863 (EA) Follow-up: 1460/12,995 (EA)	ADAMTSL3	1.35×10^{-7}	0.68	144
Purcell 2009 (ISC)	3322/3587 (EA)	MHC region[a] MYO18B	9.5×10^{-9} 3.4×10^{-7}	0.82	102
Stefansson 2009 (SGENE)	Discovery: 2663/13,498 (EA) Follow-up: 4999/15,555 (EA)	MHC region[b] NRGN[b] TCF4[b]	1.4×10^{-12} 2.4×10^{-9} 4.1×10^{-9}	1.16[c] 1.15 1.23	103
Shi 2009 (MGS)	2681/2653 (EA) 1286/973 (AA)	MHC region[a] CENTG2 (in EA only) ERBB4 (in AA only)	9.5×10^{-9} 4.59×10^{-7} 2.14×10^{-6}	0.88 1.23 0.73	89

[a] Combined analysis of ISC, SGENE-plus (GWAS set), and MGS.
[b] Combined analysis of ISC and MGS, along with SGENE-plus and follow-up samples.
[c] OR (odds ratio) is for common allele of the associated SNP, which is different from that in ISC and MGS.

fundamental. The genome-wide significance threshold for a value of 5% significance assuming tests for all common SNPs has been estimated to be around $P<5 \times 10^{-8}$.[91–93] Because of their more comprehensive coverage of the human genome, GWAS have been more successful than any previous approach to find new susceptibility loci for complex disorders. According to www.genome.gov/gwastudies (as of September 20, 2009), 732 genes were reported associated to one or more complex disease phenotypes at genome-wide significant levels ($P<5 \times 10^{-8}$),[90,94] and many of these associations have already been replicated. GWAS are based on linkage disequilibrium (LD), a nonrandom statistical association of alleles at two or more loci, which is characteristically associated with short physical distance between genetic markers.

To a large extent, GWAS was made possible by the Human Genome Project (www.ornl.gov/sci/techresources/Human_Genome/home.shtml). Major improvements in SNP genotyping and DNA sequencing were spinoffs from the human genome project, and microarrays made possible rapid and accurate genome-wide genotyping resulting in a map of common genetic variation in a reference set of individuals of European, Asian, and African descent (HapMap project). Most of the markers used for GWAS are tag SNPs; the most significant associated SNP in a GWAS may reflect an indirect association (ie, be in LD with a causative variant). The Affymetrix 6.0 and Illumina 1M SNP arrays include approximately 1-M common SNPs and probes for analysis of copy number variants (CNVs), with their SNPs assaying approximately 80% of the common variation in the genome for EA samples.[95] The estimated number of common (minor allele frequency, MAF >1%) SNPs is approximately 10 M, but the genotyping capabilities are not sufficiently developed yet to genotype every SNP in a very large clinical sample (deep resequencing technology and new arrays may soon overcome this difficulty). In the meantime imputation, the computational prediction of genotypes from nongenotyped SNPs, is used to extend GWAS map coverage.[96,97] By design, the main assumption under GWAS is the common disease–common variant hypothesis.[98,99]

Recent complex disorders GWAS show two main characteristics. First, common loci with small effects are typically reported (OR = 1.1–1.5), an empirical confirmation that a large body of epidemiological studies predicting multiple small common genetic effects for complex disorders were correct (including for schizophrenia),[100,101] because loci with larger effects are rapidly eliminated from the population through selection. Second, most studies have tended to detect new susceptibility loci, and only very large samples obtained from combining studies are powered to show robust replication. This is because the power to detect one out of many possible risk loci is much larger than the power to detect specific disorder alleles.[21] Furthermore, if only small effects are found, many genes would be predicted to underlie the pathophysiology of most complex genetic disorders. It is important to also emphasize, however, some main GWAS limitations. The reader should be aware that the statistical power of GWAS to detect an association with rare alleles (ie, SNPs or CNVs with MAF <1%) is very limited; that for the detection of rare variants resequencing is more useful than GWAS; and that the study of gene-gene interactions (epistasis), although widely expected to be a significant source of heritability, is strictly limited by the statistical power of currently existing samples contrasted to the large number of such tests.

GWAS have already yielded genome-wide significant results for schizophrenia, though the reader should note that the small individual ORs do not permit prediction of caseness from specific individual susceptibility loci. Seven GWAS for schizophrenia have been published (see **Table 1**). The sizes of the investigated discovery samples have ranged from 322 to greater than 16,161, but even the largest studies did not yield a genome-wide significant result before combined testing of independent samples. This was not unexpected. The collective experience of GWAS for complex disorders shows that a typical susceptibility locus has an OR of 1.1 to 1.3, which often necessitates extremely large samples for detection. A sample with a total number of 5334, such as the Molecular Genetics of Schizophrenia (MGS) EA sample (most investigated samples have been smaller), has adequate statistical power only to detect very common risk alleles (30%–60% frequency, log additive effects) with genotypic relative risks approximately 1.3.[89] To reach sufficient statistical power, the combined analysis of independent datasets is useful. Although the diagnostic spectrum of the final combined sample is naturally wider than for the component datasets, combining datasets has been remarkably successful for a variety of complex disorders including schizophrenia (see next).[89,102,103] Different samples often were typed with different platforms, but imputation largely overcomes the limitation that many SNPs from different platforms do not overlap. These results suggest that schizophrenia, despite the very high reported heritability, is among the most complex of human genetic disorders. An additional analysis of the International Schizophrenia Consortium (ISC) and MGS samples[102] supported a polygenic model for schizophrenia susceptibility, involving a set of hundreds of genes, each with unquantified but very small individual effects (see later, polygenic section).[100] Finally, rapidly mounting evidence shows that cases have more rare (<1%) and large (>100 kb) CNVs than controls.

META-ANALYSIS OF GWAS DATA AND THE MAJOR HISTOCOMPATIBILITY COMPLEX LOCUS

The initial attempts to map schizophrenia to the major histocompatibility complex (MHC) started in the 1970s,[104] only a few years after the discovery of the human HLA system.[105] Many attempts since then had been made, and some yielded suggestive evidence,[106] but definitive evidence of MHC involvement was only recently obtained from a combined analysis of GWAS data. Three GWAS studies published jointly in 2009 (ISC, MGS, and Schizophrenia Genetics Consortium [SGENE]), reaching a total EA sample of 8008 cases and 19,077 controls, performed a meta-analysis of schizophrenia GWAS for the first time.[89,102,103] The meta-analysis combined the P values for all imputed and genotyped SNPs from the most significant regions of each study. This analysis generated a genome-wide significant association at the MHC region on chromosome 6.

The MHC signal extends over much of the MHC region, from approximately 26 Mb to approximately 33 Mb (**Fig. 2**). The strongest evidence (rs13194053; $P = 9.54 \times 10^{-9}$) for association from the meta-analysis was observed near a cluster of histone genes and several immune-related genes, including *butyrophilin subfamily 3 member A2 and A1 (BTN3A2 and BTN3A1)* and *protease serine 16 (PRSS16)*, but each individual dataset tends to have a different location for its best findings. The MHC region has a very high gene density and long-range LD blocks[107]; the human genome is structured in many "blocklike" islands of LD generated by a great variation of recombination rates. Blocks from regions of low recombination are long and are interspersed with interblock regions of higher recombination.[108,109] The location of the causative variation remains indeterminate but it could be in one or more genes or a nongenic region within the MHC. In the MGS sample (and in the other two samples), approximately 50% of the top 1000 highest ranking GWAS SNPs were intergenic, located outside the 10 kb region on either side of a gene, although many of these may represent a genic region signal caused by LD. Even at the MHC locus, rs13194053, the SNP with the most significant association from the meta-analysis, is approximately 29 kb

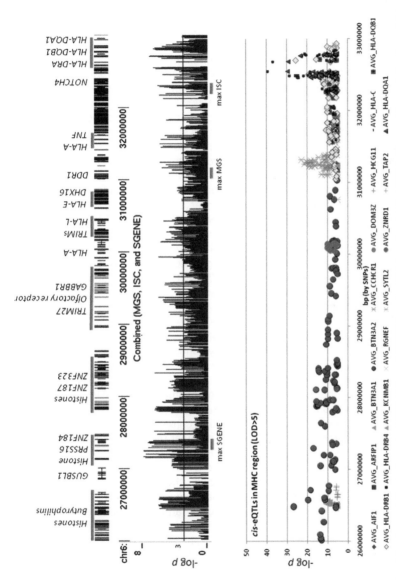

Fig. 2. The combined *P* values of three datasets (MGS, ISC, and SGENE) at the MHC region (~26–33Mb). The positions of the three histone gene clusters and *NOTCH4* are indicated in the RefSeq track (*top*). The relative location of the maximum peak in each data set is indicated by a line below the *P* value peaks. *Cis*-eQTL (with LOD >5) are shown below the graph with association -log *P* value. (*Data from* Dixon AL, Liang L, Moffatt MF, et al. A genome-wide association study of global gene expression. Nat Genet 2007;39:1202.)

away from its closest gene, *HIST1H2AH* (*histone cluster 1, H2ah*).[89,102,103] A functional role for many intergenic regions would not be surprising. Many of these regions contain highly conserved sequences believed to have a regulatory function.[110] The associated variants, or variants in LD with them, in intergenic regions may then alter expression of upstream or downstream genes. Moreover, most of the human genome is transcribed, with some transcripts serving as regulatory RNAs, but the function of most transcripts still undefined.[111]

The genes in the MHC region have many different biological functions, but genes with an immune function predominate. Histones regulate DNA transcription by chromatin modification through histone methylation or acetylation,[112–114] and have a role as antimicrobial agents; histones disrupt the bacterial cell membrane and interfere with microbial gene expression.[115] In human placenta, histones (H2A and H2B) neutralize bacterial endotoxins as part of an infection barrier.[116] This raises the possibility that genetic variation in histones might underlie a differential placental susceptibility to infections, and that one or more haplotypes spanning histones might increase the susceptibility to schizophrenia through this mechanism. A Danish registry study reported an increased risk of autoimmune disorders (thyrotoxicosis, intestinal malabsorption, acquired hemolytic anemia, chronic active hepatitis, interstitial cystitis, alopecia areata, myositis, polymyalgia rheumatica, and Sjögren syndrome) for schizophrenics, and a history of any autoimmune disorder (of 29 evaluated) was found associated with a 45% increase in risk for schizophrenia.[117] The MHC region has been implicated in many genetic disorders with immune-related abnormalities,[118] including type 1 diabetes (T1D), multiple sclerosis, Crohn disease, and rheumatoid arthritis, among many others per www.genome.gov/gwastudies.[90] It is noteworthy that rs3800307 (found on the DRB1*03-DQA1*0501-DQB1*0201 haplotype), a SNP in complete LD ($r^2 = 1$) with rs13194053, which reached genome-wide significant association with schizophrenia in the combined GWAS meta-analysis,[89,102,103] is associated with T1D.[119] In addition, rs3131296 at *NOTCH4* is in strong LD ($r^2 > 0.73$) with the classical HLA allele DRB1*03 and other SNPs that are associated with several autoimmune disorders (T1D, celiac disease, systemic lupus erythematosus, and so forth), albeit with opposite alleles.[103] Finally, the MGS GWAS showed some evidence, with $P = 3.5 \times 10^{-5}$ in the EA data set and $P = 1.9 \times 10^{-6}$ in the EA plus AA data set, for association with schizophrenia at the chromosome 1p22.1 *FAM69A-EVI-RPL5* gene cluster,[89] which has been implicated in multiple sclerosis.[120]

Other genes in the same region are involved in chromatin structure (high mobility group nucleosomal binding domain 4); transcriptional regulation (activator of basal transcription 1; zinc finger protein 322A [ZNF322A]; ZNF184); G-protein–coupled receptor signaling (FKSG83); and the nuclear pore complex (nuclear pore membrane protein 121-like 2, POM121L2). The SGENE-plus (their GWAS set) and follow-up samples (ie, an extended SGENE dataset that added a follow-up EA sample of 4999 cases and 15,555 controls) analysis reported an independent association (ie, in weak LD with rs13194053 at the histone gene cluster) at *NOTCH4* (*Notch homolog 4 [Drosophila]*, rs3131296, $P = 2 \times 10^{-8}$), located at 32.28 Mb on chromosome 6, and the combined meta-analysis of SGENE-plus and follow-up samples, along with MGS and ISC samples, gave a $P = 2.3 \times 10^{-10}$ there.[103] See **Table 2** for a list of genes mentioned in the text and their functions.

Non-MHC Loci That Have also Achieved Genome-wide Significance

The combined analysis of SGENE-plus GWAS samples and replication samples uncovered associations with *neurogranin* (*NRGN*) and with *transcription factor 4* (*TCF4*) that subsequently reached genome-wide significance in the combined analysis of

SGENE-plus and replication samples along with ISC and MGS samples (see **Table 1**).[103] *NRGN* encodes a postsynaptic protein kinase substrate that binds calmodulin, mediating *N*-methyl-D-aspartate receptor signaling that is important for learning and memory, and relevant to the proposed glutamate pathophysiology of schizophrenia.[121,122] *TCF4* is a neuronal transcriptional factor essential for brain development, specifically neurogenesis.[123] Mutations in *TCF4* cause Pitt-Hopkins syndrome, a neurodevelopmental disorder characterized by severe motor and mental retardation, including absent language development, microcephaly, epilepsy, and facial dysmorphisms.[124–126] It is also of interest that homozygous and compound-heterozygote deletions and mutations in *CNTNAP2* and *NRXN1* can symptomatically resemble Pitt-Hopkins syndrome along with autistic behavior,[127] and both *NRXN1* (by the 2p16.3 CNV, **Table 3**) and *CNTNAP2* (a rarer CNV)[128] have previously been implicated in schizophrenia (and also autism spectrum disorders and epilepsy).[127] Another new schizophrenia susceptibility gene from schizophrenia GWAS is *ZNF804A*, which was identified by a two-stage study, with a GWAS discovery phase using 479 cases and 2937 controls, followed with 6829 cases and 9897 controls for loci with a discovery $P<10^{-5}$.[129] A combined $P = 1.61 \times 10^{-7}$ was obtained for SNP rs1344706 in the initial report, and the association evidence was supported in later large GWAS of schizophrenia.[89,102,103] Subsequently, rs1344706 in *ZNF804A* was reported to be associated with altered neuronal connectivity in the dorsolateral prefrontal cortex in a functional MRI study of healthy controls.[130]

POLYGENIC CONTRIBUTIONS TO SCHIZOPHRENIA

Many genetic variants, each with a very small effect, combined together, make substantial contributions to disorder risk under a polygenic model, first hypothesized for schizophrenia four decades ago.[100] Simulations show that even a disorder with 1000 risk loci with low mean relative risks (RR = 1.04), when evaluated in a large scale (10,000 cases and 10,000 controls), GWAS still allows prediction of individual disorder risk with an accuracy greater than 0.75 by using 75 loci explaining approximately 50% of the risk variance.[131] The first empirical test of the polygenic hypothesis of schizophrenia by the ISC used their GWAS (discovery data set) to define a large set of very small effect common variants as "score" alleles with increasingly liberal association significance thresholds.[102] With the set of score alleles, the ISC generated an aggregate risk score for each individual in independent target GWAS data sets of schizophrenia, using the MGS EA and AA data sets and a United Kingdom sample.[89,129] Aggregate risk scores in cases were found to be significantly higher than in controls in each of the GWAS data sets of schizophrenia, and also in GWAS data sets of bipolar disorder,[132,133] but not in control GWAS data sets of nonpsychiatric disorders: T1D; type 2 diabetes; hypertension; Crohn disease; rheumatoid arthritis; and coronary artery disease.[102,133] Collectively, ISC concluded that thousands of common polygenic variants with very small individual effects explain about one third of the total variation in genetic liability to schizophrenia.[102] In an independent bioinformatics-based study,[134] schizophrenia candidate genes selected from literature mining were found to be enriched in the list of genes with small *P* values from independent schizophrenia GWAS data sets. The polygenic model under the assumption of less common (MAF <5%) causal alleles did not fit well with the observed schizophrenia GWAS data[102]; however, both simulated and empirical data indicate that the spectrum of risk alleles for common disorders includes both common and rare variants.[98,135] Furthermore, despite the substantial variation in liability to schizophrenia possibly explained by polygenic variants (approximately 30%), coupled with

Table 2
Genes mentioned in review, and their functions

Gene Symbol	Gene Description	Chromosome	Function
ABT1	Activator of basal transcription 1	6	Transcriptional regulation
AKT1	v-akt murine thymoma viral oncogene homolog 1	14	Critical mediator of growth factor–induced neuronal survival
ARVCF	Armadillo repeat gene deletes in VCFS	22	Catenin family member (adherens junction complex formation)
BTN3A1	Butyrophilin subfamily 3 member A1	6	Immunoglobulin superfamily
BTN3A2	Butyrophilin subfamily 3 member A2	6	Immunoglobulin superfamily
CACNA1C	Calcium channel, voltage-dependent, L type, α_{1C} subunit	12	Regulates muscle contraction, hormone or neurotransmitter release, cell cycle
CENTG2	Centaurin gamma 2	2	Protein trafficking in the endosomal-lysosomal system
CHRNA7	Cholinergic receptor, nicotinic, alpha 7	15	Ligand-gated ion channel mediating synaptic transmission
CNTNAP2	Contactin-associated protein-like 2	7	A member of the neurexin family, which functions in the vertebrate nervous system as cell adhesion molecules and receptors
COMT	Catechol O-methyltransferase	22	Catecholamine neurotransmitter metabolism; VCFS region (22q deletion syndrome)
DAOA	D-amino acid oxidase activator	13	Activator of the enzyme DAAO, which degrades D-serine
DISC1	Disrupted in schizophrenia 1	1	Neurite outgrowth and cortical development; disrupted in t(1;11)(q42.1;q14.3)
DRD2	Dopamine receptor D_2	11	G-protein coupled receptor for dopamine; inhibits adenylyl cyclase
DRD4	Dopamine receptor D_4	11	G-protein coupled receptor for dopamine; inhibits adenylyl cyclase
DTNBP1	Dystrobrevin binding protein 1	6	Component of the biogenesis of lysosome-related organelles complex 1
ERBB4	v-erb-a erythroblastic leukemia viral oncogene	2	Receptors for neuregulins; cell differentiation
EVI	Ecotropic viral integration site 5	1	Cell cycle progression
FAM69A	Family with sequence similarity 69, member A	1	Unknown; implicated in multiple sclerosis
FKSG83	Hypothetical protein	6	G-protein-coupled receptor signaling

Symbol	Gene name	Chr	Function
FMR1	Fragile X mental retardation 1	23	May be involved in nucleus → cytoplasm mRNA trafficking
FXR1	Fragile X mental retardation, autosomal homolog 1	3	RNA-binding protein; embryonic and postnatal development of muscle tissue
HIST1H2AH	Histone cluster 1, H2ah	6	Chromatin modification, transcription regulation, host defense
HTR2A	5-Hydroxytryptamine (serotonin) receptor 2A	13	G-protein coupled receptor for serotonin; activates phosphoinositide hydrolysis
HMGN4	High-mobility group nucleosomal binding domain 4	6	Involved in chromatin structure
MYO18B	Myosin XVIIIB	22	Regulate muscle-specific genes; intracellular trafficking
NOTCH4	Notch homolog 4 (Drosophila)	6	Receptor for Jagged1, Jagged2, and Delta1; cell-fate determination
NRG1	Neuregulin 1	8	Signaling protein that mediates cell-cell interactions; roles in growth and development
NRGN	Neurogranin	11	Postsynaptic protein kinase substrate; learning and memory; glutamate signaling
POM121L2	Nuclear pore membrane protein 121-like 2	6	Nuclear pore complex
PPP3CC	Protein phosphatase 3 (formerly 2B), catalytic subunit, gamma isoform	8	Ca^{++}-dependent modifier of phosphorylation status
PRSS16	Protease serine 16	6	Alternative antigen presenting
RGS4	Regulator of G-protein signaling 4	1	GTPase activating protein for G alpha subunits of G proteins
RPL5	Ribosomal protein L5	1	rRNA maturation and formation of the 60S ribosomal subunits
STX7	Syntaxin 7	6	Endosomal soluble N-ethylmaleimide-sensitive factor attachment protein receptors
TAAR6	Trace amine associated receptor 6	6	Trace amines are endogenous amine compounds, chemically similar to classic biogenic amines, such as dopamine
TCF4	Transcription factor 4	18	Neuronal transcriptional factor; neurogenesis
ZNF184	Zinc finger protein 18	6	Transcriptional regulation
ZNF322A	Zinc finger protein 322A	6	Transcriptional regulation
ZNF804A	Zinc finger protein 804A	2	Transcription factor; neuronal connectivity in the dorsolateral prefrontal cortex

Genes are listed alphabetically by symbol. All chromosome 6 genes are in the MHC except DTNBP1.

Table 3
Summary of recent genome-wide CNV studies of schizophrenia

Study	Sample	Major Findings	1q21.1	2p16.3 (NRXN1)	15q11.2	15q13.2	16p11.2	22q11.21	References
Kirov 2008	93 trios	Two CNVs likely to be pathogenic	NA	1 del (1.08)	NA	1 dup (1.08)	NA	NA	138
Walsh 2008	150 cases/268 controls; 92 childhood onset cases	Rare CNVs in 15% cases versus 5% controls	1:0 del (0.41:0)	1:0 del (0.41:0)	NA	NA	2:0 dup (0.83:0)	NA	139
Xu 2008	359 trios as screening sample; 152 cases/159 controls	In sporadic cases, frequency of rare de novo CNVs was 10% versus 1.3% in controls	1:0 del (0.20:0)	NA	NA	NA	NA	3:0 del (0.59:0)	140
Stefansson 2008	1433 cases/33,250 controls; 3 CNVs (1q21.1, 15q11.2, and 15q13.3) were followed-up in 3285 cases/7951 controls	Three rare CNVs (1q21.1, 15q11.2, and 15q13.3) showed nominal association	11:8 del (0.23:0.02)	0:2 del (0:0.01)	26:79 del (0.55:0.19)	7:8 del (0.15:0.02)	2:11 del (0.14:0.03)	8:0 del (0.56:0)	141
Stone 2008	3391 cases/3181 controls	Rare (<1%) and large CNVs (>100 kb) are enriched in cases (1.15-fold); 3 regions (1q21.1, 15q13.2, and 22q11.21) showed significant association	10:1 del (0.29:0.03)	5:6 del (0.15:0.19)	26:11 del (0.77:0.35)	9:0 del (0.27:0)	5:1 dup (0.15:0.03)	13:0 del (0.38:0)	142

Study							
Kirov 2009 471 cases/ 2792 controls	Large CNVs (>1 Mb) were 2.26 times overrepresented in cases	0:2 del (0:0.07)	1:3 del (0.21:0.11)	4:14 del (0.85:0.5)	0:0 del (0:0)	NA	2:0 del (0.42:0) [143]
Need 2009 1013 cases/ 1084 controls	Large CNVs (>2 Mb) are enriched in cases	1:0 del (0.1:0)	3:1 del (0.3:0.09)	NA	NA	NA	4:0 del (0.39:0) [144]
Summary frequency of most implicated CNV in schizophrenia (case versus control)	CNV case control	del 0.23% 0.02%	del 0.17% 0.03%	del 0.65% 0.22%	del 0.18% 0.02%	dup 0.19% 0.00%	del 0.44% 0.00%
Other disorders reported in schizophrenia CNV carriers of the most implicated CNV in the studies above		ASD, LD			MR		LD [141–143]
Other disorders reported associated with these CNVs in other studies		ASD, MR, epilepsy, microcephaly, cardiac abnormalities	ASD, MR	ASD, MR, epilepsy	ASD, MR, epilepsy	ASD, MR, bipolar disorder	ASD, MR, VCFS [159,194–204]

Study lists first author and year. The summary frequency for 16p11.2 also includes an unlisted study that only examined 16p11.2 CNV (ie, not genome-wide) and found 21 dup in 4551 schizophrenia cases and 2 dup in 6391 controls (the sample included MGS-GAIN samples used in the authors' GWAS).
Epilepsy includes seizures.
The 22q11.21 CNV deletion also includes DiGeorge or velocardiofacial syndrome.
CNVs in case:control.
Abbreviations: ASD, autism or autism spectrum disorders; LD, learning disability (dyslexia and others); MR, mental retardation; VCSF, velocardiofacial syndrome.

contributions from common and small-effect variants individually detectable in GWAS (eg, MHC variants, *TCF4*, and so forth) and rare and large-effect CNVs (see later), the problem of how to explain the substantial missing heritability remains fundamental. Missing heritability here refers to heritability that is unexplained after well-powered GWAS have been conducted. Although it has been argued that the heritability of some behavioral traits and disorders may have been overestimated,[136] this seems unlikely for schizophrenia given the large body of high-quality evidence that is available, and other reasons seem more plausible.[137]

RARE CNVS AND SCHIZOPHRENIA

CNVs are stretches of genomic deletions and duplications ranging from 1 kb to several Mb, and are likely to have larger phenotypic effects than SNPs. Only rare (<1%) and large (>100 kb) CNVs have been implicated in schizophrenia,[138–144] as reflected by overall CNV burden and individual CNV loci. Supporting evidence for association of specific rare and large CNVs with schizophrenia is emerging at 1q21.1, 2p16.3 (*NRXN1*), 15q11.2, 15q13.2, 16p11.2, and 22q11.21 (see **Table 3**).[138–144] The 3 Mb deletion at 22q11.21 (22qDS) has been known to cause velocardiofacial syndrome, and increases the risk for schizophrenia.[145–147] An epidemiological study found that more than 30% of 22qDS carriers develop psychosis, about 80% of this manifesting as schizophrenia,[147] which represents the largest known individual risk factor for the development of schizophrenia, besides having an identical twin with schizophrenia. The 22q11.21 CNV was the only CNV reaching genome-wide significance in some schizophrenia GWAS[142] and the only one not found in controls (case%/control% was 0.30/0.00). Each of these other CNVs was found overrepresented in schizophrenia cases in at least one study (see **Table 3**), with the supporting evidence remaining consistent for CNVs at the 1q21.1 deletion (0.24/0.02), 2p16.3 (*NRXN1*) deletion (0.10/0.02), 15q13.2 deletion (0.20/0.02), and 16p11.2 duplication (0.35/0.03), and plausible for the 15q11.2 deletion (0.65/0.22). All the CNVs (except for 22q11.21) initially found only in schizophrenia cases were also found in healthy controls in later studies, suggesting that the penetrance of these rare CNVs may be relatively low (see **Table 3**). The deletions at *NRXN1*, which only involve this single gene, suggest that exon disruptions rather than deletions of other parts of *NRXN1* are associated with schizophrenia.[148] With the rest of the rare and large CNVs implicated in schizophrenia spanning multiple genes, specific gene effects, including possibly genes presenting pleiotropy (see next section), are difficult to disentangle.

PLEIOTROPY AND OVERLAP WITH BIPOLAR DISORDER AND AUTISM

Pleiotropy refers to the common phenomenon of variation in a gene simultaneously affecting different phenotypes. Although examples abound in model organisms (eg, flies),[149] evidence for pleiotropy in humans is also available, such as genes for body weight and height,[150] and also for such disorders as type 2 diabetes[151] and prostate cancer.[152] The molecular genetic overlaps between schizophrenia and bipolar disorder and between schizophrenia and autism are consistent with pleiotropy; but shared genetic loci may actually determine an aspect (somewhat in isolation from the overall phenotype) shared by two disorders, such as psychosis in schizophrenia and in bipolar disorder.[153]

Although schizophrenia and bipolar disorder are classified as different psychiatric disorders in most contemporary classifications,[154] a distinction historically referred to as the "Kraepelinian dichotomy,"[7] they share some similarities, such as peak onset in early adulthood; prevalence around 1% generally similar worldwide; psychotic symptoms in more than half of bipolar disorder type 1 subjects and the same treatment of psychosis (in both cases with antipsychotic medications); substance use comorbidity; increased suicide risk (and common severe mood disorder in schizophrenia); and sometimes a difficult differential diagnosis with schizoaffective disorder. Overlap of susceptibility genes has been postulated[155–157] for more circumscribed aspects, such as psychosis proneness,[153,158] especially for "positive symptoms," such as hallucinations and delusions, or might reflect a wider range of susceptibility to higher brain dysfunction, such as pleiotropy found with CNVs (an overlapping CNV for schizophrenia and bipolar disorder has been reported for the 16p11.2 duplication in a meta-analysis with an association $P = 4.8 \times 10^{-7}$ for schizophrenia and $P = 0.017$ for bipolar disorder).[159] Family studies have shown that schizoaffective disorder is more common in families ascertained from probands with schizophrenia or with bipolar disorder type 1 than in the general population.[9–14] A recent meta-analysis of family studies found familial coaggregation of schizophrenia and bipolar disorder.[160] The largest family study reported to date, comprised of almost 36,000 schizophrenia and over 40,000 bipolar disorder Swedish probands, concluded that familial coaggregation between schizophrenia and bipolar disorder was approximately 63% because of additive genetic effects common to both disorders.[161] Recent GWAS SNP data strongly support a genetic overlap between schizophrenia and bipolar disorder, which were shown to share polygenic common variants with very small effect sizes (see polygenic section previously).[102] A gene-wide analysis found a significant excess of genes showing associations with both disorders.[162] ZNF804A and CACNA1C (calcium channel, voltage-dependent, L type, α_{1C} subunit) are two such genes that are shared by both disorders: ZNF804A was initially identified as a schizophrenia susceptibility gene, and CACNA1C was initially identified as a bipolar disorder susceptibility gene, in respective GWAS.[129,163]

Interestingly, the strongest SNP association of $P = 4.6 \times 10^{-7}$ in the MGS GWAS EA data set was found with centaurin gamma 2 (CENTG2, also known as AGAP1), a gene that has been implicated in autism.[164] It is also noteworthy that exploratory analysis of MGS GWAS data combining both EA and AA ancestries (3967 cases and 3626 controls) showed a $P = 1.9 \times 10^{-6}$ association with fragile X mental retardation, autosomal homolog 1 (FXR1),[89] and the association reached genome-wide significance when the ISC and SGENE-plus GWAS datasets were included in the analysis along with MGS EA plus AA (data not shown). FXR1 is a paralog of fragile X mental retardation 1 (FMR1), dysfunction of which causes the fragile X syndrome that includes autism as a common feature.[165] Schizophrenia and autism also share some clinical features, such as social interaction and communication impairments, and some negative and deficit symptoms.[166] This is more noticeable for childhood-onset schizophrenia where developmental delays may be more marked than in adult-onset schizophrenia with subtler such findings.[167] Autism remains an exclusion criterion for schizophrenia in the Diagnostic and Statistical Manual of Mental Disorders-IV unless prominent hallucinations and delusions are present for at least a month.[154] A study of 129 adults with autism spectrum disorders found that 7% had psychotic bipolar disorder and 8% had schizophrenia or other psychotic disorders.[168] The current diagnostic hierarchy, which largely treats autism spectrum disorders and schizophrenia as mutually exclusive, could mask some autism spectrum disorders and schizophrenia comorbidity because an autism case might be less likely to be diagnosed with schizophrenia in adulthood,[167] even in the presence of overt and chronic psychosis. A twofold increase of schizophrenia in the parents of autism cases,[169] a risk ratio of 3.44 for autism when prenatal parental history of a schizophrenia-like psychosis was present in a nationwide Danish study,[170] and an increased risk of schizophrenia in autism patients[168,171] suggest overlapping risk factors between schizophrenia and autism. Genetic overlap of schizophrenia and autism (and other conditions) has recently received indirect support because a number of schizophrenia cases carrying rare and large CNVs have comorbidities, such as learning disabilities, mental retardation, autism and autism spectrum disorders, and seizures or epilepsy, or such disorders' own CNV scans have implicated the same CNV loci (see **Table 3**). Besides the aforementioned conditions, others are overrepresented in schizophrenia cases in general, such as seizures.[172,173]

CHALLENGES FOR THE FIELD OF SCHIZOPHRENIA GENETICS

After over a quarter century of molecular genetics work in schizophrenia, advances in biotechnology and statistics applied to the study of large and well-characterized clinical samples have made possible the discovery of individual susceptibility loci with subsequent replication. A comprehensive discussion of what comes next after a successful GWAS is outside the scope of this article. Selected for discussion are a handful of issues that have been instrumental to generate progress until now, and are a foundation for further progress. First, the social environment where science is conducted has deeply changed during the last years. Of fundamental importance is the accentuated stance of new openness in the field of schizophrenia genetics in consonance with the instituted National Institutes of Health (NIH) policy of wide GWAS data sharing. Deidentified phenotypic and genotypic data from GWAS studies funded by NIH are to be submitted to a centralized NIH GWAS data repository, the database of Genotypes and Phenotypes (www.ncbi.nlm.nih.gov/gap) hosted by the National Center for Biotechnology Information, and studies supported the Wellcome Trust Case-Control Consortium are also deposited at a database (www.wtccc.org. uk). Data, in both cases, are accessible by application to access committees. The new NIH policy (grants.nih.gov/grants/gwas) has already created extraordinary opportunities to access data from independent research groups before publication.[174] For example, the MGS Genetic Association Information Network genotypic/phenotypic sample (www.genome.gov/19518582) has been accessed 140 times for a large diversity of genetics research projects as of November 17, 2009. The Psychiatric GWAS Consortium[175,176] continues this new tradition of openness. The Psychiatric GWAS Consortium is comprised of five groups: (1) schizophrenia, (2) bipolar disorder, (3) major depressive disorder, (4) attention deficit hyperactivity disorder, and (5) autism. A primary goal of the Psychiatric GWAS Consortium is to perform disease-specific and cross-disorder analyses from combined GWAS datasets composed of all qualifying samples for each of the disorders.

The method for following-up GWAS results needs to be thorough; replication and fine mapping of associated regions are necessary for further progress.[177] The preferred approach is to combine GWAS data from independent studies, but when some of the samples do not have GWAS data, focused genotyping is still useful, although less informative. The analysis of combined data is important because most clinical samples do not carry the power to detect effect sizes typically uncovered in well-powered GWAS,[178] and the estimated ORs tend to be inflated because only top-ranking associations are reported[179]; a less biased estimation of ORs requires the systematic combination of GWAS and focused replication studies. Data can be meta-analyzed with a variety of methods.[177] For example, three consortia[89,102,103] meta-analyzed a set of their most significant P values ($P<.001$) from their independent GWAS uncovering a genome-wide significant locus at the MHC. SNPs other than genome-wide significant ($P<5 \times 10^{-8}$) ones merit inclusion in confirmation experiments: although some genome-wide significant SNPs from a single study might not be confirmed in replication studies, other SNPs very highly ranking in the primary study, although not achieving genome-wide significance (eg, SNPs with $P < 1 \times 10^{-5}$), might surpass that threshold in a replication experiment. Association signals in an extended LD block that spans many genes (eg, the MHC locus implicated in schizophrenia) make it hard to disentangle which genes are likely to be causal. Populations of non-European ancestry might have some nonoverlapping susceptibility loci and it is fundamental to investigate these differences, because they can also be informative about different environmental risk factors. An important characteristic of African populations (eg, AA) is reduced LD, which facilitates the narrowing of the associated genomic intervals; existing limitations of CNV and SNP map coverage, and imputation of AA datasets are currently being addressed.[180,181]

It is important to bear in mind that given the GWAS SNP design (where SNPs are selected because they are common and are informative of many other SNPs, not because of their functional properties) in most cases the associated SNPs are probably not the causal SNPs. It has been noted that in the MGS GWAS and in the combined sample (MGS, ISC, and SGENE-plus),[89,102,103] most of the strongest common SNP associations were not located in coding sequences where such a signal is easier to interpret, but are in intergenic regions (over half of these SNPs >10 kb from a gene, almost all with no clear association to any known gene [ie, by LD]) or of unclear function (eg, intronic, but not near a splice site), or known or putative regulatory site. Although the causal SNPs should be in LD with the GWAS-associated SNPs, the causative genes may be close to the statistically associated locus, but may also be farther removed, even on a different chromosome. For example, if the causal variant was a *trans*-acting factor that regulates transcription, the regulated genes might be located on a different chromosome. The integration of genome-wide transcription data (expression quantitative trait loci [eQTL], currently detected by microarray expression data) and GWAS data (DNA variation data) can help close this gap by linking the GWAS statistical results and biology and is expected to lead to discoveries of mechanisms of disease susceptibility otherwise obscured to either method in isolation. The approach has been proved successful in asthma.[182] Interestingly, within the MHC region implicated in schizophrenia, there are more than 10 *cis*-eQTL (*cis* meaning nearby on the same chromosome) in the eQTL database, which uses expression data from lymphoblastoid cell lines of asthma patients (see **Fig. 2**),[183] and the SNP showing the most significant association with schizophrenia, rs13194053 with $P = 9.54 \times 10^{-9}$, is in strong LD ($r^2 = 0.43$) with a SNP showing the strongest association with BTN3A2 expression (see **Fig. 2**).

The selection of tissue for gene expression study is critical, and brain is not always necessarily the best choice of tissue. Epidemiological evidence strongly suggests that some of the primary genetic mechanisms leading to schizophrenia might reside in other tissues than brain (eg, an autoimmune mechanism that would compromise the brain); in such a case, the symptoms of schizophrenia still reflect brain dysfunction, but are removed from the primary noxae (investigations of these leads remain to be thoroughly explored). A more explicit example is if a genetic abnormality affecting an immunological response to a virus contributed to schizophrenia risk, studying the brain transcription characteristics of a neurotransmitter system only reflects secondary (or even terminal) neural changes to the primary immune response (which might be more apparent in immune tissue, such as lymphocytes).

Establishing causal mechanisms may require, in addition to statistical testing of association, the functional characterization of implicated genes and variants in simple cell models (and in model organisms) targeting phenotypes with a high probability of association with the studied disorder. Among other potential advantages, in the absence of buffering effects present in multicellular systems, in vitro effects are expected to be amplified (which may make detectable an effect that is very small in the whole or intact organism). Dendrou and colleagues[184] studied cell-specific protein phenotypes for *IL2RA*, a locus associated with T1D. By taking advantage of a large collection of normal donors from whom fresh, primary cells could be analyzed (the experimental subjects can be recalled for repeated measurements; this resource is known as the "Cambridge BioResource") it was very elegantly demonstrated that elevated CD25 expression is associated with *IL2RA* haplotypes that protect from T1D.[184]

It is still premature to conclude whether the genetic architecture of schizophrenia is like mental retardation where thousands of individual genetic disorders have been cataloged, or whether some widely speculated on but still little investigated mechanism, such as epigenetics (which influences phenotypes through the regulation of gene expression) or gene-environment interactions, explains the bulk of the missing heritability for the disorder. Basic genomics research has produced major breakthroughs during recent years, such as discovery of microRNAs, long-range promoters, epigenetic factors, and variable copy number variations, and many more will probably be made because knowledge of the genome is rapidly increasing. It should not be surprising if still unknown genetic mechanisms explain a substantial proportion of the heritability of schizophrenia. Nonetheless, the task of defining the spectrum of molecular genetic mechanisms in schizophrenia is now at the forefront of the field. Some immediate research efforts focus on whole genome resequencing and genome-wide gene transcription and epigenetic analyses. Rapid progress in biotechnology[185] is making the study of rare variants in many genes or large genomic regions in larger samples increasingly feasible; proof of principle is provided by the 1000 genomes project (www.1000genomes.org), which is designed to build a deep catalog of human genetic variation. The design of experiments aimed at fine mapping of regions of association and the precision of imputation will both benefit from this project.

It is anticipated that as genetic discoveries accumulate, the application of a myriad of tools from systems biology (eg, genomics, transcriptomics, proteomics, and so forth) will lead to a delineation of biological pathways involved in the pathophysiology of schizophrenia, and eventually to new therapies (developments in treatment still lag compared with discoveries of new genetic associations for complex disorders,[186] but this situation is expected to change as biological research makes inroads into still purely statistical associations). There is, however, a strong temptation to accept the simplest observations (ie, those with immediate biological connotation) as the most meaningful and the only ones that merit follow-up. For example, Mitchell and Porteous[187] stated: "Occam's razor and statistical probability both argue that the co-inheritance of one or just a few risk genes by any individual case is the more likely explanation for the majority of incidence." They continued: "Haven't we learnt more about disease mechanism and potential routes to the treatment of Alzheimer's disease from the rare variant examples of amyloid beta (A4) precursor protein (APP), presenilin-1 (PS1) and presenilin-2 (PS2) than from the archetypal common variant example of apolipoprotein E, isoform 4 (ApoE4)?" These arguments seem necessarily true at first sight, however, as previously discussed,[188] an explanation may superficially appear more complicated than need to be, but only if considered apart from its evolutionary context.[189] Research in model organisms (eg, *Drosophila*) shows that most phenotypes are the result of complicated genetic architectures: multiple genes, often showing pleiotropy (likely associated with multiple traits) and epistasis, and even single mutation effects differing with genetic background and environment,[190,191] and this landscape is probably also true for complex human behavioral traits. Explanations relying on single genes are unlikely to capture the fundamental complexity of most human complex traits, and all the associated genetic variation needs to be pursued to understand the pathophysiology of a complex disorder. A task of utmost importance is the integration of the spectrum of mutations found in schizophrenia into a system that takes into account constantly changing environments and evolution.

REFERENCES

1. Gejman PV, Owen MJ, Sanders AR. Psychiatric genetics. In: Tasman A, Kay J, Lieberman J, editors. Psychiatry. Hoboken (NJ): Wiley; 2003. p. 234–53.
2. McGrath J, Saha S, Chant D, et al. Schizophrenia: a concise overview of incidence, prevalence, and mortality. Epidemiol Rev 2008;30:67.
3. Messias EL, Chen CY, Eaton WW. Epidemiology of schizophrenia: review of findings and myths. Psychiatr Clin North Am 2007;30:323.
4. Girard C, Simard M. Clinical characterization of late- and very late-onset first psychotic episode in psychiatric inpatients. Am J Geriatr Psychiatry 2008;16:478.
5. Remschmidt H, Theisen FM. Schizophrenia and related disorders in children and adolescents. J Neural Transm Suppl 2005;121.
6. Leung A, Chue P. Sex differences in schizophrenia, a review of the literature. Acta Psychiatr Scand Suppl 2000;401:3.
7. Kraepelin E. Manic-depressive insanity and paranoia. Edinburgh: E. & S. Livingstone; 1899. [English translation 1921.]
8. Kasanin J. The acute schizoaffective psychoses. Am J Psychiatry 1933;90:97.
9. Maier W, Lichtermann D, Minges J, et al. Continuity and discontinuity of affective disorders and schizophrenia: results of a controlled family study. Arch Gen Psychiatry 1993;50:871.
10. Maier W, Lichtermann D, Franke P, et al. The dichotomy of schizophrenia and affective disorders in extended pedigrees. Schizophr Res 2002;57:259.
11. Gershon ES, DeLisi LE, Hamovit J, et al. A controlled family study of chronic psychoses: schizophrenia and schizoaffective disorder. Arch Gen Psychiatry 1988;45:328.
12. Gershon ES, Hamovit J, Guroff JJ, et al. A family study of schizoaffective, bipolar I, bipolar II, unipolar, and normal control probands. Arch Gen Psychiatry 1982;39:1157.
13. Kendler KS, McGuire M, Gruenberg AM, et al. The Roscommon family study. I. Methods, diagnosis of probands, and risk of schizophrenia in relatives. Arch Gen Psychiatry 1993;50:527.
14. Valles V, Van Os J, Guillamat R, et al. Increased morbid risk for schizophrenia in families of in-patients with bipolar illness. Schizophr Res 2000;42:83.
15. Heckers S. Is schizoaffective disorder a useful diagnosis? Curr Psychiatry Rep 2009;11:332.
16. Spitzer RL, Endicott J, Robins E. Research diagnostic criteria: rationale and reliability. Arch Gen Psychiatry 1978;35:773.
17. Nurnberger JI Jr, Blehar MC, Kaufmann CA, et al. Diagnostic interview for genetic studies: rationale, unique features, and training. NIMH Genetics Initiative. Arch Gen Psychiatry 1994;51:849.
18. Ng MY, Levinson DF, Faraone SV, et al. Meta-analysis of 32 genome-wide linkage studies of schizophrenia. Mol Psychiatry 2009;14:774.

19. Sporns O, Tononi G, Kotter R. The human connectome: a structural description of the human brain. PLoS Comput Biol 2005;1:e42.
20. Drachman DA. Do we have brain to spare? Neurology 2004;64:2005.
21. Kraft P, Hunter DJ. Genetic risk prediction: are we there yet? N Engl J Med 2009; 360:1701.
22. Schadt EE. Molecular networks as sensors and drivers of common human diseases. Nature 2009;461:218.
23. Petronis A. The origin of schizophrenia: genetic thesis, epigenetic antithesis, and resolving synthesis. Biol Psychiatry 2004;55:965.
24. Roth TL, Lubin FD, Sodhi M, et al. Epigenetic mechanisms in schizophrenia. Biochim Biophys Acta 2009;1790:869.
25. Byrne M, Agerbo E, Bennedsen B, et al. Obstetric conditions and risk of first admission with schizophrenia: a Danish national register based study. Schizophr Res 2007;97:51.
26. Mittal VA, Ellman LM, Cannon TD. Gene-environment interaction and covariation in schizophrenia: the role of obstetric complications. Schizophr Bull 2008;34: 1083.
27. Malaspina D, Harlap S, Fennig S, et al. Advancing paternal age and the risk of schizophrenia. Arch Gen Psychiatry 2001;58:361.
28. Torrey EF, Buka S, Cannon TD, et al. Paternal age as a risk factor for schizophrenia: how important is it? Schizophr Res 2009;114:1.
29. Clarke MC, Harley M, Cannon M. The role of obstetric events in schizophrenia. Schizophr Bull 2006;32:3.
30. Cannon M, Jones PB, Murray RM. Obstetric complications and schizophrenia: historical and meta-analytic review. Am J Psychiatry 2002;159:1080.
31. Susser ES, Lin SP. Schizophrenia after prenatal exposure to the Dutch Hunger Winter of 1944-1945. Arch Gen Psychiatry 1992;49:983.
32. St Clair D, Xu M, Wang P, et al. Rates of adult schizophrenia following prenatal exposure to the Chinese famine of 1959–1961. JAMA 2005;294:557.
33. Brown AS, Susser ES. Prenatal nutritional deficiency and risk of adult schizophrenia. Schizophr Bull 2008;34:1054.
34. James WP. The epidemiology of obesity: the size of the problem. J Intern Med 2008;263:336.
35. Wild S, Roglic G, Green A, et al. Global prevalence of diabetes: estimates for the year 2000 and projections for 2030. Diabetes Care 2004;27:1047.
36. Munk-Jorgensen P, Mortensen PB. Is schizophrenia really on the decrease? Eur Arch Psychiatry Clin Neurosci 1993;242:244.
37. Neill J. Whatever became of the schizophrenogenic mother? Am J Psychother 1990;44:499.
38. Gejman PV. Ernst Rudin and Nazi euthanasia: another stain on his career. Am J Med Genet 1997;74:455.
39. Rüdin E. Zur vererbung und neuenstehung der dementia praecox. Berlin: Springer; 1916.
40. Gottesman II, Shields J. Schizophrenia: the epigenetic puzzle. Cambridge (UK): Cambridge University Press; 1982.
41. Risch N. Linkage strategies for genetically complex traits. I. Multilocus models. Am J Hum Genet 1990;46:222.
42. Birren B, Green ED, Klapholz S, et alIn: Genome analysis: a laboratory manual: mapping genome, vol. 4. Cold Spring Harbor (NY): Cold Spring Harbor Laboratory Press; 1998.

43. Smalley SL. Genetic influences in childhood-onset psychiatric disorders: autism and attention-deficit/hyperactivity disorder. Am J Hum Genet 1997;60:1276.
44. Yang J, Visscher PM, Wray NR. Sporadic cases are the norm for complex disease. Eur J Hum Genet 2009 [Epub ahead of print].
45. Kendler KS. Sporadic vs familial classification given etiologic heterogeneity: I. Sensitivity, specificity, and positive and negative predictive value. Genet Epidemiol 1987;4:313.
46. Cardno AG, Gottesman I. Twin studies of schizophrenia: from bow-and-arrow concordances to Star Wars Mx and functional genomics. Am J Med Genet 2000;97:12.
47. Sullivan PF, Kendler KS, Neale MC. Schizophrenia as a complex trait: evidence from a meta-analysis of twin studies. Arch Gen Psychiatry 2003;60:1187.
48. Rees J. Complex disease and the new clinical sciences. Science 2002;296:698.
49. Klaning U, Mortensen PB, Kyvik KO. Increased occurrence of schizophrenia and other psychiatric illnesses among twins. Br J Psychiatry 1996;168:688.
50. Cannon TD, Kaprio J, Lonnqvist J, et al. The genetic epidemiology of schizophrenia in a Finnish twin cohort: a population-based modeling study. Arch Gen Psychiatry 1998;55:67.
51. Franzek E, Beckmann H. Different genetic background of schizophrenia spectrum psychoses: a twin study. Am J Psychiatry 1998;155:76.
52. Cardno AG, Marshall EJ, Coid B, et al. Heritability estimates for psychotic disorders: the Maudsley twin psychosis series. Arch Gen Psychiatry 1999;56:162.
53. Gottesman II, Bertelsen A. Confirming unexpressed genotypes for schizophrenia. Risks in the offspring of Fischer's Danish identical and fraternal discordant twins. Arch Gen Psychiatry 1989;46:867.
54. Kringlen E, Cramer G. Offspring of monozygotic twins discordant for schizophrenia. Arch Gen Psychiatry 1989;46:873.
55. Mill J, Tang T, Kaminsky Z, et al. Epigenomic profiling reveals DNA-methylation changes associated with major psychosis. Am J Hum Genet 2008;82:696.
56. Ellman LM, Susser ES. The promise of epidemiologic studies: neuroimmune mechanisms in the etiologies of brain disorders. Neuron 2009;64:25.
57. Ingraham LJ, Kety SS. Adoption studies of schizophrenia. Am J Med Genet 2000;97:18.
58. Heston LL. Psychiatric disorders in foster home reared children of schizophrenic mothers. Br J Psychiatry 1966;112:819.
59. Higgins J. Effects of child rearing by schizophrenic mothers: a follow-up. J Psychiatr Res 1976;13:1.
60. Wender PH, Rosenthal D, Kety SS, et al. Crossfostering: a research strategy for clarifying the role of genetic and experiential factors in the etiology of schizophrenia. Arch Gen Psychiatry 1974;30:121.
61. Rosenthal D, Wender PH, Kety SS, et al. Schizophrenics' offspring raised in adoptive homes. J Psychiatr Res 1968;6:377.
62. Tienari P. Interaction between genetic vulnerability and family environment: the Finnish adoptive family study of schizophrenia. Acta Psychiatr Scand 1991;84:460.
63. Tienari P, Sorri A, Lahti I, et al. The Finnish Adoptive Family Study of Schizophrenia. Yale J Biol Med 1985;58:227.
64. Tienari P, Wynne LC, Moring J, et al. The Finnish adoptive family study of schizophrenia: implications for family research. Br J Psychiatry Suppl 1994;20.
65. Wahlberg KE, Wynne LC, Oja H, et al. Gene-environment interaction in vulnerability to schizophrenia: findings from the Finnish Adoptive Family Study of Schizophrenia. Am J Psychiatry 1997;154:355.

66. Kendler KS, Gruenberg AM, Kinney DK. Independent diagnoses of adoptees and relatives as defined by DSM-III in the provincial and national samples of the Danish Adoption Study of Schizophrenia. Arch Gen Psychiatry 1994;51:456.

67. Kendler KS, Gruenberg AM, Strauss JS. An independent analysis of the Copenhagen sample of the Danish adoption study of schizophrenia. II. The relationship between schizotypal personality disorder and schizophrenia. Arch Gen Psychiatry 1981;38:982.

68. Kety SS, Wender PH, Jacobsen B, et al. Mental illness in the biological and adoptive relatives of schizophrenic adoptees. Replication of the Copenhagen study in the rest of Denmark. Arch Gen Psychiatry 1994;51:442.

69. Kety SS, Rosenthal D, Wender PH, et al. The types and prevalence of mental illness in the biological and adoptive families of adopted schizophrenics. In: Rosenthal D, Kety SS, editors. The transmission of schizophrenia. Oxford, England (UK): Pergamon Press; 1968. p. 345.

70. Kety SS, Rosenthal D, Wender PH, et al. Mental illness in the biological and adoptive families of adopted individuals who have become schizophrenic: a preliminary report based upon psychiatric interviews. In: Fieve R, Rosenthal D, Brill H, editors. Genetic research in psychiatry. Baltimore (MD): The Johns Hopkins University Press; 1975. p. 147.

71. Kallmann FJ. The genetics of schizophrenia: a study of heredity and reproduction in the families of 1,087 schizophrenics. New York: J.J. Augustin Publisher; 1938.

72. Svensson AC, Lichtenstein P, Sandin S, et al. Fertility of first-degree relatives of patients with schizophrenia: a three generation perspective. Schizophr Res 2007;91:238.

73. Haukka J, Suvisaari J, Lonnqvist J. Fertility of patients with schizophrenia, their siblings, and the general population: a cohort study from 1950 to 1959 in Finland. Am J Psychiatry 2003;160:460.

74. Keller MC, Miller G. Resolving the paradox of common, harmful, heritable mental disorders: which evolutionary genetic models work best? Behav Brain Sci 2006; 29:385.

75. Fananas L, Bertranpetit J. Reproductive rates in families of schizophrenic patients in a case-control study. Acta Psychiatr Scand 1995;91:202.

76. MacCabe JH, Koupil I, Leon DA. Lifetime reproductive output over two generations in patients with psychosis and their unaffected siblings: the Uppsala 1915-1929 Birth Cohort multigenerational study. Psychol Med 2009;39:1667.

77. Allison AC. Notes on sickle-cell polymorphism. Ann Hum Genet 1954;19:39.

78. Gottesman II, Gould. TD. The endophenotype concept in psychiatry: etymology and strategic intentions. Am J Psychiatry 2003;160:636.

79. Greenwood TA, Braff DL, Light GA, et al. Initial heritability analyses of endophenotypic measures for schizophrenia: the consortium on the genetics of schizophrenia. Arch Gen Psychiatry 2007;64:1242.

80. Book JA. Schizophrenia as a gene mutation. Acta Genet Stat Med 1953;4:133.

81. Friedman JM. Genetic disease in the offspring of older fathers. Obstet Gynecol 1981;57:745.

82. Sipos A, Rasmussen F, Harrison G, et al. Paternal age and schizophrenia: a population based cohort study. BMJ 2004;329:1070.

83. Crow JF. The origins, patterns and implications of human spontaneous mutation. Nat Rev Genet 2000;1:40.

84. Allen NC, Bagade S, McQueen MB, et al. Systematic meta-analyses and field synopsis of genetic association studies in schizophrenia: the SzGene database. Nat Genet 2008;40:827.

85. Sanders AR, Duan J, Levinson DF, et al. No significant association of 14 candidate genes with schizophrenia in a large European ancestry sample: implications for psychiatric genetics. Am J Psychiatry 2008;165:497.

86. Ioannidis JP. Why most discovered true associations are inflated. Epidemiology 2008;19:640.

87. McCarthy MI, Abecasis GR, Cardon LR, et al. Genome-wide association studies for complex traits: consensus, uncertainty and challenges. Nat Rev Genet 2008;9:356.

88. Richter SH, Garner JP, Wurbel H. Environmental standardization: cure or cause of poor reproducibility in animal experiments? Nat Methods 2009;6:257.

89. Shi J, Levinson DF, Duan J, et al. Common variants on chromosome 6p22.1 are associated with schizophrenia. Nature 2009;460:753.

90. Hindorff LA, Sethupathy P, Junkins HA, et al. Potential etiologic and functional implications of genome-wide association loci for human diseases and traits. Proc Natl Acad Sci U S A 2009;106:9362.

91. Dudbridge F, Gusnanto A. Estimation of significance thresholds for genomewide association scans. Genet Epidemiol 2008;32:227.

92. Hoggart CJ, Clark TG, De Iorio M, et al. Genome-wide significance for dense SNP and resequencing data. Genet Epidemiol 2008;32:179.

93. Pe'er I, Yelensky R, Altshuler D, et al. Estimation of the multiple testing burden for genomewide association studies of nearly all common variants. Genet Epidemiol 2008;32:381.

94. Manolio TA, Collins FS, Cox NJ, et al. Finding the missing heritability of complex diseases. Nature 2009;461:747.

95. Li M, Li C, Guan W. Evaluation of coverage variation of SNP chips for genome-wide association studies. Eur J Hum Genet 2008;16:635.

96. Halperin E, Stephan DA. SNP imputation in association studies. Nat Biotechnol 2009;27:349.

97. Nothnagel M, Ellinghaus D, Schreiber S, et al. A comprehensive evaluation of SNP genotype imputation. Hum Genet 2009;125:163.

98. Pritchard JK. Are rare variants responsible for susceptibility to complex diseases? Am J Hum Genet 2001;69:124.

99. Reich DE, Lander ES. On the allelic spectrum of human disease. Trends Genet 2001;17:502.

100. Gottesman II, Shields J. A polygenic theory of schizophrenia. Proc Natl Acad Sci U S A 1967;58:199.

101. Risch N. Genetic linkage and complex diseases, with special reference to psychiatric disorders. Genet Epidemiol 1990;7:3.

102. Purcell SM, Wray NR, Stone JL, et al. Common polygenic variation contributes to risk of schizophrenia and bipolar disorder. Nature 2009;460:748.

103. Stefansson H, Ophoff RA, Steinberg S, et al. Common variants conferring risk of schizophrenia. Nature 2009;460:744.

104. Worden FG, Childs B, Matthysse S, et al. Frontiers of psychiatric genetics. Neurosci Res Program Bull 1976;14:8.

105. Bach ML, Bach FH, Joo P. Leukemia-associated antigens in the mixed leukocyte culture test. Science 1969;166:1520.

106. Wei J, Hemmings GP. The NOTCH4 locus is associated with susceptibility to schizophrenia. Nat Genet 2000;25:376.

107. Traherne JA. Human MHC architecture and evolution: implications for disease association studies. Int J Immunogenet 2008;35:179.

108. Daly MJ, Rioux JD, Schaffner SF, et al. High-resolution haplotype structure in the human genome. Nat Genet 2001;29:229.

109. Gabriel SB, Schaffner SF, Nguyen H, et al. The structure of haplotype blocks in the human genome. Science 2002;296:2225.

110. Kleinjan DA, van Heyningen V. Long-range control of gene expression: emerging mechanisms and disruption in disease. Am J Hum Genet 2005;76:8.

111. Birney E, Stamatoyannopoulos JA, Dutta A, et al. Identification and analysis of functional elements in 1% of the human genome by the ENCODE pilot project. Nature 2007;447:799.

112. Adegbola A, Gao H, Sommer S, et al. A novel mutation in JARID1C/SMCX in a patient with autism spectrum disorder (ASD). Am J Med Genet A 2008;146:505.

113. Costa E, Dong E, Grayson DR, et al. Reviewing the role of DNA (cytosine-5) methyltransferase overexpression in the cortical GABAergic dysfunction associated with psychosis vulnerability. Epigenetics 2007;2:29.

114. Shi Y. Histone lysine demethylases: emerging roles in development, physiology and disease. Nat Rev Genet 2007;8:829.

115. Kawasaki H, Iwamuro S. Potential roles of histones in host defense as antimicrobial agents. Infect Disord Drug Targets 2008;8:195.

116. Kim HS, Cho JH, Park HW, et al. Endotoxin-neutralizing antimicrobial proteins of the human placenta. J Immunol 2002;168:2356.

117. Eaton WW, Byrne M, Ewald H, et al. Association of schizophrenia and autoimmune diseases: linkage of Danish national registers. Am J Psychiatry 2006;163:521.

118. Shiina T, Inoko H, Kulski JK. An update of the HLA genomic region, locus information and disease associations: 2004. Tissue Antigens 2004;64:631.

119. Viken MK, Blomhoff A, Olsson M, et al. Reproducible association with type 1 diabetes in the extended class I region of the major histocompatibility complex. Genes Immun 2009;10:323.

120. Oksenberg JR, Baranzini SE, Sawcer S, et al. The genetics of multiple sclerosis: SNPs to pathways to pathogenesis. Nat Rev Genet 2008;9:516.

121. Wang H, Feng R, Phillip Wang L, et al. CaMKII activation state underlies synaptic labile phase of LTP and short-term memory formation. Curr Biol 2008;18:1546.

122. Harrison PJ, Weinberger DR. Schizophrenia genes, gene expression, and neuropathology: on the matter of their convergence. Mol Psychiatry 2005;10:40.

123. Gulacsi AA, Anderson SA. Beta-catenin-mediated Wnt signaling regulates neurogenesis in the ventral telencephalon. Nat Neurosci 2008;11:1383.

124. Flora A, Garcia JJ, Thaller C, et al. The E-protein Tcf4 interacts with Math1 to regulate differentiation of a specific subset of neuronal progenitors. Proc Natl Acad Sci U S A 2007;104:15382.

125. Kalscheuer VM, Feenstra I, Van Ravenswaaij-Arts CM, et al. Disruption of the TCF4 gene in a girl with mental retardation but without the classical Pitt-Hopkins syndrome. Am J Med Genet A 2008;146:2053.

126. Brockschmidt A, Todt U, Ryu S, et al. Severe mental retardation with breathing abnormalities (Pitt-Hopkins syndrome) is caused by haploinsufficiency of the neuronal bHLH transcription factor TCF4. Hum Mol Genet 2007;16:1488.

127. Zweier C, de Jong EK, Zweier M, et al. CNTNAP2 and NRXN1 are mutated in autosomal-recessive Pitt-Hopkins-like mental retardation and determine the level of a common synaptic protein in drosophila. Am J Hum Genet 2009;85:655.

128. Friedman JI, Vrijenhoek T, Markx S, et al. CNTNAP2 gene dosage variation is associated with schizophrenia and epilepsy. Mol Psychiatry 2008;13:261.

129. O'Donovan MC, Craddock N, Norton N, et al. Identification of loci associated with schizophrenia by genome-wide association and follow-up. Nat Genet 2008;40:1053.

130. Esslinger C, Walter H, Kirsch P, et al. Neural mechanisms of a genome-wide supported psychosis variant. Science 2009;324:605.
131. Wray NR, Goddard ME, Visscher PM. Prediction of individual genetic risk to disease from genome-wide association studies. Genome Res 2007;17:1520.
132. Sklar P, Smoller JW, Fan J, et al. Whole-genome association study of bipolar disorder. Mol Psychiatry 2008;13:558.
133. Wellcome Trust Case Control Consortium. Genome-wide association study of 14,000 cases of seven common diseases and 3,000 shared controls. Nature 2007;447:661.
134. Sun J, Jia P, Fanous AH, et al. A multi-dimensional evidence-based candidate gene prioritization approach for complex diseases-schizophrenia as a case. Bioinformatics 2009;25:2595.
135. Kathiresan S, Willer CJ, Peloso GM, et al. Common variants at 30 loci contribute to polygenic dyslipidemia. Nat Genet 2009;41:56.
136. Kamin LJ, Goldberger AS. Twin studies in behavioral research: a skeptical view. Theor Popul Biol 2002;61:83.
137. Herold C, Steffens M, Brockschmidt FF, et al. INTERSNP: genome-wide interaction analysis guided by A priori information. Bioinformatics 2009;5:3275–81.
138. Kirov G, Gumus D, Chen W, et al. Comparative genome hybridization suggests a role for NRXN1 and APBA2 in schizophrenia. Hum Mol Genet 2008;17:458.
139. Walsh T, McClellan JM, McCarthy SE, et al. Rare structural variants disrupt multiple genes in neurodevelopmental pathways in schizophrenia. Science 2008;320:539.
140. Xu B, Roos JL, Levy S, et al. Strong association of de novo copy number mutations with sporadic schizophrenia. Nat Genet 2008;40:880.
141. Stefansson H, Rujescu D, Cichon S, et al. Large recurrent microdeletions associated with schizophrenia. Nature 2008;455:232.
142. ISC. Rare chromosomal deletions and duplications increase risk of schizophrenia. Nature 2008;455:237.
143. Kirov G, Grozeva D, Norton N, et al. Support for the involvement of large copy number variants in the pathogenesis of schizophrenia. Hum Mol Genet 2009;18:1497.
144. Need AC, Ge D, Weale ME, et al. A genome-wide investigation of SNPs and CNVs in schizophrenia. PLoS Genet 2009;5:e1000373.
145. Shprintzen RJ, Goldberg R, Golding-Kushner KJ, et al. Late-onset psychosis in the velo-cardio-facial syndrome. Am J Med Genet 1992;42:141.
146. Pulver AE, Nestadt G, Goldberg R, et al. Psychotic illness in patients diagnosed with velo-cardio-facial syndrome and their relatives. J Nerv Ment Dis 1994;182:476.
147. Murphy KC, Jones LA, Owen MJ. High rates of schizophrenia in adults with velo-cardio-facial syndrome. Arch Gen Psychiatry 1999;56:940.
148. Rujescu D, Ingason A, Cichon S, et al. Disruption of the neurexin 1 gene is associated with schizophrenia. Hum Mol Genet 2009;18:988.
149. Mackay TF. The genetic architecture of complex behaviors: lessons from *Drosophila*. Genetica 2009;136:295.
150. Weedon MN, Lango H, Lindgren CM, et al. Genome-wide association analysis identifies 20 loci that influence adult height. Nat Genet 2008;40:575.
151. Zeggini E, Scott LJ, Saxena R, et al. Meta-analysis of genome-wide association data and large-scale replication identifies additional susceptibility loci for type 2 diabetes. Nat Genet 2008;40:638.

152. Thomas G, Jacobs KB, Yeager M, et al. Multiple loci identified in a genome-wide association study of prostate cancer. Nat Genet 2008;40:310.
153. Schulze TG, Hedeker D, Zandi P, et al. What is familial about familial bipolar disorder? Resemblance among relatives across a broad spectrum of phenotypic characteristics. Arch Gen Psychiatry 2006;63:1368.
154. American Psychiatric Association. Diagnostic and statistical manual of mental disorders. 4th edition. (DSM-IV). Washington, DC: American Psychiatric Association; 1994.
155. Berrettini WH. Are schizophrenic and bipolar disorders related? A review of family and molecular studies. Biol Psychiatry 2000;48:531.
156. Craddock N, Owen MJ. Rethinking psychosis: the disadvantages of a dichotomous classification now outweigh the advantages. World Psychiatry 2007;6:84.
157. van Os J, Kapur S. Schizophrenia. Lancet 2009;374:635.
158. Goes FS, Zandi PP, Miao K, et al. Mood-incongruent psychotic features in bipolar disorder: familial aggregation and suggestive linkage to 2p11-q14 and 13q21-33. Am J Psychiatry 2007;164:236.
159. McCarthy SE, Makarov V, Kirov G, et al. Microduplications of 16p11.2 are associated with schizophrenia. Nat Genet 2009;41:1223.
160. Van Snellenberg JX, de Candia T. Meta-analytic evidence for familial coaggregation of schizophrenia and bipolar disorder. Arch Gen Psychiatry 2009;66:748.
161. Lichtenstein P, Yip BH, Bjork C, et al. Common genetic determinants of schizophrenia and bipolar disorder in Swedish families: a population-based study. Lancet 2009;373:234.
162. Moskvina V, Craddock N, Holmans P, et al. Gene-wide analyses of genome-wide association data sets: evidence for multiple common risk alleles for schizophrenia and bipolar disorder and for overlap in genetic risk. Mol Psychiatry 2009;14:252.
163. Green EK, Grozeva D, Jones I, et al. The bipolar disorder risk allele at CACNA1C also confers risk of recurrent major depression and of schizophrenia. Mol Psychiatry 2009 [Epub ahead of print].
164. Wassink TH, Piven J, Vieland VJ, et al. Evaluation of the chromosome 2q37.3 gene CENTG2 as an autism susceptibility gene. Am J Med Genet B Neuropsychiatr Genet 2005;136B:36.
165. Bassell GJ, Warren ST. Fragile X syndrome: loss of local mRNA regulation alters synaptic development and function. Neuron 2008;60:201.
166. Konstantareas MM, Hewitt T. Autistic disorder and schizophrenia: diagnostic overlaps. J Autism Dev Disord 2001;31:19.
167. Rapoport J, Chavez A, Greenstein D, et al. Autism spectrum disorders and childhood-onset schizophrenia: clinical and biological contributions to a relation revisited. J Am Acad Child Adolesc Psychiatry 2009;48:10.
168. Stahlberg O, Soderstrom H, Rastam M, et al. Bipolar disorder, schizophrenia, and other psychotic disorders in adults with childhood onset AD/HD and/or autism spectrum disorders. J Neural Transm 2004;111:891.
169. Daniels JL, Forssen U, Hultman CM, et al. Parental psychiatric disorders associated with autism spectrum disorders in the offspring. Pediatrics 2008;121:e1357.
170. Larsson HJ, Eaton WW, Madsen KM, et al. Risk factors for autism: perinatal factors, parental psychiatric history, and socioeconomic status. Am J Epidemiol 2005;161:916.
171. Mouridsen SE, Rich B, Isager T, et al. Psychiatric disorders in individuals diagnosed with infantile autism as children: a case control study. J Psychiatr Pract 2008;14:5.

172. Cascella NG, Schretlen DJ, Sawa A. Schizophrenia and epilepsy: is there a shared susceptibility? Neurosci Res 2009;63:227.
173. Hyde TM, Weinberger DR. Seizures and schizophrenia. Schizophr Bull 1997;23:611.
174. Manolio TA, Rodriguez LL, Brooks L, et al. New models of collaboration in genome-wide association studies: the genetic association information network. Nat Genet 2007;39:1045.
175. Cichon S, Craddock N, Daly M, et al. Genomewide association studies: history, rationale, and prospects for psychiatric disorders. Am J Psychiatry 2009;166:540.
176. Psychiatric GWAS Consortium Steering Committee. A framework for interpreting genome-wide association studies of psychiatric disorders. Mol Psychiatry 2009; 14:10.
177. Ioannidis JP, Thomas G, Daly MJ. Validating, augmenting and refining genome-wide association signals. Nat Rev Genet 2009;10:318.
178. Spencer CC, Su Z, Donnelly P, et al. Designing genome-wide association studies: sample size, power, imputation, and the choice of genotyping chip. PLoS Genet 2009;5:e1000477.
179. Bowden J, Dudbridge F. Unbiased estimation of odds ratios: combining genomewide association scans with replication studies. Genet Epidemiol 2009; 33:406.
180. Hao K, Chudin E, McElwee J, et al. Accuracy of genome-wide imputation of untyped markers and impacts on statistical power for association studies. BMC Genet 2009;10:27.
181. McElroy JP, Nelson MR, Caillier SJ, et al. Copy number variation in African Americans. BMC Genet 2009;10:15.
182. Moffatt MF, Kabesch M, Liang L, et al. Genetic variants regulating ORMDL3 expression contribute to the risk of childhood asthma. Nature 2007;448:470.
183. Dixon AL, Liang L, Moffatt MF, et al. A genome-wide association study of global gene expression. Nat Genet 2007;39:1202.
184. Dendrou CA, Plagnol V, Fung E, et al. Cell-specific protein phenotypes for the autoimmune locus IL2RA using a genotype-selectable human bioresource. Nat Genet 2009;41:1011.
185. Mardis ER. New strategies and emerging technologies for massively parallel sequencing: applications in medical research. Genome Med 2009;1:40.
186. O'Rahilly S. Human genetics illuminates the paths to metabolic disease. Nature 2009;462:307.
187. Mitchell KJ, Porteous DJ. GWAS for psychiatric disease: is the framework built on a solid foundation? Mol Psychiatry 2009;14:740.
188. Sullivan PF, Gejman PV. Response to Mitchell & Porteus. Mol Psychiatry, in press.
189. Crick F. What mad pursuit: a personal view of scientific discovery. New York: Basic Books; 1988.
190. Mackay TF, Anholt RR. Of flies and man: drosophila as a model for human complex traits. Annu Rev Genomics Hum Genet 2006;7:339.
191. Ayroles JF, Carbone MA, Stone EA, et al. Systems genetics of complex traits in *Drosophila melanogaster.* Nat Genet 2009;41:299.
192. Lencz T, Morgan TV, Athanasiou M, et al. Converging evidence for a pseudoautosomal cytokine receptor gene locus in schizophrenia. Mol Psychiatry 2007;12:572.
193. Sullivan PF, Lin D, Tzeng JY, et al. Genomewide association for schizophrenia in the CATIE study: results of stage 1. Mol Psychiatry 2008;13:570.

194. Sebat J, Lakshmi B, Malhotra D, et al. Strong association of de novo copy number mutations with autism. Science 2007;316:445.
195. Weiss LA, Shen Y, Korn JM, et al. Association between microdeletion and micro-duplication at 16p11.2 and autism. N Engl J Med 2008;358:667.
196. Christian SL, Brune CW, Sudi J, et al. Novel submicroscopic chromosomal abnormalities detected in autism spectrum disorder. Biol Psychiatry 2008;63:1111.
197. Kumar RA, KaraMohamed S, Sudi J, et al. Recurrent 16p11.2 microdeletions in autism. Hum Mol Genet 2008;17:628.
198. Marshall CR, Noor A, Vincent JB, et al. Structural variation of chromosomes in autism spectrum disorder. Am J Hum Genet 2008;82:477.
199. Brunetti-Pierri N, Berg JS, Scaglia F, et al. Recurrent reciprocal 1q21.1 deletions and duplications associated with microcephaly or macrocephaly and developmental and behavioral abnormalities. Nat Genet 2008;40:1466.
200. de Kovel CG, Trucks H, Helbig I, et al. Recurrent microdeletions at 15q11.2 and 16p13.11 predispose to idiopathic generalized epilepsies. Brain 2010;133(Pt 1):23–32.
201. Dibbens LM, Mullen S, Helbig I, et al. Familial and sporadic 15q13.3 microdeletions in idiopathic generalized epilepsy: precedent for disorders with complex inheritance. Hum Mol Genet 2009;18:3626.
202. Helbig I, Mefford HC, Sharp AJ, et al. 15q13.3 microdeletions increase risk of idiopathic generalized epilepsy. Nat Genet 2009;41:160.
203. Mefford HC, Sharp AJ, Baker C, et al. Recurrent rearrangements of chromosome 1q21.1 and variable pediatric phenotypes. N Engl J Med 2008;359:1685.
204. Sharp AJ, Mefford HC, Li K, et al. A recurrent 15q13.3 microdeletion syndrome associated with mental retardation and seizures. Nat Genet 2008;40:322.

Genetic Research into Bipolar Disorder: The Need for a Research Framework that Integrates Sophisticated Molecular Biology and Clinically Informed Phenotype Characterization

Thomas G. Schulze, MD[a,b,c],*

KEYWORDS

• Manic-depressive illness • Schizophrenia • Depression
• Classification • Linkage • Association

This review of the basic principles and recent advances in genetic research into bipolar disorder (BD) could take advantage of a large, already extant body of work reviewing the evolution of findings from early family, twin, and adoption studies to linkage and association studies in BD.[1–16] However, rather than reviewing these findings again in a chronological and detailed manner, this article describes where we

Disclosure: This work was supported by the Intramural Research Program of the National Institute of Mental Health. Dr Schulze reports no conflicts of interest or other sources of funding.
[a] Unit on the Genetic Basis of Mood and Anxiety Disorders, National Institute of Mental Health (NIMH), National Institutes of Health (NIH), 35 Convent Drive, Bldg. 35, Rm 1A205, MSC 3719, Bethesda, MD 20892-3719, USA
[b] Department of Psychiatry and Behavioral Sciences, The Johns Hopkins University, Baltimore, MD, USA
[c] Department of Genetic Epidemiology in Psychiatry, Central Institute of Mental Health, Mannheim, Germany
* Unit on the Genetic Basis of Mood and Anxiety Disorders, National Institute of Mental Health (NIMH), National Institutes of Health (NIH), 35 Convent Drive, Bldg. 35, Rm 1A205, MSC 3719, Bethesda, MD 20892-3719.
E-mail address: schulzet@mail.nih.gov

Psychiatr Clin N Am 33 (2010) 67–82
doi:10.1016/j.psc.2009.10.005
0193-953X/10/$ – see front matter. Published by Elsevier Inc.

psych.theclinics.com

have come from, where we stand right now, how we can use the knowledge gleaned over the course of nearly a century, and how we can incorporate novel molecular and analytical techniques into our quest to unravel the genetics of BD.

FORMAL GENETICS, LINKAGE, AND ASSOCIATION STUDIES

To summarize some well-known facts, BD is a highly heritable disorder. Early twentieth-century family and twin studies observed that BD and other mental disorders aggregate in families, and that they have a heritable basis.[17–19] Whereas the lifetime prevalence of BD in the general population is around 1% to 2%, multiple studies have reported that the lifetime morbidity risk for BD in a first-degree relative of an individual with BD lies between 10 to 20%.[13] Furthermore, twin studies have repeatedly cemented the heritable component of BD, with heritability estimates ranging between 80% and 90%. Adoption studies similarly support the notion that genetic factors contribute substantially more to the etiology of BD than environmental factors (for a comprehensive review of family, twin, and adoption studies, see Shih and colleagues).[13] This large body of evidence, established over several decades, across changing diagnostic concepts of BD, and in populations of varying ethnic backgrounds, laid the foundation for gene mapping via linkage and association studies.

The early days of this molecular era of genetic research into BD were frustrating,[20] as most linkage findings were not supported by subsequent studies.[11] Problems associated with these early linkage studies were manifold: limited sample sizes, sparse genetic maps, and the use of the standard parametric logarithm-of-the-odds score method; in this method, originally designed for Mendelian disorders with monogenic inheritance, such parameters as mode of inheritance, penetrance, or the clinically unaffected status of probands' relatives need to be specified, which is not possible for complex phenotypes.

With the advent of larger, multicenter studies, the availability of denser maps, and the use of nonparametric linkage algorithms (eg, affected-sib-pair design), many of these early problems were addressed. Half a decade ago, I argued that large-scale linkage studies would in the end succeed in gene identification, or at least serve as the starting point for systematic molecular genetic research in BD.[11] Since then, however, even the largest studies or meta-analyses have left us with a void. Some consistencies of linkage findings hold up in large meta-analyses (eg, for chromosomes 6q and 8q),[21] but most of the reported linkages on virtually every chromosome remain isolated findings. The importance of this lack of replicability is significant. For instance, does it imply that the linkage findings are false? If so, linkage analysis as a tool to pinpoint susceptibility genes might be considered a thing of the past. The genetic (or locus) heterogeneity of BD may be so high that we will not be able to dissect it by linkage analysis alone, even with very large sample sizes. Nevertheless, incorporating the information gained from linkage studies into future analyses, as well as continuing to collect exact phenotype data of families, might still be very valuable and should not be dismissed.[22]

As with linkage analysis, positional cloning efforts by means of candidate-gene association mapping have not lived up to their promise. Although several studies, particularly systematic linkage disequilibrium mapping in linkage regions, have identified potential susceptibility genes for BD,[3,7–9] these findings have been difficult to replicate. While replication at the gene level has been reached for some of these genes, replications at the allelic level (ie, association with the identical allele of a particular single nucleotide polymorphism [SNP] across studies) are rare (**Table 1**).[23]

Table 1
Potential susceptibility genes for bipolar disorder

Gene	Symbol	Individual Study or Meta-Analysis	Evidence
Candidate gene association studies			
Serotonin Transporter	SLC6A3	Anguelova et al 2003 (MA)	+++
D-amino acid oxidase activator (G72)	DAOA	Detera-Wadleigh and McMahon 2006 (MA)	+++
Brain-derived neurotrophic factor	BDNF	Kanazawa et al 2007 (MA); Fan and Sklar 2008 (MA)	+++
Disrupted-in-schizophrenia-1	DISC1	Hodgkinson et al 2004; Thomson et al 2005; WTCCC 2007; Perlis et al 2008	++
Tryptophan hydroxilase 2	TPH2	Harvey et al 2004; Van den Bogaert et al 2006; Lopez et al 2007; Harvey et al 2007; Cichon et al 2007	++
Aryl hydrocarbon receptor nuclear translocatorlike	ARNTL/CLOCK	Mansour et al 2006; Nievergelt et al 2006	+
Cadherin gene (homolog of the *Drosophila* tumor suppressor gene *fat*)	FAT	Blair et al 2006; Abou Jamra et al 2008	+
Genome-wide association studies			
Diacylglycerol kinase eta	DGKH	Baum et al 2008a	++++
Alpha-1 subunit of a voltage-dependent calcium channel	CACNA1C	Sklar et al 2008; Ferreira et al 2008	++++
Ankyrin 3	ANK3	Baum et al 2008a; Ferreira et al 2008; Smith et al 2009; Scott et al 2009	++++

Abbreviations: MA, meta-analysis; WTCCC, Wellcome Trust Case Control Consortium.
Symbols: +, supported by two studies; ++, supported by several studies; +++, supported by meta-analysis of three or more samples; ++++, genome-wide level of significance (in at least one of the studies).

GENOME-WIDE ASSOCIATION STUDIES OF BIPOLAR DISORDER

Despite these rather disheartening experiences, researchers in the field of complex genetics entered the twenty-first century with great aspirations based on an ever-advancing technology that made genome-wide association studies (GWAS) a practical reality. The first two articles of this special issue present this method in detail. GWAS have been performed in the study of several complex disease and physiological trait phenotypes, including type I and type II diabetes,[24–28] lung cancer,[29–31] body mass index and obesity,[32–35] coronary heart disease,[24,36,37] hypertension,[24] rheumatoid arthritis,[24] age-related macular degeneration,[38,39] Crohn disease,[24,40,41] prostate cancer,[42,43] height,[44–47] and pigmentation and hair color.[48–50] Thus, the study of GWAS in complex disorders has successfully identified and replicated several susceptibility genes.[51]

With regards to GWAS of BD, several studies have been published or are in the pipeline.[24,52–56] These have highlighted several novel susceptibility genes. Among these, *DGKH*, *CACNA1C*, and *ANK3* have been found at robust levels of genome-wide significance and have notably been replicated across samples (see **Table 1**).[52–58] *DGKH* is located within the BD linkage region on chromosome 13q14, and encodes di-acylglycerol kinase eta, a key protein in the lithium-sensitive phosphatidyl inositol pathway. *CACNA1C* encodes an alpha-1 subunit of a voltage-dependent calcium channel. *ANK3* encodes ankyrin-G, a large protein whose neural-specific isoforms, localized at the axonal initial segment and nodes of Ranvier, may help maintain ion channels and cell adhesion molecules.

GWAS in BD have taught us several important lessons, which can be easily generalized to genetic research into other complex psychiatric or somatic disorders:

- BD is a polygenic disorder. That means that the contribution of each locus to risk of disease is modest, that cases carry significantly more risk alleles than controls, and that disease risk increases substantially with the total burden of risk alleles carried.
- The best findings from GWAS do not necessarily fall within those genes that have previously been widely studied. These "usual suspects" typically included candidate genes studied on the basis of either hypothetical reasoning concerning neurotransmission or linkage findings.
- Pursuing a "top-hits-only" strategy may prevent us from understanding the genetic complexity of BD and polygenic disorders in general. Stringent levels of statistical significance, such as genome-wide significance, are indispensible for confirming any risk gene or polymorphism identified through a GWAS. However, meta-analyses may reveal several points of agreement between independent studies and highlight genes that do not make it to the *P*-value-defined top of an individual study. A detailed consideration of the wider distribution of association signals across studies may thus prove to be a valuable strategy in complex genetics.[59]
- Allelic heterogeneity may be an important factor in complex disorders, such as BD. Allelic heterogeneity means that different alleles within a gene can cause a phenotype; this phenomenon has been extensively observed in monogenic disorders, such as cystic fibrosis,[60] as well as in *BRCA1/2*-associated breast cancer.[61] In the case of *ANK3* and BD, various alleles and haplotypes appear to be independent risk factors.[56,58]
- Finally, as with other complex phenotypes, GWAS in BD have brought to light the fact that the identified variants only account for a small fraction of genetic variability. This phenomenon has become known as the "case of the missing heritability."[62]

CONSEQUENCES FOR FUTURE APPROACHES IN THE GENETICS OF BIPOLAR DISORDER

The information detailed above might lead one to believe that GWAS have failed, and that the genetics of a complex disorder, such as BD, may be too complex to ever be understood. However, in the scientific community, there is broad consensus that GWAS results are only a starting point rather than an end point, that many more steps need to be taken to put the pieces together, and that GWAS need to be embedded in a framework of complementary approaches.[63–65] These include studies focusing on genomic, epigenomic, phenomic, neurobiological, and environmental aspects (**Fig. 1**).

Genomics and Epigenomics

Most of the world's largest data collections of individuals with BD and controls have already been analyzed by GWAS, and the results published. Compared to many GWAS of nonpsychiatric phenotypes, sample sizes in psychiatric GWAS—usually totaling around 2000 to 4000 cases and controls—are still not large enough to detect risk variants with small effect sizes. Thus, the psychiatric genetic research community has embraced the idea of bringing together all available samples for joint mega- and meta-analyses through a collaborative effort known as the Psychiatric GWAS Consortium.[66] While this will most certainly help to identify further common vulnerability variants, validate existing findings, and enable the study of allelic heterogeneity and gene-gene interaction, increasing sample size is only one of many necessary steps.

Such collaborative GWAS focusing on common SNP variations (ie, GWAS to date have typically studied HapMap-SNPs [http://www.hapmap.org/] with a minor allele

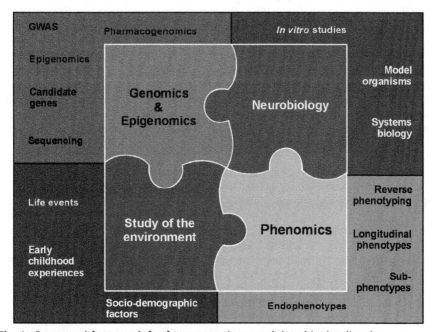

Fig. 1. Conceptual framework for future genetic research into bipolar disorder.

frequency above 5%) will need to be complemented by studies investigating uncommon (ie, in the 1%–5% range) and rare (ie, <1%) genetic variations. This includes the genome-wide study of copy number variants presenting with deletions or duplication of variably sized segments of DNA. The study of copy number variants has proven pivotal for identifying structural chromosomal variation as rare sources of genetic susceptibility to psychiatric disorders,[67] such as schizophrenia[68,69] and autism.[70–72] With regards to BD, it was recently shown that singleton deletions—deletions that appear only once in the dataset of more than 100 kilobase in length—were present in 16.2% of BD cases, in contrast to 12.3% of controls, and that this effect was more pronounced in patients with an age at onset of mania at or below 18 years of age. This suggests that BD can result from the effects of multiple rare structural variants.[73]

The notion that current GWAS designs fail to assess the impact of uncommon or rare variations has led to the development of several resequencing strategies. In contrast to GWAS approaches that use SNP markers derived from HapMap and thus miss rare or idiosyncratic variations, resequencing determines an individual's DNA sequence. Large-scale international resequencing projects, such as the 1000 Genomes Project (www.1000genomes.org) or the ClinSeq project,[74] are well under way. While the latter study focuses on disease traits, it is hoped that both will contribute to the hunt for the lost heritability.

The field of pharmacogenomics may also emerge as an important part of the process of discovery in BD, and especially the discovery of genetic variation relevant to the management of patients. While the high heritability of psychiatric disorders is well known, evidence for the heritability of response or side-effect susceptibility to psychiatric medications is less well established; systematic formal genetic studies, such as twin studies, have not been performed.[75] However, in addition to clinical observations supporting the notion that response to treatment is familial, ample justification exists for pursuing pharmacogenetic studies in psychiatry, as reviewed by Peter Zandi in this special issue. Over the last decades, progress has been made in understanding the genetics of pharmacokinetics—broadly defined as mechanisms regarding the blood and tissue concentrations of a drug. As a result, quantitative dose adjustments based on genotype can be calculated for many medications, including antidepressants and antipsychotics. In marked contrast, translation of genetic findings on pharmacodynamic phenotypes (ie, drug effects) into psychiatric clinical practice is still not feasible.[76,77] However, recent findings on the genetics of response or susceptibility to adverse events to pharmacotherapy in depression have yielded relatively large effect sizes, illustrating that the availability of large and adequately characterized samples will be key to success in this line of research.[75,78–85]

Overall, little research has been done on the genetics of response or susceptibility to adverse events in the treatment of BD. Despite lithium's proven efficacy, and evidence suggesting that there is a genetic basis of response to lithium treatment,[86] pharmacogenetic studies in this area have so far been confined to small sample sizes and varying phenotype definitions.[87] Using data from the Systematic Treatment Enhancement Program for Bipolar Disorder study sample and collaborators from the United Kingdom, Perlis and colleagues[88] performed a GWAS on lithium response that included more than 800 lithium-treated patients. They identified multiple regions of interest but none met the threshold for genome-wide significance.[88] Recently, researchers from the International Study Group of Lithium Treated Patients (www.igsli.org) and the National Institute of Mental Health spearheaded the creation of the Consortium on Lithium Genetics (ConLiGen; www.ConLiGen.org). ConLiGen is a worldwide effort to harmonize phenotype definition of response to lithium treatment and to perform GWAS of response and adverse events to lithium in adequately sized samples.[89] Efforts like this will be needed to move towards a personalized medicine approach in the treatment of BD. The potential pharmacogenetic target phenotypes are plentiful. They include, for example, acute depressive and manic episodes, prophylaxis, and characteristic acute and long-term side effects of mood stabilizers.

The field of epigenomics has recently drawn increased attention, given ample evidence for the involvement of epigenetic mechanisms and of their interplay with environmental factors in the etiology of somatic disorders, such as cancer.[90] With regards to mental illness, postmortem studies suggest that epigenetic factors play a role in the etiology of schizophrenia and BD.[91,92] Stress-induced imbalances of histone acetylation may also be involved in the transition from acute adaptive response to chronic psychiatric illness.[93]

Phenomics

To date, psychiatric genetic studies, including GWAS, have mainly focused on categorical diagnoses, such as BD, for phenotype definitions. While the use of diagnostic systems, such as the *Diagnostic and Statistical Manual of Mental Disorders* (Fourth Edition), has increased diagnostic reliability, categorical diagnoses are by definition artificial constructs. The psychiatric genetic community has thus embraced the idea of thorough genotype-phenotype studies. Here, investigators hope that focusing on phenotypic dissection will help decrease phenotypic—and hence genotypic—heterogeneity; this would enable the delineation of characteristic genotype-phenotype signatures.[94-98] Thorough genotype-phenotype studies may also deliver clues in dissecting the phenotypic and genotypic overlap between schizophrenia and BD.

Subphenotype approaches have proven successful in elucidating the genetics of breast cancer[99] and nonsyndromal deafness.[100] Thus, they may prove valuable in psychiatric genetics. To avoid an insurmountable multiple testing problem, investigators should carefully choose the subphenotypes to be studied out of the plethora of phenotypic variables potentially amenable to phenotypic dissection approaches. This could be done by focusing on well-formulated hypotheses, or by concentrating on variables that show some evidence of heritability or at least familiality. As regards BD, considerable research has established the familiality of clinical variables for subphenotypic analyses. For instance, the following familial phenotypic characteristics have been identified: episode frequency, comorbid panic disorder, comorbid obsessive compulsive disorder, comorbid anorexia nervosa, comorbid substance abuse, comorbid alcoholism, psychosis, a history of suicide attempts, a history of missed work, a history of psychiatric hospitalizations, (early) age of onset, polarity of onset, puerperal trigger of onset, temperament, rapid cycling, and level of social functioning.[97,101-108] For some of these, heritability has also been established. Most of these variables are currently being used in subphenotype analyses of large GWAS datasets.

One major motivation behind these analyses is the notion that subphenotyping may help define more homogenous subgroups of the disorder, and that this increased homogeneity will improve chances of identifying susceptibility genes. Furthermore, both case-control and cases-only strategies can be pursued in these subphenotype analyses. In the case-control design, cases with (or without) a specific subphenotype are compared to control individuals. In the cases-only design, cases with a specific subphenotype are compared to cases without this subphenotype. These different strategies are believed capable of better disentangling the underlying genetic architecture, as they may help to differentiate between factors, such as genetic heterogeneity (eg, gene A may increase the risk of developing BD with psychosis while gene B may increase the risk of developing BD without psychosis) and modifier genes (eg, gene A may increase risk of developing BD only in the presence of gene B, which by itself confers no risk for BD).

Reverse phenotyping, originally proposed by Schulze and McMahon[109] (2004), is a particular form of subphenotyping. Here, genetic marker data are used to drive, or form, the basis of new phenotype definitions. In the case of association studies, reverse phenotyping aims to define phenotypic groupings distinguished by more deviant allele frequencies than are seen in traditional diagnostic categories. For instance, we demonstrated that the association between a haplotype in *G72* and BD in a large German and Polish sample was driven by an association with the subphenotype "history of persecutory delusions."[98] Furthermore, in the Polish sample, the association was only revealed through this approach, as the overall sample of BD patients showed no association. Thus, the subphenotype "history of persecutory delusions" helped to homogenize the samples. Reverse phenotyping has now also been successfully applied to research in nonmental illnesses.[110]

As outlined below, applying phenotypic dissection approaches, such as reverse phenotyping, to the study of the longitudinal course of psychiatric illness might be another fruitful—though so far largely untraveled—road in psychiatric genetics. To fully understand the phenomic expression of genetic liability to disease, phenomic studies should include the study of endophenotypes, comprising neurophysiological, biochemical, endocrine, neuroanatomical, cognitive, or neuropsychological measurements.[111] The joint consideration of endophenotypes and genetic factors may hold promise for understanding the actual mechanisms leading from genetic variation to phenotypic expression.[112] The prerequisite for phenomic studies is the availability of large and adequately characterized samples, as well as sophisticated data management strategies.[107,113]

For decades, biological psychiatric research, in particular psychiatric genetics, has been based on cross-sectional datasets but has not paid much attention to a phenotype that is of utmost relevance to the clinician, the patient, and the patient's family: the longitudinal course. In the case of schizophrenia, epidemiological studies have shown that there are characteristic subtypes of longitudinal courses in schizophrenia,[114] and that these are defined by both relapse pattern and level of impairment. In BD, there is broad consensus that BD is a severe, usually lifelong, chronic condition, as suggested by longitudinal studies like the McLean-Harvard First Episode Project.[115–117] According to these data, full recovery from initial episodes is uncommon. When full symptomatic recovery does happen, it occurs much more slowly than early syndromal recovery. Furthermore, initial depression or mixed states predict more depressive episodes and overall morbidity during later stages of the disorder, while initial mania or psychotic features predict more manic episodes and a better prognosis. Characteristic polymorphic patterns with mood-dominated, schizo-affective-dominated and schizo-dominated course have also been described for BD.[118] Again, switching between mania and depression within one episode has been suggested to predict poor prognosis,[119] and rapid cycling is associated with substantial depressive morbidity and high risk for serious suicide attempts.[120] Nevertheless, data are still lacking on the course of BD across the life cycle, encompassing aspects of phenomenology, severity, and impairment.[121]

In their recent review on the course and outcome of BD, Treuer and Tohen[122] (2009) urged more research to establish better and more reliable course predictors for individual patients. This need is reflected by current efforts for a paradigmatic change in the upcoming *Diagnostic and Statistical Manual of Mental Disorders* (Fifth Edition) and the *International Classification of Diseases, Eleventh Revision*; notably, measures of longitudinal course along with dimensional aspects will be core elements of the new classification systems.[123] Surprisingly, integrating longitudinal aspects into future classification systems has not yet been paralleled by a similar move in the field of biological, mainly genetic, research in psychiatry; rather, current efforts focus on increasing sample sizes of cross-sectional diagnoses, not in establishing longitudinal cohorts. In the future, genetic studies of BD and other psychiatric disorders should target the longitudinal course of the illness as an important phenotype of interest. This, of course, will require patience as well as a trained clinician's eye. Such efforts will have to be paralleled by the establishment of phenotypic databases, such as the Bipolar Phenome Project,[107] as well as by the development of mathematical algorithms that allow for the robust delineation of phenomic profiles and their genomic signatures. Finally, it is important to note that these genomic, epigenomic, and phenomic approaches outlined above need to be embedded in a framework of "neurobiological vetting," and that environmental influences must also be modeled.

Neurobiology

Once genetic susceptibility to psychiatric disorders has been identified and, more crucially, robustly replicated, the variants in question become prime targets for focused neurobiological studies to further elucidate their relevance to the mode of action in the pathway leading up to disease presentation.[124–127] Such studies should include gene-expression studies and the development and testing of animal models. Ideally, phenotype and endophenotype studies in humans (eg, brain imaging) can be paralleled with identical approaches in animals (eg, brain imaging in animals).

Study of Environment

As noted previously, classic formal genetic studies demonstrated that heritability estimates in BD range up to 80% to 90%. Given this high heritability, it is easy to forget that nongenetic factors are also part of the equation describing phenotypic variance. Psychiatric geneticists have long wanted to study the complex interplay between genes and environment. The crucial question, however, has always been how best to do it. A recent, large-scale, meta-analysis of the widely reported interaction between variation in the serotonin transporter gene and stressful life events[128] found little substance to this finding. Inconsistency of study designs, measures, and analyses proved to be main explanatory factors in this sobering but much-needed finding. Therefore, the question remains whether we will ever be able to account for environmental factors in a robust way. Plugging in retrospectively collected environmental data as covariates into an analysis may prove to be a futile endeavor. Instead, prospective studies may be key to success in this area. Furthermore, we may see a renaissance of studies targeting multiply affected families, this time not to conduct linkage studies but rather for in-depth sequencing within the framework of longitudinal observation. Families from populations with similarly shared patterns of idiosyncratic environmental exposures (eg, Amish or Hutterite communities in the Americas) might prove ideal for gene-environment studies.

SUMMARY

Over the last decade, the psychiatric genetics research community has made considerable progress and has learned much. Indeed, our most important lesson has been that the complexity of a complex disorder like BD is always a little more complex than we think. As our technological advances become progressively more sophisticated, new layers of complexity will undoubtedly arise; this is, in essence, the nature of science. That said, we should not shy away from these new challenges because we have made some headway. Our research efforts have demonstrated that BD is a truly polygenic disorder and have revealed potential mechanisms beyond those tradition- ally hypothesized pathophysiological pathways, as illustrated by replicated GWAS findings of susceptibility genes involved in the architecture of calcium and sodium channels. Furthermore, we now know that we will not find one specific gene or a few specific genes for BD. We may have to settle for a scenario where we can only sufficiently characterize the joint effect of several hundreds or even thousands of genes on disease presentation. However, recent replicated findings that only explain a fraction of phenotypic variability should not discourage us, but should stim- ulate thinking. After all, GWAS in somatic phenotypes may have produced smaller P- values, but they do not fare better in terms of providing an explanation. Thus, many areas of research still need to be explored. If explored systematically and in a harmo- nized way, they will shed more light on the genetics of disorders such as BD.

ACKNOWLEDGMENTS

The author is greatly indebted to Francis J. McMahon for highly inspirational discus- sions and gratefully acknowledges the support of the Intramural Research Program of the National Institute of Mental Health. Ioline Henter provided outstanding editorial assistance. The author gratefully acknowledges Daniela Reich-Erkelenz for assistance in designing graphical presentations.

REFERENCES

1. Baron M. Manic-depression genes and the new millennium: poised for discovery. Mol Psychiatry 2002;7(4):342–58.
2. Berrettini WH. Molecular linkage studies of bipolar disorders. Bipolar Disord 2001;3(6):276–83.
3. Craddock N, Forty L. Genetics of affective (mood) disorders. Eur J Hum Genet 2006;14(6):660–8.
4. Craddock N, Jones I. Molecular genetics of bipolar disorder. Br J Psychiatry Suppl 2001;41:s128–33.
5. Craddock N, Sklar P. Genetics of bipolar disorder: successful start to a long journey. Trends Genet 2009;25(2):99–105.
6. Detera-Wadleigh SD, McMahon FJ. Genetic association studies in mood disor- ders: issues and promise. Int Rev Psychiatry 2004;16(4):301–10.
7. Farmer A, Elkin A, McGuffin P. The genetics of bipolar affective disorder. Curr Opin Psychiatry 2007;20(1):8–12.
8. Hayden EP, Nurnberger JI Jr. Molecular genetics of bipolar disorder. Genes Brain Behav 2006;5(1):85–95.
9. Kato T. Molecular genetics of bipolar disorder and depression. Psychiatry Clin Neurosci 2007;61(1):3–19.
10. Prathikanti S, McMahon FJ. Genome scans for susceptibility genes in bipolar affective disorder. Ann Med 2001;33(4):257–62.
11. Schulze TG, McMahon FJ. Genetic linkage and association studies in bipolar affective disorder: a time for optimism. Am J Med Genet C Semin Med Genet 2003;123C(1):36–47.
12. Schumacher J, Cichon S, Rietschel M, et al. [Genetics of bipolar affective disor- ders. Current status of research for identification of susceptibility genes]. Nerve- narzt 2002;73(7):581–92 [quiz: 593–4] [in German].

13. Shih RA, Belmonte PL, Zandi PP. A review of the evidence from family, twin and adoption studies for a genetic contribution to adult psychiatric disorders. Int Rev Psychiatry 2004;16(4):260–83.

14. Sklar P. Linkage analysis in psychiatric disorders: the emerging picture. Annu Rev Genomics Hum Genet 2002;3:371–413.

15. Taylor L, Faraone SV, Tsuang MT. Family, twin, and adoption studies of bipolar disease. Curr Psychiatry Rep 2002;4(2):130–3.

16. Tsuang MT, Faraone SV. The genetics of mood disorders. Baltimore (MD): Johns Hopkins University Press; 1990.

17. Luxenburger H. Psychiatrisch-neurologische Zwillingspathologie. Zbl Ges Neurol Psychiat 1930;56:145–80 [in German].

18. Rosanoff AJ, Handy LM, Plessett IR. The etiology of manic-depressive syndromes with special reference to their occurrence in twins. Am J Psychiatry 1934;91:247–86.

19. Schulze TG, Fangerau H, Propping P. From degeneration to genetic susceptibility, from eugenics to genethics, from Bezugsziffer to LOD score: the history of psychiatric genetics. Int Rev Psychiatry 2004;16(4):246–59.

20. Risch N, Botstein D. A manic depressive history. Nat Genet 1996;12(4):351–3.

21. McQueen MB, Devlin B, Faraone SV, et al. Combined analysis from eleven linkage studies of bipolar disorder provides strong evidence of susceptibility loci on chromosomes 6q and 8q. Am J Hum Genet 2005;77(4):582–95.

22. Clerget-Darpoux F, Elston RC. Are linkage analysis and the collection of family data dead? Prospects for family studies in the age of genome-wide association. Hum Hered 2007;64(2):91–6.

23. Detera-Wadleigh SD, McMahon FJ. G72/G30 in schizophrenia and bipolar disorder: review and meta-analysis. Biol Psychiatry 2006;60(2):106–14.

24. Wellcome Trust Case Control Consortium. Genome-wide association study of 14,000 cases of seven common diseases and 3,000 shared controls. Nature 2007;447(7145):661–78.

25. Saxena R, Voight BF, Lyssenko V, et al. Genome-wide association analysis identifies loci for type 2 diabetes and triglyceride levels. Science 2007;316(5829):1331–6.

26. Scott LJ, Mohlke KL, Bonnycastle LL, et al. A genome-wide association study of type 2 diabetes in Finns detects multiple susceptibility variants. Science 2007; 316(5829):1341–5.

27. Sladek R, Rocheleau G, Rung J, et al. A genome-wide association study identifies novel risk loci for type 2 diabetes. Nature 2007;445(7130):881–5.

28. Zeggini E, Scott LJ, Saxena R, et al. Meta-analysis of genome-wide association data and large-scale replication identifies additional susceptibility loci for type 2 diabetes. Nat Genet 2008;40(5):638–45.

29. Amos CI, Wu X, Broderick P, et al. Genome-wide association scan of tag SNPs identifies a susceptibility locus for lung cancer at 15q25.1. Nat Genet 2008; 40(5):616–22.

30. Hung RJ, McKay JD, Gaborieau V, et al. A susceptibility locus for lung cancer maps to nicotinic acetylcholine receptor subunit genes on 15q25. Nature 2008;452(7187):633–7.

31. Thorgeirsson TE, Geller F, Sulem P, et al. A variant associated with nicotine dependence, lung cancer and peripheral arterial disease. Nature 2008; 452(7187):638–42.

32. Frayling TM, Timpson NJ, Weedon MN, et al. A common variant in the FTO gene is associated with body mass index and predisposes to childhood and adult obesity. Science 2007;316(5826):889–94.

33. Loos RJ, Lindgren CM, Li S, et al. Common variants near MC4R are associated with fat mass, weight and risk of obesity. Nat Genet 2008;40(6):768–75.
34. Thorleifsson G, Walters GB, Gudbjartsson DF, et al. Genome-wide association yields new sequence variants at seven loci that associate with measures of obesity. Nat Genet 2009;41(1):18–24.
35. Willer CJ, Speliotes EK, Loos RJ, et al. Six new loci associated with body mass index highlight a neuronal influence on body weight regulation. Nat Genet 2009; 41(1):25–34.
36. Helgadottir A, Thorleifsson G, Manolescu A, et al. A common variant on chromosome 9p21 affects the risk of myocardial infarction. Science 2007;316(5830): 1491–3.
37. McPherson R, Pertsemlidis A, Kavaslar N, et al. A common allele on chromosome 9 associated with coronary heart disease. Science 2007;316(5830): 1488–91.
38. Klein RJ, Zeiss C, Chew EY, et al. Complement factor H polymorphism in age-related macular degeneration. Science 2005;308(5720):385–9.
39. Maller J, George S, Purcell S, et al. Common variation in three genes, including a noncoding variant in CFH, strongly influences risk of age-related macular degeneration. Nat Genet 2006;38(9):1055–9.
40. Hampe J, Franke A, Rosenstiel P, et al. A genome-wide association scan of non-synonymous SNPs identifies a susceptibility variant for Crohn disease in ATG16L1. Nat Genet 2007;39(2):207–11.
41. Rioux JD, Xavier RJ, Taylor KD, et al. Genome-wide association study identifies new susceptibility loci for Crohn disease and implicates autophagy in disease pathogenesis. Nat Genet 2007;39(5):596–604.
42. Gudmundsson J, Sulem P, Manolescu A, et al. Genome-wide association study identifies a second prostate cancer susceptibility variant at 8q24. Nat Genet 2007;39(5):631–7.
43. Yeager M, Orr N, Hayes RB, et al. Genome-wide association study of prostate cancer identifies a second risk locus at 8q24. Nat Genet 2007;39(5):645–9.
44. Lettre G, Jackson AU, Gieger C, et al. Identification of ten loci associated with height highlights new biological pathways in human growth. Nat Genet 2008; 40(5):584–91.
45. Sanna S, Jackson AU, Nagaraja R, et al. Common variants in the GDF5-UQCC region are associated with variation in human height. Nat Genet 2008;40(2): 198–203.
46. Weedon MN, Lango H, Lindgren CM, et al. Genome-wide association analysis identifies 20 loci that influence adult height. Nat Genet 2008;40(5):575–83.
47. Weedon MN, Lettre G, Freathy RM, et al. A common variant of HMGA2 is associated with adult and childhood height in the general population. Nat Genet 2007;39(10):1245–50.
48. Han J, Kraft P, Nan H, et al. A genome-wide association study identifies novel alleles associated with hair color and skin pigmentation. PLoS Genet 2008; 4(5):e1000074.
49. Sulem P, Gudbjartsson DF, Stacey SN, et al. Two newly identified genetic determinants of pigmentation in Europeans. Nat Genet 2008;40(7):835–7.
50. Sulem P, Gudbjartsson DF, Stacey SN, et al. Genetic determinants of hair, eye and skin pigmentation in Europeans. Nat Genet 2007;39(12):1443–52.
51. Lango H, Weedon MN. What will whole genome searches for susceptibility genes for common complex disease offer to clinical practice? J Intern Med 2008;263(1):16–27.

52. Baum AE, Akula N, Cabanero M, et al. A genome-wide association study implicates diacylglycerol kinase eta (DGKH) and several other genes in the etiology of bipolar disorder. Mol Psychiatry 2008a;13(2):197–207.
53. Ferreira MA, O'Donovan MC, Meng YA, et al. Collaborative genome-wide association analysis supports a role for ANK3 and CACNA1C in bipolar disorder. Nat Genet 2008;40(9):1056–8.
54. Scott LJ, Muglia P, Kong XQ, et al. Genome-wide association and meta-analysis of bipolar disorder in individuals of European ancestry. Proc Natl Acad Sci U S A 2009;106(18):7501–6.
55. Sklar P, Smoller JW, Fan J, et al. Whole-genome association study of bipolar disorder. Mol Psychiatry 2008;13(6):558–69.
56. Smith EN, Bloss CS, Badner JA, et al. Genome-wide association study of bipolar disorder in European American and African American individuals. Mol Psychiatry 2009;14(8):755–63.
57. Ollila HM, Soronen P, Silander K, et al. Findings from bipolar disorder genome-wide association studies replicate in a Finnish bipolar family-cohort. Mol Psychiatry 2009;14(4):351–3.
58. Schulze TG, Detera-Wadleigh SD, Akula N, et al. Two variants in Ankyrin 3 (ANK3) are independent genetic risk factors for bipolar disorder. Mol Psychiatry 2009;14(5):487–91.
59. Baum AE, Hamshere M, Green E, et al. Meta-analysis of two genome-wide association studies of bipolar disorder reveals important points of agreement. Mol Psychiatry 2008;13(5):466–7.
60. O'Sullivan BP, Freedman SD. Cystic fibrosis. Lancet 2009;373(9678):1891–904.
61. Narod SA, Foulkes WD. BRCA1 and BRCA2: 1994 and beyond. Nat Rev Cancer 2004;4(9):665–76.
62. Maher B. Personal genomes: the case of the missing heritability. Nature 2008; 456(7218):18–21.
63. Cordell HJ. Genome-wide association studies: detecting gene-gene interactions that underlie human diseases. Nat Rev Genet 2009 [Epub ahead of print].
64. Ioannidis JP, Thomas G, Daly MJ. Validating, augmenting and refining genome-wide association signals. Nat Rev Genet 2009;10(5):318–29.
65. McCarthy MI, Abecasis GR, Cardon LR, et al. Genome-wide association studies for complex traits: consensus, uncertainty and challenges. Nat Rev Genet 2008; 9(5):356–69.
66. Psychiatric GWAS Consortium Steering Committee. A framework for interpreting genome-wide association studies of psychiatric disorders. Mol Psychiatry 2009; 14(1):10–7.
67. Cook EH Jr, Scherer SW. Copy-number variations associated with neuropsychiatric conditions. Nature 2008;455(7215):919–23.
68. Stefansson H, Rujescu D, Cichon S, et al. Large recurrent microdeletions associated with schizophrenia. Nature 2008;455(7210):232–6.
69. Walsh T, McClellan JM, McCarthy SE, et al. Rare structural variants disrupt multiple genes in neurodevelopmental pathways in schizophrenia. Science 2008;320(5875):539–43.
70. Mefford HC, Sharp AJ, Baker C, et al. Recurrent rearrangements of chromosome 1q21.1 and variable pediatric phenotypes. N Engl J Med 2008;359(16):1685–99.
71. Sebat J, Lakshmi B, Malhotra D, et al. Strong association of de novo copy number mutations with autism. Science 2007;316(5823):445–9.
72. Weiss LA, Shen Y, Korn JM, et al. Association between microdeletion and microduplication at 16p11.2 and autism. N Engl J Med 2008;358(7):667–75.

73. Zhang D, Cheng L, Qian Y, et al. Singleton deletions throughout the genome increase risk of bipolar disorder. Mol Psychiatry 2009;14(4):376–80.
74. Biesecker L, Mullikin JC, Facio F, et al. The ClinSeq Project: piloting large-scale genome sequencing for research in genomic medicine. Genome Res 2009; 19(9):1665–74.
75. Perlis RH. Pharmacogenetic studies of antidepressant response: how far from the clinic? Psychiatr Clin North Am 2007;30(1):125–38.
76. Kirchheiner J, Fuhr U, Brockmoller J. Pharmacogenetics-based therapeutic recommendations–ready for clinical practice? Nat Rev Drug Discov 2005;4(8):639–47.
77. Kirchheiner J, Nickchen K, Bauer M, et al. Pharmacogenetics of antidepressants and antipsychotics: the contribution of allelic variations to the phenotype of drug response. Mol Psychiatry 2004;9(5):442–73.
78. Binder EB, Salyakina D, Lichtner P, et al. Polymorphisms in FKBP5 are associated with increased recurrence of depressive episodes and rapid response to antidepressant treatment. Nat Genet 2004;36(12):1319–25.
79. Hu XZ, Rush AJ, Charney D, et al. Association between a functional serotonin transporter promoter polymorphism and citalopram treatment in adult outpatients with major depression. Arch Gen Psychiatry 2007;64(7):783–92.
80. Laje G, Paddock S, Manji H, et al. Genetic markers of suicidal ideation emerging during citalopram treatment of major depression. Am J Psychiatry 2007;164(10):1530–8.
81. Lekman M, Laje G, Charney D, et al. The FKBP5-gene in depression and treatment response–an association study in the Sequenced Treatment Alternatives to Relieve Depression (STAR*D) Cohort. Biol Psychiatry 2008;63(12):1103–10.
82. McMahon FJ, Buervenich S, Charney D, et al. Variation in the gene encoding the serotonin 2A receptor is associated with outcome of antidepressant treatment. Am J Hum Genet 2006;78(5):804–14.
83. Paddock S, Laje G, Charney D, et al. Association of GRIK4 with outcome of antidepressant treatment in the STAR*D cohort. Am J Psychiatry 2007;164(8):1181–8.
84. Perlis RH, Moorjani P, Fagerness J, et al. Pharmacogenetic analysis of genes implicated in rodent models of antidepressant response: association of TREK1 and treatment resistance in the STAR(*)D study. Neuropsychopharmacology 2008;33(12):2810–9.
85. Uher R, Huezo-Diaz P, Perroud N, et al. Genetic predictors of response to antidepressants in the GENDEP project. Pharmacogenomics J 2009;9(4):225–33.
86. Grof P, Duffy A, Cavazzoni P, et al. Is response to prophylactic lithium a familial trait? J Clin Psychiatry 2002;63(10):942–7.
87. Mamdani F, Groisman IJ, Alda M, et al. Pharmacogenetics and bipolar disorder. Pharmacogenomics J 2004;4(3):161–70.
88. Perlis RH, Smoller JW, Ferreira MA, et al. A genomewide association study of response to lithium for prevention of recurrence in bipolar disorder. Am J Psychiatry 2009;166(6):718–25.
89. Schulze TG, Alda M, Adli M, et al. The international Consortium on Lithium Genetics (ConLiGen)—an initiative by the NIMH and IGSLI to study the genetic basis of response to lithium treatment. Neuropsychobiology, in press.
90. Esteller M. Epigenetics in cancer. N Engl J Med 2008;358(11):1148–59.
91. Connor CM, Akbarian S. DNA methylation changes in schizophrenia and bipolar disorder. Epigenetics 2008;3(2):55–8.
92. Sharma RP, Grayson DR, Gavin DP. Histone deactylase 1 expression is increased in the prefrontal cortex of schizophrenia subjects: analysis of the

National Brain Databank microarray collection. Schizophr Res 2008;98(1–3): 111–7.

93. Tsankova N, Renthal W, Kumar A, et al. Epigenetic regulation in psychiatric disorders. Nat Rev Neurosci 2007;8(5):355–67.

94. Craddock N, Owen MJ. Rethinking psychosis: The disadvantages of a dichotomous classification now outweigh the advantages. World Psychiatry. 2007;6(2): 84–91.

95. Potash JB. Carving chaos: genetics and the classification of mood and psychotic syndromes. Harv Rev Psychiatry 2006;14(2):47–63.

96. Rietschel M, Beckmann L, Strohmaier J, et al. G72 and its association with major depression and neuroticism in large population-based groups from Germany. Am J Psychiatry 2008;165(6):753–62.

97. Schulze TG, Hedeker D, Zandi P, et al. What is familial about familial bipolar disorder? Resemblance among relatives across a broad spectrum of phenotypic characteristics. Arch Gen Psychiatry 2006;63(12):1368–76.

98. Schulze TG, Ohlraun S, Czerski PM, et al. Genotype-phenotype studies in bipolar disorder showing association between the DAOA/G30 locus and persecutory delusions: a first step toward a molecular genetic classification of psychiatric phenotypes. Am J Psychiatry 2005;162(11):2101–8.

99. Wooster R, Neuhausen SL, Mangion J, et al. Localization of a breast cancer susceptibility gene, BRCA2, to chromosome 13q12-13. Science 1994; 265(5181):2088–90.

100. Tekin M, Arnos KS, Pandya A. Advances in hereditary deafness. Lancet 2001; 358(9287):1082–90.

101. Evans L, Akiskal HS, Keck PE Jr, et al. Familiality of temperament in bipolar disorder: support for a genetic spectrum. J Affect Disord 2005;85(1–2):153–68.

102. Fisfalen ME, Schulze TG, DePaulo JR Jr, et al. Familial variation in episode frequency in bipolar affective disorder. Am J Psychiatry 2005;162(7):1266–72.

103. Jones I, Craddock N. Familiality of the puerperal trigger in bipolar disorder: results of a family study. Am J Psychiatry 2001;158(6):913–7.

104. Kassem L, Lopez V, Hedeker D, et al. Familiality of polarity at illness onset in bipolar affective disorder. Am J Psychiatry 2006;163(10):1754–9.

105. MacKinnon DF, Zandi PP, Cooper J, et al. Comorbid bipolar disorder and panic disorder in families with a high prevalence of bipolar disorder. Am J Psychiatry 2002;159(1):30–5.

106. O'Mahony E, Corvin A, O'Connell R, et al. Sibling pairs with affective disorders: resemblance of demographic and clinical features. Psychol Med 2002;32(1): 55–61.

107. Potash JB, Toolan J, Steele J, et al. The bipolar disorder phenome database: a resource for genetic studies. Am J Psychiatry 2007;164(8):1229–37.

108. Saunders EH, Scott LJ, McInnis MG, et al. Familiality and diagnostic patterns of subphenotypes in the National Institutes of Mental Health bipolar sample. Am J Med Genet B Neuropsychiatr Genet 2008;147B(1):18–26.

109. Schulze TG, McMahon FJ. Defining the phenotype in human genetic studies: forward genetics and reverse phenotyping. Hum Hered 2004;58(34):131–8.

110. Iannuzzi MC, Baughman RP. Reverse phenotyping in sarcoidosis. Am J Respir Crit Care Med 2007;175(1):4–5.

111. Gottesman II, Gould TD. The endophenotype concept in psychiatry: etymology and strategic intentions. Am J Psychiatry 2003;160(4):636–45.

112. Meyer-Lindenberg A, Weinberger DR. Intermediate phenotypes and genetic mechanisms of psychiatric disorders. Nat Rev Neurosci 2006;7(10):818–27.

113. Fangerau H, Ohlraun S, Granath RO, et al. Computer-assisted phenotype characterization for genetic research in psychiatry. Hum Hered 2004;58(3–4): 122–30.
114. Watt DC, Katz K, Shepherd M. The natural history of schizophrenia: a 5-year prospective follow-up of a representative sample of schizophrenics by means of a standardized clinical and social assessment. Psychol Med 1983;13(3): 663–70.
115. Baca-Garcia E, Perez-Rodriguez MM, Basurte-Villamor I, et al. Diagnostic stability and evolution of bipolar disorder in clinical practice: a prospective cohort study. Acta Psychiatr Scand 2007;115(6):473–80.
116. Salvatore P, Baldessarini RJ, Tohen M, et al. McLean-Harvard International First-Episode Project: two-year stability of DSM-IV diagnoses in 500 first-episode psychotic disorder patients. J Clin Psychiatry 2009;70(4):458–66.
117. Salvatore P, Khalsa HM, Hennen J, et al. Psychopathology factors in first-episode affective and non-affective psychotic disorders. J Psychiatr Res 2007;41(9):724–36.
118. Marneros A, Roettig S, Roettig D, et al. The longitudinal polymorphism of bipolar I disorders and its theoretical implications. J Affect Disord 2008;107(1–3): 117–26.
119. Turvey CL, Coryell WH, Solomon DA, et al. Long-term prognosis of bipolar I disorder. Acta Psychiatr Scand 1999;99(2):110–9.
120. Coryell W, Solomon D, Turvey C, et al. The long-term course of rapid-cycling bipolar disorder. Arch Gen Psychiatry 2003;60(9):914–20.
121. Goodwin GM, Anderson I, Arango C, et al. ECNP consensus meeting. Bipolar depression. Nice, March 2007. Eur Neuropsychopharmacol 2008;18(7):535–49.
122. Treuer T, Tohen M. Course and outcome of bipolar disorder—focusing on depressive aspects. In: Zarate CA, Manji H, editors. Bipolar depression: molecular neurobiology, clinical diagnosis and pharmacotherapy. Basel, Switzerland: Birkhauser; 2009. p. 29–46.
123. Regier DA, Narrow WE, Kuhl EA, et al. The conceptual development of DSM-V. Am J Psychiatry 2009;166:645–50.
124. Mei L, Xiong WC. Neuregulin 1 in neural development, synaptic plasticity and schizophrenia. Nat Rev Neurosci 2008;9(6):437–52.
125. Newberg AR, Catapano LA, Zarate CA, et al. Neurobiology of bipolar disorder. Expert Rev Neurother 2008;8(1):93–110.
126. Ross CA, Margolis RL, Reading SA, et al. Neurobiology of schizophrenia. Neuron 2006;52(1):139–53.
127. Sawamura N, Sawa A. Disrupted-in-schizophrenia-1 (DISC1): a key susceptibility factor for major mental illnesses. Ann N Y Acad Sci 2006;1086:126–33.
128. Risch N, Herrell R, Lehner T, et al. Interaction between the serotonin transporter gene (5-HTTLPR), stressful life events, and risk of depression: a meta-analysis. JAMA 2009;301(23):2462–71.

The Genetics of Autism: Key Issues, Recent Findings, and Clinical Implications

Paul El-Fishawy, MD, JD[a,b], Matthew W. State, MD, PhD[a,b,c,d],*

KEYWORDS

- Autism genetics • Rare variants
- Copy number variation • Association

Autism is an often debilitating disorder of development with a worldwide prevalence of approximately 0.1%.[1] The clinical hallmarks include fundamental deficits in social functioning and language development and the presence of narrowed or repetitive interests and behaviors.[2] Autism is the most prevalent syndrome in a spectrum of disorders that are currently grouped together in the *Diagnostic and Statistical Manual of Mental Disorders* (Fourth Edition, Text Revision) under the rubric of pervasive developmental disorders (PDD); these include pervasive developmental disorder not otherwise specified (PDD-NOS) (0.15% prevalence), Rett disorder (0.006% prevalence), Asperger disorder (ASP) (0.025% prevalence), and childhood disintegrative disorder (0.001% prevalence).[1,3] In addition, it is has become commonplace to refer to PDDs as autism spectrum disorders (ASD) and within this group to include individuals with so-called not quite autism, that is, persons who fall just below the threshold for diagnosis in one of the key domains.

Autism affects predominately males with a male-to-female ratio of approximately 4.3:1.[1] The male predominance identified in ASP may be as high as 14:1.[4] The oft-cited prevalence in the lay literature of 1 per 166 individuals includes the entire spectrum of disorders, which makes accurate comparisons with rates determined before the development of diagnostic criteria for PDD-NOS and ASP highly problematic.

[a] Child Study Center, Yale University School of Medicine, 230 South Frontage Road, New Haven, CT 06520, USA
[b] Department of Genetics, Yale University School of Medicine, 230 South Frontage Road, New Haven, CT 06520, USA
[c] Department of Psychiatry, Yale University School of Medicine, 300 George Street, New Haven, CT 06511, USA
[d] Program on Neurogenetics, Yale University School of Medicine, 230 South Frontage Road, New Haven, CT 06520, USA
* Corresponding author. Department of Genetics, Yale University School of Medicine, 230 South Frontage Road, New Haven, CT 06520.
E-mail address: matthew.state@yale.edu (M.W. State).

Psychiatr Clin N Am 33 (2010) 83–105
doi:10.1016/j.psc.2009.12.002
0193-953X/10/$ – see front matter © 2010 Elsevier Inc. All rights reserved.
psych.theclinics.com

The question of whether or not, using consistent diagnostic approaches, there is an increasing prevalence of ASD remains a subject of debate, and a detailed treatment is beyond the scope of this review. The best epidemiological evidence to date suggests, however, that there may be as much as a threefold increase in the prevalence of individuals meeting full diagnostic criteria for autism over the past 4 decades.[1] If this reflects a true increase in incidence, it has implications for understanding of potential genetic mechanisms (discussed later).

Whether or not the prevalence or the sensitivity of detection of ASD (or both) has increased over the past approximately 40 years, the numbers of individuals seeking care have grown markedly. This increase will continue to pose significant societal challenges: disorders within the spectrum typically result in marked social, cognitive, and behavioral impairments that are lifelong, and current treatment approaches are palliative at best. The public health burden, reflected in annual costs, was recently estimated at $35 billion in the United States alone.[5]

Although there is currently intense interest in ASD in the public and the scientific community and dramatic progress has been made in a variety of areas of research, the underlying pathophysiology of these syndromes remains largely a mystery.[6,7] As ASDs are thought to be among the most heritable of all developmental neuropsychiatric conditions, the identification of susceptibility genes would seem to hold tremendous promise for elucidating the underlying cellular and molecular mechanisms of disease and for paving the way for improvements in diagnosis and the development of novel therapeutic strategies. At the same time, despite strong evidence (reviewed later) for a genetic contribution and some notable recent findings,[8,9] the rate of progress in gene discovery has not been as rapid as hoped. As a result, there has been mounting skepticism regarding the wisdom of continued investment in genetic approaches and the ability of investigators in this area to make tangible contributions to the lives of affected individuals and their families.

Such concerns warrant serious consideration. There is little doubt that the promise of genetic investigation of social disability has not yet been fully realized. It is also the case that studies of the genetics of polygenic disorders in general, including ASD, have just begun to reach maturity. The slope of the discovery curve over the past 4 to 5 years has become increasingly steep, and it is no longer hyperbole to suggest that recent findings are offering the first glimpses of the biology underlying common conditions. There is an extraordinary convergence of factors that is driving a rapidly accelerating rate of return on investment in the area of ASD. The combination of public and private interest in supporting research efforts, highly effective advocacy groups, the rapid evolution of genomic tools and methodologies, and a long-term investment in developing large DNA collections has already resulted in key findings and promises a flurry of discoveries over the next several years.

This article reviews the genetics of ASD with a particular focus on the steep part of the discovery curve, that is, studies published over the past 5 years. The discussion is divided into four sections: the first addresses broad conceptual issues that help explain the early difficulties with gene discovery in ASD; the second turns to a discussion of key controversies regarding the nature of the genetic contribution to ASD, which continue to enliven debate in the field; in the third, major recent advances are highlighted; and finally, this article addresses the clinical implications of recent findings, including recommendations for the genetic evaluation of newly presenting patients with ASD.

THE HERITABILITY OF AUTISM SPECTRUM DISORDERS

Autism is one of the most familial of all psychiatric disorders, with heritability estimated at approximately 90%.[10] The twin studies on which such estimates are based note that the concordance rate for monozygotic twins is between 70% and 90% compared with the corresponding value for dizygotic twins of no more than 10%.[10,11] The spread of concordance estimates for a given twin type reflects a degree of diagnostic uncertainty, with the lower bound based on strict diagnostic criteria and the upper bound reflecting siblings who both fall within the PDD spectrum. Given evolving diagnostic nosology and methods, it would not be surprising if ongoing twin studies lead to some modest downward adjustment of heritability estimates. The risk to siblings of autistic individuals is at least 20 times higher than in the general population,[12] which is similar to findings for ASDs in general.[13]

THE ALLELIC ARCHITECTURE OF AUTISM SPECTRUM DISORDERS

Although twin and family studies demonstrate the contribution of genes to ASDs, they do not address some of the questions for researchers interested in discovering the specific character and identity of these risks. These include key questions, such as (1) How many genes may be involved in an individual and in the affected population at large? (2) Do variations in the genetic code need occur only within a single gene (ie, simple/mendelian inheritance) in a given individual to dramatically increase the risk for ASD or must simultaneous variations in multiple genes occur alone or in combination with nongenetic factors (complex/nonmendelian inheritance) to result in pathology? (3) What is the magnitude of the risk carried by individual transcripts? and (4) Are the sequence variations associated with ASDs common or rare in the general population? These questions, which center on the underlying allelic architecture of ASDs, are critical for study design. Consequently, a brief review of the topics is a prelude to a discussion of recent findings.

Over the past decade, large-scale gene discovery efforts have shown that autism is not a simple/mendelian disorder converging on a single gene at the level of the population (reviewed elsewhere).[14] This fact, however, should not be mistakenly taken to suggest certainty regarding the other issues (discussed previously), which remain far less clear. At present, it seems ASD may be transmitted in a mendelian fashion within a single individual or family.[15–17] Whether or not this applies to only a tiny fraction of affected individuals or a larger proportion of ASD families, however, remains unclear. Moreover, recent studies have suggested that common genetic variation in the population may contribute to ASD in a complex/nonmendelian manner.[8] Whether or not this suggests oligogenic or polygenic inheritance in individuals and the affected population and what proportion of the overall genetic risk is transmitted in this fashion have not yet been clarified.

In addition to the issue of "How many?" a second fundamental question regarding allelic architecture revolves around the question of "How big?" As a general proposition, genetic variations that have large effects on early-onset disabling conditions tend to be rare in the population and are often observed to be transmitted in mendelian fashion. Conversely, common genetic variations associated with disease tend to carry small risks (discussed at greater length later). Given these relationships, the question of the effect size of a genetic variation closely relates to the rate at which it is likely to observed within the population (Fig. 1). Traditionally, rare disease alleles were defined as having a frequency of less than 1%. It is now common in the literature, however, to define those with a frequency of 5% or less as rare and those with a frequency of 1% or less as very rare. Conversely, common alleles are those found in the population at a frequency of greater than 5%.

The foregoing brief discussion outlines some of the key basic issues that remain not only for autism genetics but also for many other common, complex disorders.

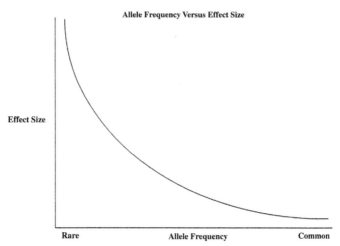

Fig. 1. This graph illustrates the anticipated relationship between allele frequency and effect size for common and rare disorders. Mendelian (or simple genetic) syndromes fall to the leftmost aspect of the X axis. To date, most GWAS across all of medicine have demonstrated that common alleles carry very small risks (far right side of the graph). Recent findings with regard to common risk variants in ASD have followed this pattern. Many of the rare mutations so far identified in ASD appear to fall somewhere in the middle of this graph, showing low allele frequency and effect sizes that are not as great as those found in single gene disorders.

Determining whether or not disease-related alleles are common or rare in the population, whether or not they are transmitted in a mendelian or complex fashion, and the degree to which a syndrome or disease displays locus heterogeneity (that is, genetic variations in multiple different genes leading to the same phenotype) are not simply points of academic interest. Because available genetic and genomic tools and analytic approaches tend to be specialized in the sense that they are optimal for studying rare or common variation, but typically not both, study design currently must take into account hypotheses about the allelic architecture of ASD, and the success or failure of an investigation may rest heavily on these assumptions.

THE COMMON DISEASE–COMMON VARIANT HYPOTHESIS

Over the past decade, one of the leading theories regarding the allelic architecture of common disorders (by definition, those that affect >1%–5% of the population) is the so-called common disease–common variant (CDCV) hypothesis. Building on previous work by Chakravarti,[18] an influential article by Reich and Lander published in 2001[19] summarizes the underlying reasoning: archeological data and evolutionary genetics support the out of Africa theory of evolution, which posits that all humans descended from a small population over a brief period of time. Specifically, it is thought that approximately 10,000 individuals grew into the current world population in approximately 100,000 years. The original, ancestral population, owing to its small size, could not have supported a large variety of disease alleles at any particular locus. Thus, by definition, disease alleles for common diseases in that original population must have been common, and disease alleles for rare diseases must have been rare. The hypothesis goes on to posit that due to rapid population expansion, common disease alleles massively proliferated. Rare disease alleles also spread, but, as they were rare in the original population, not as widely as their common counterparts.

In addition to the dynamics of human population expansion, a second key aspect of the CDCV hypothesis rests on the rate of new mutation in the genome: new alleles are constantly introduced into the population with the result that novel variations will dilute out rare and common disease alleles. The rate of introduction of new mutations is slow relative to the dramatic expansion described by the out of Africa theory, however. Thus, the fraction of new mutation in the population is predicted to be small relative to widely proliferated common variants but may represent a considerable proportion of the disease burden for initially rare disorders. In short, it is supposed that in today's population, alleles causing rare diseases still are individually rare and that new mutations have not yet had time to dilute out common variants sufficiently, such that common diseases are predicted still to be mostly due to common variation in today's population.

The proponents of the theory cite empiric evidence from rare monogenic disorders, pointing out that for rare diseases, such as Wilson disease (prevalence 1/30,000), there are more than 50 disease-causing alleles so far identified. Moreover, as expected, based on the CDCV hypothesis, each allele is individually rare, with the most common variant explaining only 11% of the population risk.[19] Based on similar logic, it could be predicted that the rarer the disease, the greater the number of disease-causing alleles present and the lower the percentage of population risk explained by the most common allele. This appears to hold true in many cases, including with regard to aniridia (prevalence of 1/100,000), which has greater than 250 disease-causing alleles, the most common of which explains only 5% of the population risk.[19]

A few of early findings from the study of common diseases also lent support to the theory. For example, APOE4 is a common allele found in approximately 15% of individuals of European descent and explains a significant amount of the interindividual genetic variation and approximately 50% of the population risk for Alzheimer disease.[20] Moreover, it has been determined to be an ancient allele, dating back at least as far as the original population described in the CDCV hypothesis.[20] A similar situation has been identified with respect to macular degeneration.[21,22]

These findings engendered confidence that similar common alleles of large effect would explain much of the genetic variation in all or nearly all common complex diseases. Despite significant recent methodological advances in the study of common variation (discussed later) and studies of hundreds of disorders, however, alleles similar to APOE 4 have been by far the exception rather than the rule, with most discoveries identifying alleles with effects that are an order of magnitude less than anticipated and accounting for a small fraction of interindividual genetic risk.

Type 2 diabetes mellitus provides a case in point. Many studies of this common disorder have identified a variety of common alleles. The effect sizes of these alleles have been small compared with APOE4, however, explaining only a small percentage of the interindividual risk and each one, individually, explaining only a very small portion of the overall variance—0.04% to 0.5%.[23] In one of the earliest large-scale studies employing what have turned out to be powerful genome-wide methods to study common variants, eight disease-related risk alleles explained only 2.3% of the overall variance.[24] Moreover, the majority of the alleles discovered have been in regions of DNA that are intergenic, making the transition from gene discovery to an understanding of pathophysiology difficult.

In short, although recent studies have been strikingly successful in providing reproducible evidence for the contribution of common variants to common disease, the findings so far have simultaneously raised questions as to how much of the allelic architecture of these disorders will be explained by the CDCV hypothesis. This has led to a glass half-full situation in which those interested in common variants rightfully tout the tremendous recent progress in gene discovery in complex genetics, whereas many others in the scientific community have viewed the same results as evidence of the potentially flawed theoretical underpinnings of the theory. For example, the CDCV hypothesis relies heavily on the out of Africa theory of evolution, which, although widely accepted, is challenged by a competing theory, the multimodal theory of evolution, which, if correct, would result in markedly different predictions regarding the dynamics of disease-allele proliferation.[25] Perhaps a more important point is that the CDCV hypothesis also assumes that diseases that were common in the original population did not have a negative on impact reproductive fitness, such that associated disease alleles were not selected out of the population.[25]

The small effect sizes of the genetic variants so far identified for most common disorders may be viewed as calling this last assumption into question. The inability to identify risk alleles with more than modest effects raises the possibility that this observation is a signature of natural selection at work. There is increasing speculation that the findings in Alzheimer disease and macular degeneration may be special cases, as these diseases affect the truly aged, and, consequently, are relatively immune from purifying selection. This point is further supported by evidence from early-onset Alzheimer disease where all familial forms of the disease so far identified are monogenic disorders caused by heterogeneous and rare alleles.[26]

The reliance of the CDCV hypothesis on risk alleles not having an impact on reproductive fitness warrants particular attention in the case of autism. Although it is possible that individual alleles in a highly polygenic disorder might carry such small risks so as to escape purifying selection, or that so-called balancing selection may be operating (ie, a risk allele results in reproductive advantages in one context or environment while leading to a negative impact on fitness in another), it also seems logical that an allele carrying large risks for a syndrome that has a fundamental impact on social communication might sufficiently reduce reproductive fitness as to drive the frequency of the mutation down to low levels in the population. And if purifying selection has been at work with regard to autism genes from early in human history, this suggests that there would be a greater proportion of rare alleles contributing to autism than predicted by the CDCV hypothesis. Finally, there are other reasons to question the applicability of the CDCV hypothesis with regard to ASD. Given the concern over the increasing prevalence of ASD, there is a tendency to consider this a spectrum of common diseases with a single underlying biology. ASD might well reflect a collection of rare disorders resulting from hundreds of different genetic defects but leading to a shared phenotype, similar to the case of mental retardation.[27]

STUDYING RARE VARIATION

Although the CDCV hypothesis has been a leading school of thought, particularly in psychiatric genetics, there have nonetheless been strongly held alternate views of the likely genetic architecture of common diseases and autism, in particular. Not surprisingly, these have focused on the potential contribution of rare variation. With respect to ASD, gene discovery efforts focusing on low-frequency alleles can be conceptualized as falling into three broad categories: (1) studies aimed directly at the CDCV hypothesis, namely investigation of whether or not rare as opposed to common variation accounts for the lion's share of population risk for PDD; (2) studies aimed at investigating extreme outliers, that is, presumed unusual families that the phenotype in a mendelian fashion—these are of interest regardless of whether or not they represent only a small fraction of cases of so-called idiopathic autism; and (3) studies of known rare monogenic syndromes that share features with ASD.

The first of these alternatives, the rare variant–common disease approach, supposes that common disease and autism, in particular, may reflect the convergence of multiple, rare variations in the same gene (allelic heterogeneity) or multiple genes (locus heterogeneity) leading to a common/shared phenotype. Given a sufficiently large number of genomic targets, individually rare mutations could accumulate in the population so as to account for a significant proportion of a commonly occurring disorder.[28,29] Such variation could be transmitted from generation to generation or de novo. In the latter case, a large number of apparently sporadic cases (in which only the proband in the family was affected) and a high rate of monozygotic concordance versus dizygotic concordance (both of which have been suggested with regard to ASD; discussed later) would be expected.

Regardless of whether or not rare variants account for the majority of genetic risk for ASD, a focus on identifying low-frequency alleles nonetheless represents an avenue of study. The investigation of extreme outliers has played a central role in illuminating the pathophysiology of a range of common complex disorders, from hypercholesterol-emia[30] to hypertension.[31] In these cases, identifying rare mutations has less to do with accounting for population risk and rather focuses on the importance of gaining a foothold in the molecular and cellular mechanisms of disease. Rare mendelian mutations may be particularly valuable, even if extremely rare, because the methods of gene discovery for this type of variation are powerful and well elaborated and because the identified alleles are likely to carry large effects and correspond to coding regions of the genome, changes in the genetic code that are, at present, typically easier to investigate in the laboratory than those variations that correspond to noncoding, regulatory, or intergenic and intragenic regions.

Finally, a particularly relevant rare variant approach with regard to social disability involves the study of monogenic syndromes, such as fragile X, neurofibromatosis, and tuberous sclerosis, that show phenotypic overlap with ASD. Such examples of so-called syndromic autism have often been relegated to the sidelines in the study of the genetics of ASD by those interested in "pure" social disability. Recent findings in the study of these conditions have provided remarkable insights into the developing central nervous system, however, and promise to transform understanding of the pathophysiology and treatment of developmental delay and ASD.[32–34]

RECENT FINDINGS IN AUTISM GENETICS

The foregoing discussion has outlined conceptual issues in the study of the genetics of common disease in general and autism in particular. This discussion turns to a consideration of the past 5 years in the genetics of ASD and outlines recent progress with regard to rare and common variants. As discussed later, the weight of the empirical evidence highlights the critical role already played by the discovery of rare variation in ASD and suggests that common and rare variant approaches will continue to be highly relevant to the understanding of this potentially debilitating spectrum of syndromes.

Studies Geared to Finding Common Autism Alleles

Several study designs have been geared largely to investigating the contribution of common disease alleles to autism. The first of these types of studies are nonparametric linkage studies, the most common of which is the affected sib-pair design (ASP) (see O'Roak and State for a more in depth description of this method[6]). Briefly, this approach studies the transmission of genetic variation from one generation to another in an effort to identify regions of the genome carrying disease risk. The analysis specifically avoids specifying the mode of transmission of a disorder, an approach that is intended to increase the ability to identify alleles contributing to risk in a complex fashion. Although theoretically the ASP approach may identify common or rare variations, it is not particularly robust in the face of high locus heterogeneity, making its application most useful in a practical sense to studying common risk alleles.

So far, more than a dozen such studies have been completed using genome-wide nonparametric approaches. The largest and most recent of these involved 1181 multiplex families and 10,000 markers.[35] Taking all of these into account, nearly every chromosome has shown some evidence in favor of linkage, but no single region has been found to be highly significant, and no disease-related variation/mutation has been identified yet within any of the most promising intervals. Nonetheless, attempts at further replication, studies of endophenotypes, and intensive fine mapping of some of these intervals have yielded some interesting findings (discussed later).[36,37]

Candidate gene association has also been a mainstay of methods aimed at identifying common alleles contributing to ASD. In these studies, variations in or near a gene or genes of interest are examined. Unlike linkage studies that evaluate the transmission of genomic segments from generation to generation, this type of analysis typically relies on evaluation of the frequency of previously identified common variation in cases versus controls. Such studies are practical in that evaluation of known common alleles is inexpensive compared with rare variant discovery and many of the relevant study designs allow for the use of all probands whether or not additional family members are available, affected, or willing to participate in genetic research. The latter considerations are relevant to the feasibility of recruiting large numbers of patients for study, something increasingly appreciated as an aspect of common variant studies.

Although these approaches are attractive due to their relative ease of implementation and their utility in hypothesis-driven investigations, they have by and large not been reliable. A comprehensive review several years ago looking across all of medicine, including psychiatry, found that of 603 different reported gene-disease associations, of which 166 had been studied three or more times, only six were consistently replicated, with none in autism or other psychiatric disorders (with the exception of APOE4).[38]

With the development of genome-wide as opposed to candidate gene–based association studies and a related explosion of reproducible findings, several explanations for the poor track record of candidate approaches have emerged. These include (but are not limited to) a tendency to underestimate the sample size needed to identify risk (based on an initial overestimation of effect size of common risk alleles), often a failure to account sufficiently for the confound of ethnic variation (also known as population stratification), the low prior probability of picking the right variations to study, and overly permissive statistical thresholds.

Although these potential flaws are found in many studies of ASD (as they are across all of medicine), several recent candidate gene investigations have employed more rigorous methodologies and have provided some evidence for replication, which ultimately is the gold standard for genetic findings. Although not an exhaustive list, the genes engrailed 2 (*EN2*), *MET*, and contactin-associated protein-like 2 (*CNTNAP2*) have emerged as strong candidates from these recent single locus association studies.

EN2 is a homeobox transcription factor that maps to the long arm of chromosome 7 and plays a key role in the development of the midbrain and cerebellum. Benayed and colleagues[39] in the Millonig laboratory reported significant association of this gene with autism in an initial sample and added additional support by showing that misexpression of mouse *En2* in primary cortical cultures impairs neuronal differentiation.

Although the initial study was notable for the use of an internal replication sample before publication, the results of subsequent genetic studies have not been as clear. Zhong and colleagues[40] found no association between autism and single-nucleotide polymorphisms (SNPs) in the *EN2* region, and a second small study in the Chinese population was not able to replicate the initially reported SNP but did find some evidence for association of haplotypes in the region.[41] Given these results, *EN2* must still be considered a candidate for involvement in ASD, although so far it has not been independently replicated in a fashion that confers it clear disease risk status.

The potential explanations for this are myriad. It is possible that the initial result represents type 1 error despite the investigators' best efforts to avoid this. Alternatively, the initial study may have simply overestimated the effect size of the risk allele, suggesting that the aforementioned efforts at replication have been underpowered. As discussed later, the failure to identify this or any of the other candidate genes discussed in this section in the first genome-wide association study (GWAS) of autism tend to supports either alternative. To the extent that the effect sizes have been overestimated, one would have to conclude that the total sample sizes studied to date with regard to ASD have not been nearly sufficient to rule out the contribution of these transcripts.

A similar story has evolved with regards to the *MET* oncogene, also located on chromosome 7 in a region that was found to show suggestive linkage to ASD in an ASP study.[42] Campbell and colleagues[43] performed a rigorous analysis that included an internal replication sample and functional assays leading to the identification of a significant association between a regulatory SNP upstream of the *MET* gene and autism. Additional genetic and biological studies have lent support to this initial observation, including work from the same laboratory.[44] In addition, in an independent study of 185 cases and 88 controls, Sousa and colleagues found[45] significant association but to different markers than those implicated in the Campbell study.

A third gene also on chromosome 7 (7q35), *CNTNAP2*, has emerged recently as a candidate for involvement in a range of developmental disorders, including autism, language development, and seizure, based on common and rare variant findings. The rare variant findings are discussed later with the rare variant research.

In 2002, Alarcón and colleagues in Geschwind's laboratory implicated the 7q35 region in two nonparametric linkage studies focusing on an age at first word language phenotype in individuals with ASD.[36,46] In 2008, these investigators reported a follow-up fine mapping association study using the same measures and evaluating 1172 trios from the Autism Genetic Resource Exchange (AGRE). This was a two-stage study in which genes meeting an initial nominally significant cutoff were investigated in a second independent set of 304 AGRE trios.[47] The only marker that remained significant through both rounds of analysis corresponded to *CNTNAP2*.

At the same time, Arking and colleagues[37] in Charkravarti's laboratory conducted an analysis of linkage in 72 multiplex families and identified a suggestive peak at 7q35. Subsequently, they performed a follow-up transmission disequilibrium test (TDT) in this interval, showing association with a single SNP at *CNTNAP2* (permutation $P<.006$). This was a different SNP from that reported by Alarcón and colleagues.[47] An internal replication using TDT analysis on an additional set of 1295 trios, however, supported the identified association based on the broader autism diagnosis.

Vernes and colleagues[48] subsequently studied *CNTNAP2* in relation to specific language impairment. Using chromatin immunoprecipitation, they first demonstrated that the protein product of *FOXP2*, a gene causing a monogenic form of speech and language disorder, binds to *CNTNAP2* and regulates its expression.[48] They then went on to demonstrate a positive association between SNPs in *CNTNAP2* and an endo-phenotype of specific language disorder in a small sample[48] but in the same region identified as associated in the Alarcón study (described previously).[47]

The aforementioned analyses are among the most rigorous contemporary candidate gene association studies to date. The first large-scale GWAS of autism was recently completed and identified significant association of ASD to an intergenic region on chromosome 5—5p14.1, mapping between the neuronal adhesion molecules cadherin 9 and cadherin 10.[8] As suggested previously, the transition from candidate gene to genome-wide approaches in general has represented a key methodological shift in common variant studies. The latter have been shown to have considerable advantages with regard to reproducibility. Most likely this has resulted from the unbiased nature of the initial investigation (essentially all genes are queried simultaneously); the tendency to study somewhat larger sample sizes, which have allowed identification of common variants carrying small risks; the use of genome-wide genotyping data and sophisticated methods to guard against population stratification; and a general agreement within the scientific community with regard to an appropriate statistical threshold for genome-wide significance that accounts for the large number of tests inherent in such studies.

This recent finding must be viewed as a major success for the common variant approach to ASD. At the same time, it is consistent with studies of other complex conditions that have suggested that such variation is likely to be only a part of the overall story. For example, despite a sample size of 10,000 individuals, only a single significant locus was identified. Moreover, the most significantly associated SNP showed an odds ratio of 1.19, again consistent with the general findings of modest effects for common variants in other complex disorders.[8] Finally, the identification of association with a marker mapping approximately 1 million base pairs from cadherin 9 or cadherin 10 (either or both of which are plausible candidates) presents a significant challenge for follow-up studies aimed at understanding the biology of this variation.[49–53]

In sum, with regard to common variants, the results of the nonparametric linkage studies remain uncertain as do the majority of promising candidate gene associations. The GWAS finding provides additional support for the contribution of common alleles but makes the future identification of a common variant carrying even moderate risks for autism unlikely.

Studies Geared to Finding Rare Autism Alleles

Cytogenetic studies
The study of abnormalities in chromosomal structure, cytogenetics, has proved a source of rare variant findings in a variety of disorders, including ASD. Traditionally, these abnormalities have been detected via microscopic examination of chromosomes. More recently, submicroscopic structural changes have been detectable using the analysis of copy number variation (CNV).[54]

Rare microscopic chromosomal abnormalities occur at a mean rate of up to 7.4% in autism versus less than 1% in the general population.[55] Moreover, multiple studies have converged on particular chromosomal abnormalities in autism, the most common of which are maternally inherited duplications at 15q11–13. These duplications are found in as many as 1% to 3% of patients diagnosed with idiopathic autism.[56,57]

Several studies have originated from or been strongly supported by traditional cytogenetic evidence leading to a number of key findings. For example, Thomas and colleagues[58] in 1999 reported de novo deletions or translocations that affected the same region on the X chromosome at Xp22.3 in three girls with autism confirmed by the Autism Diagnostic Interview.

Jamain and colleagues[59,60] in 2003 looked for rare deleterious mutations in genes mapping to this interval and came across the first example of a clear functional mutation in a case of otherwise idiopathic autism which corresponded to the gene neuroligin 4X (NLGN4X), a neuronal adhesion molecule subsequently found to be important for the specification of excitatory versus inhibitory synapses. The identified frameshift mutation in NLGN4X led to a premature termination of the protein with the loss of the critical transmembrane domain. This was found in two affected brothers (one with autism and one with ASP). The mutation was also found to be de novo in the unaffected mother, a finding that is not unexpected for a deleterious X-linked mutation. As expected, the mutation was not found in an unaffected brother nor was it present in 350 unrelated controls.[59]

Jamain and colleagues[59] also screened NLGN3 and NLGN4Y in 158 subjects with autism or ASP and found a single suspect missense mutation in NLGN3. NLGN3 is a homolog of NLGN4 but is located on a different region of the X chromosome at Xq13. The finding was again identified in two affected brothers, one with autism and the other with ASP.[59] Although this substitution was present in a highly conserved region of the protein and was later found to alter synaptic function in the mouse, its relationship to disease was less clear initially, and, unlike the mutation in NLGN4X, has not been replicated in other human genetic studies.[61]

Shortly after publication of the Jamain and colleagues' article, Laumonnier and colleagues[62] reported on the study of a large family with X-linked mental retardation. Three of the 13 children with mental retardation also had autism or PDD. Parametric analysis supported linkage to the Xp22.3 region corresponding to the NLGN4X, and subsequent sequencing of this transcript in affected individuals revealed a two-base pair deletion leading to a frameshift and premature stop codon. Similar to the independent mutation observed by Jamain and colleagues,[59] this resulted in loss of the transmembrane domain and was not found in several hundred healthy male controls.

Several mutation screenings of modest samples of patients (several hundred individuals) have not identified additional mutations in the genes NLGN4X or NLGN3 clearly carrying risks for[63-66] ASD. In addition to the convergence of findings from the Lammonier and Jamain studies (discussed previously), neurobiological and molecular evidence has accumulated supporting the importance of NLGN4X. Most importantly, genes coding for molecules that interact with NLGN4X, including SHANK3 and NRXN1, have been strongly implicated in ASD. Given the expectation of a high rate of genetic heterogeneity, this type of evidence showing multiple mutations in a relevant molecular pathway as opposed to a single gene is an avenue for confirmation of rare variant findings and autism.[17,67,68]

In this regard, the evidence for the involvement of SHANK3 is particularly compelling. Bourgeron's laboratory, initially responsible for the first NLGN4X finding, subsequently identified de novo and transmitted structural and sequence variations in this transcript that codes for a postsynaptic binding partner of NLGN4X.[17] In an independent subsequent study,[68] four de novo abnormalities and nine inherited missense variants were identified in 400 families. Three of the de novo events were large-scale deletions, encompassing 277 kilobases (kb), 3.2 megabases (Mb), and 4.36 Mb, whereas the fourth was a missense variant. The high rate of de novo mutations involving coding segments of SHANK3 in individuals with idiopathic ASD identified in independent studies, the finding of developmental delay and autistic features in patients with the 22q13 deletion syndrome (the genomic segment corresponding to where SHANK3 resides), and the interaction with NLGN4X provide strong convergent evidence for the importance of rare mutations in this transcript for ASD.

Several studies have also implicated neurexin 1 (NRXN1), a trans-synaptic binding partner for neuroligins. The Autism Genome Project Consortium reported a combined linkage and copy number analysis involving 1168 subjects.[35] This investigation, one of the first to address the issue of CNVs in autism, was confined to an analysis of only large-scale variations because it used first-generation arrays with 10,000 probes. Despite this, a family was identified in which two affected siblings shared the same 300-kb deletion, encompassing the coding region of NRXN1. This was not present in the parents, highlighting the phenomena of germline mosaicism. Rare missense variants and balanced chromosomal abnormalities disrupting NRXN1 in ASD patients also have been reported.[69,70]

The convergence of findings suggesting an ASD-related NRXN/NLGN/SHANK3 pathway may also point more broadly to the importance of other cell-adhesion molecules in ASD. In 2005, Fernandez and colleagues[71] studied a child with features of a rare deletion syndrome on the short arm of chromosome 3 who presented with social disability. Using cytogenetic techniques, they identified and mapped a balanced translocation that disrupted the coding segment of the transcript contactin 4, suggesting a potential role for these neuronal adhesion molecules in ASD. Two subsequent studies have provided additional evidence for the role of rare variation and particularly CNVs, in contactin 4.[9,72]

As discussed previously, subsequent studies involving common and rare variant findings have implicated a similar molecular, CNTNAP2, in ASD. As a general proposition, contactins bind to contactin-associated proteins to mediate their functions, at least in the peripheral nervous system. CNTNAP2 was first, and so far most convincingly, tied to ASD by Strauss and colleagues,[16] who mapped a homozygous recessive mutation in CNTNAP2 leading to intractable epilepsy, developmental delay, and autistic features. Moreover, the range of phenotypic expression of recessive mutations in this transcript have recently been expanded to include periventricular leukomalacia and hepatosplenomegaly.[73]

Subsequently, Bakkaloglu and colleagues[74] mapped a de novo chromosomal abnormality in the only affected member of a pedigree and found the rearrangement disrupted CNTNAP2. The investigators comprehensively resequenced this molecule in 635 patients and 942 controls. This large-scale resequencing effort demonstrated a twofold increase in the burden of rare variants in cases versus controls and identified a single rare variant associated with affected status. Although the cytogenetic and rare variant association findings were interesting in light of the other evidence implicating rare variants in CNTNAP2 to developmental delay, the investigators pointed out that (1) the increase in the burden of rare mutations in cases and controls did not reach statistical significance and (2) based on the methodology used in their study, they could not rule out the confound of population stratification with respect to the rare associated allele.

Parametric linkage analysis

The use of parametric linkage to study consanguineous families, as exemplified by the Strauss study (discussed previously), represents an alternative to cytogenetic approaches to the identification of extreme outlier families. Subsequent to the Strauss article (discussed previously), Morrow and colleagues[15] conducted a large-scale homozygosity mapping study in consanguineous Middle Eastern families. They identified multiple, mostly nonoverlapping regions of homozygosity, that is, regions of the genome in which a single identical chromosomal segment is inherited from mother and father due to a recent common shared ancestor. Although the study did not reach genome-wide statistical significance, several large, rare, inherited homozygous deletions were found that disrupted the coding or potential regulatory regions of brain-expressed transcripts, including deleted in autism-1 (DIA1 or c3orf58), sodium/proton exchanger 9 (NHE9), protocadherin 10 (PCDH10), and CNTN3 (contactin 3). The investigators found additional strong evidence supporting a role for the gene NHE9, the $(Na^+, K^+)/H^+$ exchanger, in ASD through the identification of a rare nonsense mutation in two male siblings with autism, one of whom has epilepsy and the other probable seizures, in a nonconsanguineous family. They found rare amino acid changes in NHE9 in nearly 6% of patients with both autism and epilepsy versus only 0.63% of controls. Further, based on an independent set of studies reported in the same publication, three of the genes located within or closest to the two largest deletions (DIA1, NHE9, and PCDH10) were found to be regulated by neural activity or were the targets of activity-induced transcription factors. This suggests that changes in activity-regulated gene expression during brain development may contribute to ASD.

Copy number variation analysis

The development of new technology has expanded the scope of cytogenetic studies. In addition to potentially identifying smaller "abnormalities" of the type that have led to outlier findings (discussed previously), CNV analysis offers researchers the first truly cost-effective tools for scanning the entire genome for rare variants, allowing for an assessment of the rare variant–common disease hypothesis. The earliest studies in this regard seemed to support an overall contribution of rare variation to the population risk of ASD, consistent with the rare variant–common disease hypothesis. The first study to suggest this found that 7% to 10% of simplex autism families, 2% to 3% of multiplex families, and only 1% of control families carried rare de novo CNVs.[54] Subsequent studies have supported this overall pattern.[75,76] Moreover, the finding of an increased rate of de novo variation is consistent with the monozygotic and dizygotic data and research suggesting that increasing paternal age at the time of conception is a risk factor for autism.[77]

These studies initially focused on large CNVs and used samples that included patients with significant developmental disability in addition to ASD. Whether or not the same overall increase in mutation burden will be as evident as the resolution of CNV analysis increases and more diverse samples (with, for example, higher IQs and less dysmorphology) are included, is not yet clear.

In addition to identifying an increase in large de novo CNVs on a population basis, several recent CNV studies have identified specific regions of the genome that appear to carry substantial risk for ASD. For example, de novo deletions and duplications at 16p11.2 have been identified in patients with ASD,[78,79] and, when evaluated together, they have been found to increase the risk of autism.[79] Weiss and colleagues found them in 1% of autism case samples versus in less than 0.1% of the general population. Statistical significance was achieved independently in three distinct populations and 15 brain-expressed genes in the region are being explored.[79] Marshall and colleagues[75] conducted a similar CNV analysis that further supported the association of CNVs at 16p.11. A more recent study, however, did not replicate the 16p11 findings due to an increased frequency of these variants seen in controls.[9] This disparity may suggest sample heterogeneity or potentially the confound of population stratification, something not explicitly explored in the initial Weiss report. Additional studies with well-characterized and fastidiously matched controls, now common in GWAS studies, will be required to further evaluate this locus. Moreover, additional biological studies will be helpful in determining whether or not the inclusion of deletions and duplications in this and other CNV association analyses makes biological sense. Recent findings in other pervasive developmental disorders support this hypothesis.[80]

Several other recent CNV studies have supported the role of this class of variation to ASD risk. For example, Marshall and colleagues,[75] in addition to finding support for the 16p.11 locus (as described previously), identified CNVs (deletions or duplications) that were over-represented in cases versus controls for SHANK3, NLGN4, and NRXN1 genes They also identified several new candidates, including DPP6 and DPP10.[75]

Bucan and colleagues[76] conducted a similar study using multiple independent samples of cases and controls. They identified 14 deletions present at least once in both groups of probands but in neither control set (N = 2539).[76] As in previous studies, some of these supported previous candidate genes, including NRXN1. Newly identified genes included BZRAP1 at 17q22 and MDGA2 at 14q21.3. The former codes for an adaptor molecule thought to regulate synaptic transmission by linking vesicular release machinery to voltage-gated Ca2+ channels.[76] The latter is less well characterized but the researchers noted that the protein structure as predicted by BLASTP is unexpectedly similar to that of contactin 4 (discussed previously).[76]

Finally, a recent large-scale study supported prior rare variant discoveries, including the relevance of CNTN4 and neurexin 1 in ASD.[9] As in the case of 16p11, the investigators have chosen at times to combine duplications and deletions in considering replication: for example, previous findings have pointed to a role for deletions or disrupting translocations in CNTN4, whereas the report of replication in this case focused on duplications present in cases and absent in controls. In addition to providing additional evidence for previously mapped regions, this recent study suggested an entirely new molecular mechanism: four of the candidate genes identified were related to the ubiquitin pathway. The investigators point out that "the ubiquitin system operates both pre and post-synaptically to regulate the range of synaptic attributes including endo and exocytosis, dendritic elaboration and the formation of the post-synaptic density."[9]

Syndromic autism

As discussed previously, another line of evidence implicating the contribution of rare alleles to autism genetics is the overlap in phenotype between autism and rare monogenic diseases. For example, "ASD may be diagnosed in 30% of males with FXS and likewise Fragile X mutations may be found among as many as 7%–8% of individuals with idiopathic ASD."[81] Similarly, mutations in MECP2, the Rett disorder gene, have been found in cases of "idiopathic autism" without the Rett phenotype. For example, 2 of 69 female patients diagnosed as having idiopathic autism were found to have MECP2 mutations in one case series.[82] Likewise, autistic patients have an increased risk for neurofibromatosis (100 fold) and other rare monogenic diseases, such as tuberous sclerosis and Joubert syndrome, and patients with these disorders are reported to have an increased risk for having autism.[83,84] The association between autism and these neuropsychiatric syndromes is reviewed in further detail elsewhere.[85-87]

Although the evidence discussed previously (and related biological studies) underscores that the study of rare monogenic syndromes may be useful in understanding idiopathic autism, the reported rates of phenotypic overlap need to be viewed with a modicum of caution. First, a distinction must be drawn between evidence that derives from the finding of rare syndromic mutations in children who are thought to represent cases of idiopathic autism versus evidence that derives from the identification of ASD features in individuals with developmental delay syndromes. With regard to the latter, many studies focusing on this question are limited in their ability to blind diagnostic assessments owing to the nature of patient recruitment and the often pathognomonic physical features of affected individuals. An additional consideration is that ASD diagnoses are not uniformly made using state-of-the-art instruments and there may be a considerable degree of diagnostic uncertainty arising in cases of severe developmental delay.[88]

CLINICAL IMPLICATIONS

What are the clinical implications of the genetic findings to date (summarized in **Table 1**)? It is worthwhile to start by restating the obvious: there is not a single gene or genetic test that definitively diagnoses autism. The diagnosis of autism remains a clinical/syndromic one. This does not preclude, however, the usefulness of genetic testing in aiding in diagnosis, family planning, or prognosis, the importance of which should not be underestimated.[89]

There are several institutional practice parameters and guidelines that provide recommendations regarding genetic testing in autism. In addition, there are scholarly articles that review the subject. On certain recommendations, there is near complete agreement. Others remain debated, and practice often differs from clinic to clinic. Moreover, many of the formal practice parameters were developed before the recent explosion of data from CNV analyses and consequently tend to underestimate the now demonstrated yield of these approaches.

The American Academy of Child and Adolescent Psychiatry's most recent practice parameter from 1999 offers broad recommendations regarding the need for genetic testing after the diagnosis of autism has been made. They state that the presence of dysmorphic features or a family history of intellectual disability may "suggest" obtaining genetic screening for metabolic disorders or chromosomal analysis or genetics consultation.[90] An updated version of these recommendations with more detailed recommendations based on current literature is forthcoming.

In 2000, the American Academy of Neurology guidelines made the following level 2 evidence-based recommendation: "Genetic testing in children with autism, specifically high-resolution chromosome studies (karyotype) and DNA analysis for [Fragile X], should be performed in the presence of mental retardation (or if mental retardation cannot be excluded), if there is a family history of [Fragile X] or undiagnosed mental retardation, or if dysmorphic features are present. However, there is little likelihood of positive karyotype or [Fragile X] testing in the presence of high-functioning autism."[91] The latter conclusion is currently a matter of some debate as ongoing studies focusing on higher functioning ASD continue to identify cases of previously undiagnosed Fragile X syndrome.

The 2007 American Academy of Pediatrics clinical report states that genetic testing, such as chromosomal analysis, subtelomeric fluorescence in situ hybridization (FISH), and specific fragile X testing, may be indicated in children with ASDs only if they have coexisting global developmental delay or intellectual disability. Newer techniques, however, such as comparative genomic hybridization–microarray analysis, that can detect submicroscopic chromosomal abnormalities may become standard of care in the future but to date are not sufficiently evaluated in children with ASDs.[92]

Thus, within the institutional guidelines, the consensus is that routine genetic screening or referral to a geneticist is not indicated for every patient diagnosed with idiopathic autism. Rather, screening or referral should be triggered only when suspicion is raised by the history or presentation. All agree that one such trigger is

Table 1
Summary evidence for selected autism spectrum disorders candidate genes

Gene/Region	Chromosome	Evidence
Neurexin 1 (NRXN1)	2	• Linkage and copy number analysis leading to the discovery of sequence variation[35] • Independent discovery of rare variants and balanced chromosomal abnormalities[69,70] • Three independent CNV analyses[9,75,76] • Binding partner for neuroligin 4X (see below)
Contactin 4	3	• Cytogenetic study of patient with deletion syndrome on the short arm of chromosome 3 who presented with social disability.[71] Two independent CNV studies,[9,72] one highlighting deletions[9] and the other duplications in this region[72]
Sodium/proton exchanger 9 (NHE9)	3	• Suggestive linkage in homozygosity mapping study, followed by the discovery of large, rare homozygous deletions encompassing the gene and the identification of a rare mutation in two nonconsanguineous brothers in an independent sample. Further support via mutation screening and the finding that three genes within or closest to the largest the deleted regions, NHE9, deleted in autism-1 (DIA1), and protocadherin 10 (PCDH10), were regulated by neuronal activity[15]
5p14.1	5	• GWAS found significant association to this intergenic region. Study included internal replication samples. Most significant SNP maps between two neuronal adhesion molecules, cadherin 9 and cadherin 10[8]
Contactin-associated protein-like 2 (CNTNAP2)	7	• Homozygous recessive mutation in CNTNAP2 demonstrated to lead to intractable epilepsy, developmental delay, cortical dysplasia, and autistic features in homozygosity mapping study[16] • Study of an autism pedigree revealed a chromosomal rearrangement in the only affected member that disrupted CNTNAP2.[74] Large-scale resequencing demonstrated twofold increase in the burden of rare variants in cases versus controls that did not reach statistical significance. Single recurrent rare variant associated with affected status[74] • Two significant nonparametric linkage studies focusing on a language phenotype among individuals with ASD.[36,46] Fine mapping association study by the same investigators with internal replication[47] • Significant transmission disequilibrium test supported by an internal replication using the broader autism diagnosis. However, identified SNP different from study above[36] • Protein product of FOXP2, a gene causing a monogenic form of speech and language disorder, binds to CNTNAP2, and regulates its expression.[48] Positive association between SNPs in CNTNAP2 and an endophenotype of specific language disorder[48]
Engrailed 2 (EN2)	7	• Significant association study with internal replication and supportive functional studies[39] • Two independent replication attempts failed to show an association with initially reported SNP but one small study did find evidence for association with haplotypes in the region[40,41]

Gene	Chromosome	Notes
MET oncogene	7	• Suggestive linkage to ASD in an ASP study[42] • Significant association between a regulatory SNP upstream of the *MET* gene and autism[43] • Similar significant association study and biological studies by the same laboratory[44] • Independent replication found significant association but to a different SNP[45]
16p11.2	16	• CNV analysis showing association. Internal replication in three populations[79] grouping deletions and duplications together • Independent replication in two other CNV analysis.[75,78] However, failure of replication in a third large CNV analysis[9]
SHANK3	22	• Independently replicated de novo and transmitted structural and sequence variations discovered in autistic patients[68] • Finding of developmental delay and autistic features in patients with the 22q13 deletion syndrome (the genomic segment corresponding to the position of *SHANK3*) • CNV analysis[75] and binds in trans to neuroligin 4X at the synapse (see below)
Neuroligin 3 (*NLGN3*)	X	• Functional[61] missense mutation identified in two brothers with autism and ASP • Neuroligin pathway genes, including *SHANK3*, implicated in autism (see above) • Subsequent mutation screenings of modest samples of patients have not identified additional clearly deleterious mutations[63-66]
Neuroligin 4X (*NLGN4X*)	X	• Cytogenetic evidence.[58] Identification of nonsense mutation not present in controls[59,60] • Significant linkage and identification of similar nonsense mutation in a pedigree with X-linked mental retardation, PDD, or autism[62] • Neuroligin pathway genes, including *SHANK3*, implicated in autism (see above) • CNV analysis[75] but subsequent mutation screenings of modest samples of patients have not identified additional deleterious mutations[63-66]

the presence of intellectual disability in the patient or a history of it in the family. Two of the guidelines suggest that another trigger should be dysmorphic features in a patient. All recommend chromosomal analysis and fragile X testing at a minimum or referral to a geneticist. Again, this article highlights that the most recent of these recommendations were published in 2007 and could not take into account the widespread dissemination of high-resolution CNV analyses.

There has been an increasing appreciation in the primary literature that more extensive genetic screening may be valuable on a more routine basis. Using a three-tiered protocol of neurogenetic evaluation of patients diagnosed with idiopathic autism, a 2006 study reported a 40% yield.[93] The first tier included the dysmorphology criteria found in the clinical guidelines (discussed previously) with these findings resulting in targeted genetics work-ups. If a diagnosis was not found in each tier, a subsequent panel of tests was undertaken. The subsequent tiers included karyotyping, fragile X testing, MECP-2 testing, 22q11 FISH, 15 interphase FISH, Prader-Willi/Angelman testing, 17p11 FISH, and subtelomeric FISH if IQ was less than 50. The investigators felt that the yield was sufficiently high to warrant more routine evaluation and testing by clinical geneticists.[93]

A 2009 review of the subject also goes beyond the institutional guidelines in its recommendations. For example, it recommends karyotype and fragile X testing for all patients with ASDs and *MECP2* testing in all girls with autism and intellectual disability, even in the absence of Rett symptoms.[89] It also points to the near future (which has now arrived) when the cost of array-based comparative genomic hybridization–microarray analysis for the detection of CNVs will be inexpensive enough that it is not restricted to patients with dysmorphology or history of intellectual disability.[89]

The definite trend in the literature over the past decade is for increased genetic testing and a decreasing threshold for obtaining such tests. This is well justified as more is learned about the genetic causes of autism and as tests become more accurate and less expensive. These changes are occurring rapidly, and it is difficult for general clinicians, such as neurologists, pediatricians, and psychiatrists, to keep abreast of the changes. Furthermore, although there is some training in observing dysmorphologies in these fields, it will fall far short of that which is routine for clinical geneticists. Thus, using dysmorphology as a criterion for work-up may lead to missed opportunities for more specific diagnosis. The cost of this is not simply academic. For example, missing a 22q11 deletion syndrome diagnosis may keep a patient with a treatable cardiac condition from receiving adequate care. Finally, increased testing, especially with high-resolution microarrays, could lead to the identification of further syndromes. Owing to these issues, the authors favor a standard work-up that includes fragile X testing and screening chromosomes with a high-resolution array, along with referral to a clinical geneticist for counseling in the case of positive results and further consultation for those who screen negative but have a history of developmental delay, regression, or evidence of dysmorphology, including macrocephaly.

SUMMARY

Autism and related conditions are highly heritable disorders. Consequently, gene discovery promises to help elucidate the underlying pathophysiology of these syndromes and, it is hoped, eventually improve diagnosis, treatment, and prognosis. The genetic architecture of autism is not yet known. What can be said from the studies to date is that writ large, autism is not a monogenic disorder with mendelian inheritance. In many, but not all, individual cases, it is likely to be a complex genetic disorder that results from simultaneous genetic variations in multiple genes. The CDCV hypothesis predicts that the risk alleles in autism and other complex disorders will be common in the population. Recent evidence with regard to autism and other complex disorders, however, raises significant questions regarding the overall applicability of the theory and the extent of its usefulness in explaining individual genetic liability. In addition, considerable evidence points to the importance of rare alleles for the overall population of affected individuals and their role in providing a foothold into the molecular mechanisms of disease. Finally, there is debate regarding the clinical implications of autism genetic research to date. Most institutional guidelines recommend genetic testing or referral only for idiopathic autism if intellectual disability and dysmorphic features are present. Recent advances suggest, however, that the combination of several routine tests combined with a low threshold for referral is well justified in cases of idiopathic autism.

REFERENCES

1. Fombonne E. Epidemiological surveys of autism and other pervasive developmental disorders: an update. J Autism Dev Disord 2003;33(4):365–82.
2. American Psychiatric Association. Diagnostic and statistical manual of mental disorders. 4th edition, text revision. Washington, DC: American Psychiatric Association; 2000.
3. Martin A, Volkmar FR, Lewis M. Lewis's child and adolescent psychiatry: a comprehensive textbook. Philadelphia (PA): Lippincott Williams & Wilkins; 2007.
4. Schopler E, Mesibov GB, Kunce LJ. Asperger syndrome or high-functioning autism? New York (NY): Plenum Pub Corp; 1998.
5. Ganz ML. The lifetime distribution of the incremental societal costs of autism. Arch Pediatr Adolesc Med 2007;161(4):343.
6. O'Roak BJ, State MW. Autism genetics: strategies, challenges, and opportunities. Autism Res 2008;1(1):4–17.
7. Abrahams BS, Geschwind DH. Advances in autism genetics: on the threshold of a new neurobiology. Nat Rev Genet 2008;9(5):341–55.
8. Wang K, Zhang H, Ma D, et al. Common genetic variants on 5p14. 1 associate with autism spectrum disorders. Nature 2009;459:528–33.
9. Glessner JT, Wang K, Cai G, et al. Autism genome-wide copy number variation reveals ubiquitin and neuronal genes. Nature 2009;459(7246):569–73.
10. Liu J, Nyholt DR, Magnussen P, et al. A genomewide screen for autism susceptibility loci. Am J Hum Genet 2001;69(2):327–40.
11. Bailey A, Le Couteur A, Gottesman I, et al. Autism as a strongly genetic disorder: evidence from a British twin study. Psychol Med 1995;25(1):63.
12. Fombonne E. Epidemiology of autistic disorder and other pervasive developmental disorders. J Clin Psychiatry 2005;66:3.
13. Bolton P, Macdonald H, Pickles A, et al. A case-control family history study of autism. J Child Psychol Psychiatry 1994;35(5):877–900.
14. Gupta AR, State MW. Recent advances in the genetics of autism. Biol Psychiatry 2007;61(4):429–37.
15. Morrow EM, Yoo SY, Flavell SW, et al. Identifying autism loci and genes by tracing recent shared ancestry. Science 2008;321(5886):218.
16. Strauss KA, Puffenberger EG, Huentelman MJ, et al. Recessive symptomatic focal epilepsy and mutant contactin-associated protein-like 2. N Engl J Med 2006;354(13):1370–7.

17. Durand CM, Betancur C, Boeckers TM, et al. Mutations in the gene encoding the synaptic scaffolding protein SHANK3 are associated with autism spectrum disorders. Nat Genet 2007;39(1):25–7.

18. Chakravarti A. Population genetics—making sense out of sequence. Nat Genet 1999;21(1 Suppl):56–60.

19. Reich DE, Lander ES. On the allelic spectrum of human disease. Trends Genet 2001;17(9):502–10.

20. Farrer L, Cupples L, Haines J, et al. Effects of age, sex, and ethnicity on the association between apolipoprotein E genotype and Alzheimer disease. A meta-analysis. APOE and Alzheimer Disease Meta Analysis Consortium. JAMA 1997; 278(16):1349–56.

21. Klein RJ, Zeiss C, Chew EY, et al. Complement factor H polymorphism in age-related macular degeneration. Science 2005;308(5720):385–9.

22. Edwards AO, Ritter R III, Abel KJ, et al. Complement factor H polymorphism and age-related macular degeneration. Science 2005;308(5720):421–4.

23. Zeggini E, Scott LJ, Saxena R, et al. Meta-analysis of genome-wide association data and large-scale replication identifies additional susceptibility loci for type 2 diabetes. Nat Genet 2008;40(5):638–45.

24. Saxena R, Voight BF, Lyssenko V, et al. Genome-wide association analysis identifies loci for type 2 diabetes and triglyceride levels. Science 2007;316(5829): 1331–6.

25. Iyengar SK, Elston RC. The genetic basis of complex traits: rare variants or "common gene, common disease"? Methods Mol Biol 2007;376:71–84.

26. Clark R, Hutton M, Fuldner M, et al. The structure of the presenilin 1(S 182) gene and identification of six novel mutations in early onset AD families. Nat Genet 1995;11(2):219–22.

27. Inlow JK, Restifo LL. Molecular and comparative genetics of mental retardation. Genetics 2004;166(2):835–81.

28. Cohen JC, Pertsemlidis A, Fahmi S, et al. Multiple rare variants in NPC1L1 associated with reduced sterol absorption and plasma low-density lipoprotein levels. Proc Natl Acad Sci U S A 2006;103(6):1810–5.

29. Ji W, Foo JN, O'Roak BJ, et al. Rare independent mutations in renal salt handling genes contribute to blood pressure variation. Nat Genet 2008;40(5):592–9.

30. Brown MS, Goldstein JL. Expression of the familial hypercholesterolemia gene in heterozygotes: mechanism for a dominant disorder in man. Science 1974; 185(4145):61–3.

31. Lifton RP, Gharavi AG, Geller DS. Molecular mechanisms of human hypertension. Cell 2001;104(4):545–56.

32. Bear MF, Dölen G, Osterweil E, et al. Fragile X: translation in action. Neuropsychopharmacology 2007;33(1):84–7.

33. Ehninger D, Han S, Shilyansky C, et al. Reversal of learning deficits in a Tsc2/− mouse model of tuberous sclerosis. Nat Med 2008;14(8):843–8.

34. Li W, Cui Y, Kushner SA, et al. The HMG-CoA reductase inhibitor lovastatin reverses the learning and attention deficits in a mouse model of neurofibromatosis type 1. Curr Biol 2005;15(21):1961–7.

35. Szatmari P, Paterson AD, Zwaigenbaum L, et al. Mapping autism risk loci using genetic linkage and chromosomal rearrangements. Nat Genet 2007;39(3): 319–28.

36. Alarcón M, Cantor RM, Liu J, et al. Evidence for a language quantitative trait locus on chromosome 7q in multiplex autism families. Am J Hum Genet 2002;70(1): 60–71.

37. Arking DE, Cutler DJ, Brune CW, et al. A common genetic variant in the neurexin superfamily member CNTNAP2 increases familial risk of autism. Am J Hum Genet 2008;82(1):160–4.
38. Hirschhorn JN, Lohmueller K, Byrne E, et al. A comprehensive review of genetic association studies. Genet Med 2002;4(2):45–61.
39. Benayed R, Gharani N, Rossman I, et al. Support for the homeobox transcription factor gene ENGRAILED 2 as an autism spectrum disorder susceptibility locus. Am J Hum Genet 2005;77(5):851–68.
40. Zhong H, Serajee F, Nabi R, et al. No association between the EN2 gene and autistic disorder. J Med Genet 2003;40(1):e4.
41. Wang L, Jia M, Yue W, et al. Association of the ENGRAILED 2 (EN2) gene with autism in Chinese Han population. Am J Med Genet B Neuropsychiatr Genet 2008;147(4):434–8.
42. Imgsac A. A genomewide screen for autism: strong evidence for linkage to chromosomes 2q, 7q, and 16p. Am J Hum Genet 2001;69:570–81.
43. Campbell DB, Sutcliffe JS, Ebert PJ, et al. A genetic variant that disrupts MET transcription is associated with autism. Proc Natl Acad Sci U S A 2006; 103(45):16834.
44. Campbell DB, Li C, Sutcliffe JS, et al. Genetic evidence implicating multiple genes in the MET receptor tyrosine kinase pathway in autism spectrum disorder. Autism Res 2008;1(3):159.
45. Sousa I, Clark TG, Toma C, et al. MET and autism susceptibility: family and case–control studies. Eur J Hum Genet 2008;17(6):749–58.
46. Alarcón M, Yonan A, Gilliam T, et al. Quantitative genome scan and ordered-subsets analysis of autism endophenotypes support language QTLs. Mol Psychiatry 2005; 10(8):747–57.
47. Alarcón M, Abrahams BS, Stone JL, et al. Linkage, association, and gene-expression analyses identify CNTNAP2 as an autism-susceptibility gene. Am J Hum Genet 2008;82(1):150–9.
48. Vernes SC, Newbury DF, Abrahams BS, et al. A functional genetic link between distinct developmental language disorders. N Engl J Med 2008; 359(22):2337.
49. Feuk L. ASHG 2008 Annual Meeting: from enormous cohorts to individual genomes. Genome Med 2009;1:9.
50. Goldstein DB. Common genetic variation and human traits. N Engl J Med 2009; 360(17):1696–8.
51. Scott LJ, Mohlke KL, Bonnycastle LL, et al. A genome-wide association study of type 2 diabetes in Finns detects multiple susceptibility variants. Science 2007; 316(5829):1341–5.
52. Sladek R, Rocheleau G, Rung J, et al. A genome-wide association study identifies novel risk loci for type 2 diabetes. Nature 2007;445(7130):881–5.
53. Zeggini E, Weedon MN, Lindgren CM, et al. Replication of genome-wide association signals in UK samples reveals risk loci for type 2 diabetes. Science 2007; 316(5829):1336–41.
54. Sebat J, Lakshmi B, Malhotra D, et al. Strong association of de novo copy number mutations with autism. Science 2007;316(5823):445.
55. Xu J, Zwaigenbaum L, Szatmari P, et al. Molecular cytogenetics of autism. Curr Genom 2004;5:347–64.
56. Cook E Jr, Lindgren V, Leventhal B, et al. Autism or atypical autism in maternally but not paternally derived proximal 15q duplication. Am J Hum Genet 1997;60(4): 928.

57. Schroer RJ, Phelan MC, Michaelis RC, et al. Autism and maternally derived aberrations of chromosome 15q. Am J Med Genet 1998;76(4):327–36.
58. Thomas NS, Sharp AJ, Browne CE, et al. Xp deletions associated with autism in three females. Hum Genet 1999;104(1):43–8.
59. Jamain S, Quach H, Betancur C, et al. Mutations of the X-linked genes encoding neuroligins NLGN3 and NLGN4 are associated with autism. Nat Genet 2003; 34(1):27–9.
60. Chih B, Afridi SK, Clark L, et al. Disorder-associated mutations lead to functional inactivation of neuroligins. Hum Mol Genet 2004;13(14):1471–7.
61. Tabuchi K, Blundell J, Etherton MR, et al. A neuroligin-3 mutation implicated in autism increases inhibitory synaptic transmission in mice. Science 2007; 318(5847):71–6.
62. Laumonnier F, Bonnet-Brilhault F, Gomot M, et al. X-linked mental retardation and autism are associated with a mutation in the NLGN4 gene, a member of the neuroligin family. Am J Hum Genet 2004;74(3):552–7.
63. Blasi F, Bacchelli E, Pesaresi G, et al. Absence of coding mutations in the X-linked genes neuroligin 3 and neuroligin 4 in individuals with autism from the IMGSAC collection. Am J Med Genet B Neuropsychiatr Genet 2006;141(3):220–1.
64. Gauthier J, Bonnel A, St-Onge J, et al. NLGN3/NLGN4 gene mutations are not responsible for autism in the Quebec population. Am J Med Genet B Neuropsy-chiatr Genetics 2005;132(1):74–5.
65. Vincent JB, Kolozsvari D, Roberts WS, et al. Brief research communication: mutation screening of X-chromosomal neuroligin genes: no mutations in 196 autism probands. Am J Med Genet B Neuropsychiatr Genet 2004;129:82–4.
66. Yan J, Oliveira G, Coutinho A, et al. Analysis of the neuroligin 3 and 4 genes in autism and other neuropsychiatric patients. Mol Psychiatry 2004;10(4): 329–32.
67. Meyer G, Varoqueaux F, Neeb A, et al. The complexity of PDZ domain-mediated interactions at glutamatergic synapses: a case study on neuroligin. Neurophar-macology 2004;47(5):724–33.
68. Moessner R, Marshall CR, Sutcliffe JS, et al. Contribution of SHANK3 mutations to autism spectrum disorder. Am J Hum Genet 2007;81(6):1289–97.
69. Feng J, Schroer R, Yan J, et al. High frequency of neurexin 1β signal peptide structural variants in patients with autism. Neurosci Lett 2006;409(1):10–3.
70. Kim HG, Kishikawa S, Higgins AW, et al. Disruption of neurexin 1 associated with autism spectrum disorder. Am J Hum Genet 2008;82(1):199–207.
71. Fernandez T, Morgan T, Davis N, et al. Disruption of contactin 4 (CNTN4) results in developmental delay and other features of 3p deletion syndrome. Am J Hum Genet 2004;74(6):1286–93.
72. Roohi J, Montagna C, Tegay DH, et al. Disruption of contactin 4 in 3 subjects with autism spectrum disorder. J Med Genet 2008;46(1):176–82.
73. Jackman C, Horn ND, Molleston JP, et al. Gene associated with seizures, autism, and hepatomegaly in an Amish girl. Pediatr Neurol 2009;40(4):310–3.
74. Bakkaloglu B, O'Roak BJ, Louvi A, et al. Molecular cytogenetic analysis and re-sequencing of contactin associated protein-like 2 in autism spectrum disorders. Am J Hum Genet 2008;82(1):165–73.
75. Marshall CR, Noor A, Vincent JB, et al. Structural variation of chromosomes in autism spectrum disorder. Am J Hum Genet 2008;82(2):477–88.
76. Bucan M, Abrahams BS, Wang K, et al. Genome-wide analyses of exonic copy number variants in a family-based study point to novel autism susceptibility genes. PLoS Genet 2009;5(6):e1000536.

77. Reichenberg A, Gross R, Weiser M, et al. Advancing paternal age and autism. Arch Gen Psychiatry 2006;63(9):1026.
78. Kumar RA, KaraMohamed S, Sudi J, et al. Recurrent 16 p 11. 2 microdeletions in autism. Hum Mol Genet 2008;17(4):628.
79. Weiss LA, Shen Y, Korn JM, et al. Association between microdeletion and micro-duplication at 16p11. 2 and autism. Obstet Gynecol Surv 2008;63(6):361.
80. Van Esch H, Bauters M, Ignatius J, et al. Duplication of the MECP2 region is a frequent cause of severe mental retardation and progressive neurological symptoms in males. Am J Hum Genet 2005;77(3):442–53.
81. Muhle R, Trentacoste SV, Rapin I. The genetics of autism. Pediatrics 2004;113(5): e472–86.
82. Carney RM, Wolpert CM, Ravan SA, et al. Identification of MeCP2 mutations in a series of females with autistic disorder. Pediatr Neurol 2003;28(3):205–11.
83. Marui T, Hashimoto O, Nanba E, et al. Association between the neurofibroma-tosis-1 (NF1) locus and autism in the Japanese population. Am J Med Genet B Neuropsychiatr Genet 2004;131:43–7.
84. Smalley SL. Autism and tuberous sclerosis. J Autism Dev Disord 1998;28(5): 407–14.
85. Zafeiriou DI, Ververi A, Vargiami E. Childhood autism and associated comorbidities. Brain Dev 2007;29(5):257–72.
86. Kumar R, Christian S. Genetics of autism spectrum disorders. Curr Neurol Neurosci Rep 2009;9(3):188–97.
87. Fombonne E, Du Mazaubrun C, Cans C, et al. Autism and associated medical disor-ders in a French epidemiological survey. J Am Acad Child Adolesc Psychiatry 1997; 36(11):1561.
88. Volkmar FR, State M, Klin A. Autism and autism spectrum disorders: diagnostic issues for the coming decade. J Child Psychol Psychiatry 2009;50(1-2):108–15.
89. Lintas C, Persico A. Autistic phenotypes and genetic testing: state-of-the-art for the clinical geneticist. Br Med J 2009;46(1):1.
90. Volkmar F, Cook E Jr, Pomeroy J, et al. Summary of the practice parameters for the assessment and treatment of children, adolescents, and adults with autism and other pervasive developmental disorders. J Am Acad Child Adolesc Psychi-atry 1999;38:32s–54s.
91. Filipek P, Accardo P, Ashwal S, et al. Practice parameter: screening and diag-nosis of autism report of the quality standards subcommittee of the American Academy of Neurology and the Child Neurology Society. Neurology 2000;55(4): 468–79.
92. Johnson CP, Myers SM. Identification and evaluation of children with autism spectrum disorders. Pediatrics 2007;120(5):1183.
93. Schaefer GB, Lutz RE. Diagnostic yield in the clinical genetic evaluation of autism spectrum disorders. Genet Med 2006;8(9):549.

Genetics of Addictions

Sarah M. Hartz, MD, PhD, Laura J. Bierut, MD*

KEYWORDS

• Genetics • Alcohol dependence • Nicotine dependence

Substance use disorders are maladaptive patterns of substance use leading to inability to control use despite significant consequences.[1] When the impairment is in multiple areas of life or the individual has significant signs of tolerance or withdrawal, the diagnosis changes to substance dependence. These general definitions apply to all drugs of abuse, including alcohol, nicotine, and cocaine. Substance use disorders are common: alcohol dependence/abuse has a prevalence of 13.5%, nicotine dependence has a prevalence of 13%, and all other drug dependence/abuse has a prevalence of 6.1%.[2,3]

Substance use disorders are highly comorbid with many other mental illnesses. In one study, the odds of having an addictive disorder not related to nicotine increased by a factor of 2.7 in the presence of a mental disorder.[3] In addition, the presence of an addictive disorder increased the risk for other mental illness. Specifically, 37% of subjects with alcohol addiction had a comorbid mental disorder, and 53% of subjects with other drug addiction had a comorbid mental disorder, compared with a baseline prevalence of non–substance-related mental disorders of 22.5%.[3] This comorbidity leads to more severe illness. In a five-state study of Medicaid recipients, the subjects with both a severe mental illness and a substance use disorder had a higher odds of using inpatient and emergency psychiatric facilities compared with subjects with the respective mental illness alone.[4]

Disclosures: Dr L Bierut is listed as an inventor on a patent "Markers of Addiction" (US 20070258898), covering the use of certain single nucleotide polymorphisms in determining the diagnosis, prognosis, and treatment of addiction. Dr Bierut acted as a consultant for Pfizer, Inc in 2008.

Funding support: Collaborative Genetic Study of Nicotine Dependence P01 CA89392 (National Cancer Institute), Study of Addiction: Genetics and Environment U01 HG004422 (National Human Genome Research Institute), Case Control Candidate Gene Study of Addiction R01 DA19963 (National Institute on Drug Abuse), Human Genetics of Addiction: A Study of Common and Specific Factors K02 DA021237 (National Institute on Drug Abuse), Collaborative Study on the Genetics of Alcoholism U10 AA008401 (National Institute on Alcohol Abuse and Alcoholism).

Department of Psychiatry, Washington University School of Medicine, Campus Box 8134, 660 South Euclid Avenue, St Louis, MO 63110-1093, USA

* Corresponding author.

E-mail address: laura@wustl.edu (L.J. Bierut).

Although many studies distinguish nicotine dependence from other substance-related disorders, nicotine dependence is also highly comorbid with mental disorders and negatively affects their severity and prognosis. There are increased rates of lifetime smoking in subjects with mental illness compared with controls (59% vs 39%, respectively, P<.001).[5] The prevalence of nicotine dependence is 13% in the general population and 30% to 70% in the presence of other psychiatric disorders.[2] Although these data indicate the strong need for smoking cessation in the psychiatrically ill population, quit rates are substantially lower for subjects with active mental illness compared with smokers without mental illness (31% quit rate vs 43% quit rate).[5]

Not only is a significant proportion of nicotine dependence comorbid with psychiatric illness but a significant portion of morbidity in psychiatric illness may be attributed to nicotine dependence. The greatest mortality risk of mental illness is premature death caused by heart disease and cancer. In an 8-state comparison of deaths of clients at public mental health clinics, public mental health clients lived 13 to 30 years less than their general public counterparts.[6,7] Although rates of suicide and accidental death are higher in this population compared with controls, the primary causes of the deaths are medical illnesses such as heart disease and cancer. Therefore, the largest modifiable risk factor for mortality in the mental health population is cigarette smoking. In addition, nicotine dependence is associated with disease-specific poor outcomes. For example, lifetime smoking in bipolar disorder is associated with earlier age of onset of symptoms, greater severity of symptoms, poorer functioning, history of suicide attempts, comorbid anxiety, and substance use disorders.[8]

The more severe course of illness and increased mortality highlights the importance of integrating the study of addiction with the study of other psychiatric and medical illnesses. This importance is emphasized by recent genetic overlap found between alcohol dependence and aerodigestive cancers, and between nicotine dependence and lung disease. This article chronicles the genetic associations found in alcohol dependence, including related findings in aerodigestive cancers, and the genetic associations found in nicotine dependence, including related findings in lung disease. The article then briefly discusses the genetic findings in cocaine dependence and psychiatric comorbidities with substance dependence.

GENETICS OF ALCOHOL DEPENDENCE

Alcohol dependence is a complex disease, with genetic and environmental risk factors. Alcohol dependence (commonly known as alcoholism) necessarily has a strong environmental component because exposure to and consumption of alcohol is required for the disorder. But, there is a substantial heritable component to the risk for alcoholism. Among first-degree relatives of alcohol-dependent individuals, the risk of alcohol dependence is 3 to 8 times the baseline population risk.[9]

Alcohol dependence was the first behavioral disorder to have validated genetic findings. In 1972, subjects of Asian descent were noted to have facial flushing and decreased alcohol tolerance compared with subjects of European origin.[10] This was hypothesized to be genetic rather than cultural, based on observations that infants of Asian descent who were exposed to a small amount of alcohol were more likely to flush than infants of European descent.[10] The flushing reaction to ingestion of alcohol was found to be secondary to a deficiency of aldehyde dehydrogenase (specifically ALDH2), an enzyme involved in the metabolism of ethanol.[11] The prevalence of ALDH2 deficiency was then examined in the Japanese population and found to be 41% in the general population and 2% in alcoholics, suggesting a protective role for the deficiency of ALDH2 in alcoholism.[12]

Since these initial findings in the early 1980s, much has been learned about the genetics of alcohol metabolism. Ethanol metabolism occurs predominantly in the liver in 2 steps: (1) oxidation to acetaldehyde catalyzed by alcohol dehydrogenases (ADHs), and (2) oxidation of acetaldehyde to acetate by ALDH. Multiple genetic variants of ADH and ALDH influence rates of alcohol metabolism and alcohol dependence.[13] The mechanism through which variants of these enzymes influence risk of alcohol dependence is believed to be related to elevation of acetaldehyde levels, leading to facial flushing, nausea, and tachycardia. It is hypothesized that people with the genetic variants of ADH and ALDH leading to increased acetaldehyde levels would be less likely to drink excessively because of the discomfort of ingesting a small amount of ethanol. This behavioral aversion to alcohol with increased acetaldehyde levels is exploited by administering disulfiram, a medication that interferes with ALDH, to alcoholics. Disulfiram blocks ALDH, leading to a build-up of acetaldehyde, causing symptoms including nausea, vomiting, flushing, shortness of breath, and headache when alcohol is ingested. It is hoped that the administration of disulfiram to alcoholics decreases cravings and discourages them from using alcohol.

There are multiple ADH and ALDH genes, and many variants of these genes have been examined for their association with alcohol dependence. Most of the studied variants involve changes of single nucleotide polymorphisms (SNPs), in coding and noncoding regions of the DNA. The ADH genes are located in a small region on chromosome 4 (**Fig. 1**). The ALDH gene associated with alcohol dependence, *ALDH2*, is on chromosome 12q24.2. This article discusses the major association findings between alcohol metabolism genes and alcoholism. For a more comprehensive review on the genetics of alcohol metabolism, see Edenberg.[13]

The *ALDH2* variant leading to decreased risk of alcohol dependence, *ALDH2*2,* has been further characterized since its initial discovery in the 1980s. *ALDH2*2* is a coding variant resulting from the substitution of lysine for glutamate at position 504, resulting in a nearly inactive ALDH2 enzyme and leading to markedly elevated acetaldehyde levels in the blood with the consumption of small amounts of alcohol. The allele is common in people of East Asian descent, but it is essentially nonexistent in people of European or African descent.[14] The protective effect of this allele is strong and has been replicated in multiple studies.[15–17] The odds ratio of alcohol dependence for subjects with 1 *ALDH2*2* allele is 0.33, and there are almost no documented cases of people with alcohol dependence who are homozygous for *ALDH2*2*.[15–17] This allele interacts with a nonsynonymous gene variant for the ADH1 enzyme, *ADH1B*1*, by further decreasing the odds ratio of alcohol dependence to 0.05 in the presence of both alleles.[15] The protective effect of the *ALDH2*2* allele is susceptible to environmental pressures. A study by Higuchi and colleagues[18] found that the fraction of Japanese alcoholics carrying the *ALDH2*2* allele increased from 3% in 1979 to 13% in 1992. This increase is believed to be due to an overall increase in alcohol consumption in Japanese society during that period.

The most robust association between a variant of an ADH gene and alcohol dependence is with the *ADH1B*2* allele (previously known as *ADH2*2*). This variant is in the *ADH1B* gene that encodes the β2 subunit of ADH, and results in histidine instead of arginine at position 48.[13] It is associated with a more rapid ethanol oxidation to acetaldehyde and is protective against alcohol dependence, with an odds ratio of 0.12 in a Chinese population.[13,15] Again, this variant is common in people of East Asian descent, and rare in people of European and African descent. The protective effect of this allele seems to be weaker in European than in Asian populations.[19] It is unclear how much of this variability is due to different social and environmental factors rather than unidentified coinherited genes that modify susceptibility.

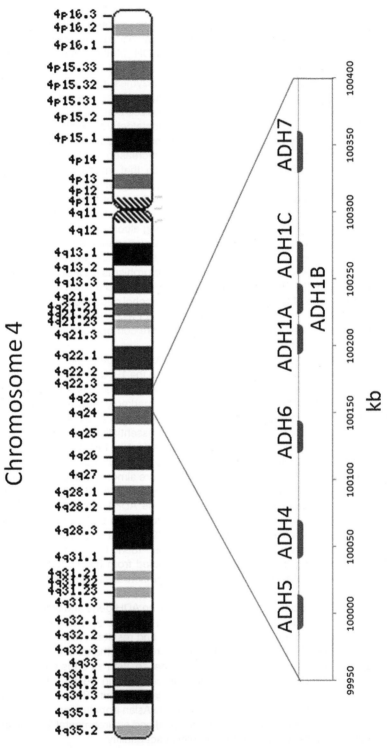

Fig. 1. Chromosome 4 region q23, including the ADH enzymes *ADH1A*, *ADH1B*, *ADH1C*, *ADH4*, *ADH5*, *ADH6*, and *ADH7*.

In addition to the association between alcohol dependence and alcohol-metabolizing enzymes, γ-aminobutyric acid (GABA) receptor genes have also been associated with alcohol dependence. This association is of particular relevance because alcohol is an agonist of the GABA receptor. This region includes the subunit genes GABRG1, GABRA2, GABRA4, and GABRB1 (**Fig. 2**). Edenberg and colleagues[20] evaluated this region in detail and found a strong association between GABRA2, encoding the α2 subunit of $GABA_A$, and alcohol dependence. This association was replicated in multiple populations, and was found to be most strong in alcohol-dependent individuals with comorbid dependence on illicit drugs.[21–24]

GABA receptor genes have a clear relationship to alcohol dependence. GABA transmission mediates effects of alcohol, including disruption of motor coordination, anxiolysis, sedation, ethanol preference, and symptoms related to withdrawal.[25] Furthermore, rat models have shown $GABA_A$ agonists increase ethanol intake and $GABA_A$ antagonists decrease ethanol intake.[26] Although GABA subunit genes and alcohol-metabolizing genes have been genetically associated with alcohol dependence, the biologic mechanism is different in each case.

The advent of the genome-wide association studies (GWAS) brought increased genomic density and large data sets. GWAS relied on the completion of the International HapMap Project in 2005, in which common SNPs were mapped tightly throughout the genome. Using a case-control design and hundreds of thousands of SNPs spanning the entire genome, GWAS looked for association between SNPs and disease. Although there are more statistical tests of association (1 test per SNP) than there are subjects (typically thousands), the combination of setting a sufficiently low threshold for P value significance and placing a high emphasis on replication of significant results in independent data sets has resulted in discovery of robust associations.

Although GWAS are a technological breakthrough in the density of markers that are tested across the genome, the genome is not completely represented by the SNP arrays used in the GWAS studies. For example, the Affymetrix Genome-Wide Human SNP Array 6.0 genotypes 906,600 SNPs out of an estimated 10,000,000 SNPs in the human genome (approximately 2,000,000 of which are known). The dense coverage in GWAS studies, although an improvement compared with previous methodology, is still not dense enough to ensure that associations are found. Nonetheless, a SNP reaching genome-wide association significance indicates that functional variation is likely to occur through this SNP or 1 of the correlated, untested SNPs.

The first GWAS for alcohol dependence was published by Treutlein and colleagues[27] in 2009. Two SNPs reached genome-wide significance, and these investigators nominated another group of candidate SNPs to evaluate in a secondary dataset. Further confirmation of their findings is necessary. The ADH and ALDH genes previously found to be associated with alcohol dependence were not significant. This finding is likely due to low-risk allele frequencies in the European population that was used for the study.

Because alcohol is related to medical illnesses such as aerodigestive cancer and variations in alcohol metabolism are related to the development of alcohol dependence, a study was designed to evaluate whether genetic variation in ADH may contribute to the development of cancer of the upper aerodigestive tract, including several types of head and neck cancer that develop in the context of heavy alcohol and tobacco exposure.[28] Based on 3800 subjects with aerodigestive cancer and 5200 controls, variants in ADH1B and ADH7 were found to be protective against aerodigestive cancer.[28] Even after stratifying for site of cancer, alcohol consumption and other covariates, the protective effects were still strong. These effects suggest that

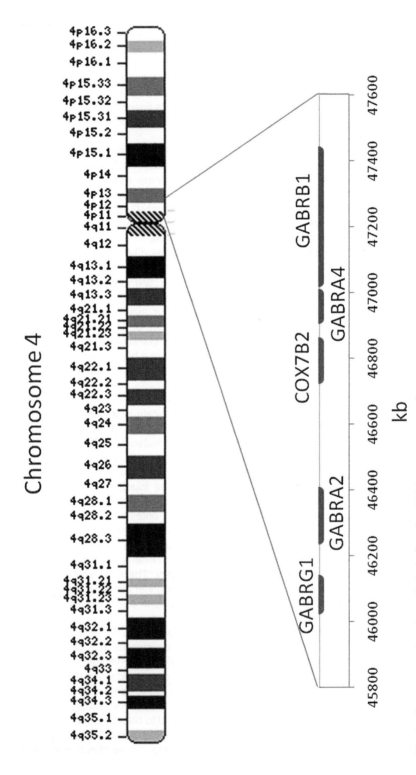

Fig. 2. Chromosome 4 region p12, including the GABA receptor gene cluster.

ADH variants not only decrease the risk for alcohol dependence but also decrease the susceptibility to cancer associated with alcohol dependence, perhaps by modifying the carcinogenic effects of alcohol.

The investigation of genetic associations in alcohol dependence started with the observation of facial flushing in an Asian subpopulation and has developed into genome-wide studies of large populations with alcohol dependence and alcohol-related cancers. Although many years of study have led to improved understanding, fundamental questions of the genetics of alcohol dependence remain unanswered.

NICOTINE DEPENDENCE

The conceptualization of the different stages of smoking is helpful in understanding the varying environmental and genetic contributions to each step in the development of smoking behaviors. To better understand smoking behavior, it is compartmentalized into (1) initiation (the period during which subjects smoke for the first time and experiment with smoking), (2) regular smoking (defined as subjects having smoked at least 100 cigarettes during their lifetime), and (3) nicotine dependence (a psychiatric disorder defined by symptoms of tolerance, withdrawal, and loss of control).[1] The heritability of smoking initiation was estimated to be 44%.[29] Conversely, the heritability of nicotine dependence was markedly higher at 75%.[29]

Although smoking initiation and nicotine dependence are related, the genetics of nicotine dependence are of primary interest because of its public health ramifications: nicotine dependence predicts difficulty with cessation and carries most of the morbidity associated with smoking. Specifically, the quantity of cigarettes smoked in a lifetime is associated with lung disease and heart disease, and smoking cessation is a positive prognostic factor for both. Individuals with nicotine dependence account for 13% of the general population but consume 58% of the cigarettes smoked in the United States.[2] Thus, understanding the genetics of nicotine dependence can lead to targeted treatments and may ultimately decrease tobacco-associated morbidity and mortality.

In the study of nicotine dependence, it is important to understand the behavioral progression to nicotine dependence when choosing a control group. Subjects who have not had adequate nicotine exposure (ie, who have not smoked enough cigarettes) have not had the opportunity to become nicotine dependent. For this reason, genetic studies of nicotine dependence carefully choose for their control group regular smokers who did not become nicotine dependent. This choice minimizes the possibility that the controls would become dependent if they had adequate nicotine exposure.

The strong heritability of nicotine dependence has led to genetic studies. The initial efforts to identify susceptibility loci primarily used linkage designs. In addition to linkage studies, isolated candidate gene case-control studies targeted various neurotransmitters and their receptors, but these generally had low power and insufficient density of genotypes.

The first GWAS on nicotine dependence was conducted by Bierut and colleagues.[30] The study compared 1050 nicotine-dependent subjects and 879 controls (who smoked but did not become dependent). Although no individual SNPs reached genome-wide significance, the data were reanalyzed for a targeted association study with 3713 SNPs in 348 candidate genes.[31] Several cholinergic nicotinic receptor genes dominated the top signals after controlling for multiple testing.

It is biologically relevant that the top genetic associations for nicotine dependence were in genes encoding for nicotinic receptor subunits. Nicotine produces its central and peripheral actions by binding to neuronal nicotinic acetylcholine receptors (nAChRs), a class of neuronal ligand-gated ion channels expressed in the nervous system. nAChRs are made of 5 combinations of α and β subunits constructed around a central pore. The subunits are encoded by 9 α ($\alpha2$–$\alpha10$) and 3 β ($\beta2$–$\beta4$) subunit genes, named *CHRNA2–CHRNA10* and *CHRNB2–CHRNB4*, respectively. The expression of the different subunits in specific anatomic areas leads to hypotheses regarding their functional relevance. The addiction of nicotine is believed to arise from the interaction between dopaminergic and nicotinic neurons in the striatum (**Fig. 3**). Multiple nicotinic subunits are involved in this interaction, including $\alpha4$, $\alpha5$, $\alpha6$, $\beta2$, and $\beta3$. This region has been implicated in the reward pathway and is important for the development of substance dependence.

CHRNA5 and *CHRNA3* are nicotinic receptor subunit genes on chromosome 15q25 coding for the $\alpha5$ nicotinic receptor subunit and the $\alpha3$ nicotinic receptor subunit, respectively (**Fig. 4**). The coding sequences are adjacent to one another, and SNPs in the 2 genes are in high linkage disequilibrium (LD). The most biologically compelling association with nicotine dependence was found in rs16969968, a nonsynonymous SNP in the $\alpha5$ nicotinic receptor subunit gene *CHRNA5*.[30,31] This association has been replicated with either rs16969968 or correlated SNPs in many other independent studies.[32–36] rs16969968 is seen in **Fig. 4** in the coding region of *CHRNA5*. rs16969968 is a nonsynonymous SNP for which the minor variant results in an amino acid change of aspartic acid to asparagine. The frequency of the minor allele varies between populations. It ranges from 0% in African populations to 37% in European populations. Although rs16969968 is in the coding sequence of *CHRNA5*, and a bio-logically plausible relationship exists between *CHRNA5* and nicotine dependence, SNPs in high LD with rs16969968 span a large area encompassing the genes *IREB2*, *PSMA4*, *CHRNA5*, *CHRNA3*, and *CHRNB4*. Although rs16969968 is a compelling candidate for a causal association with nicotine dependence, other unidentified but related markers cannot be excluded as the cause for the observed association with nicotine dependence.

The biologic importance of rs16969968 has been shown in several settings. First, the $\alpha5$ nicotinic receptor is expressed in the brain. Its expression in the striatum and direct interaction with the dopaminergic pathway is particularly relevant to addiction. Second, the protein sequences of *CHRNA5* homologs were examined in multiple species (human, chimpanzee, Bolivian squirrel monkey, domestic cow, mouse, chicken, and African clawed frog) and the aspartic acid residue was present in all species.[37] This conservation across species suggests that it has functional importance. Third, an in vitro functional study found that $\alpha4\alpha5\beta2$ receptors containing the asparagine amino acid substitution in $\alpha5$ exhibited decreased response to a nicotine agonist compared with the receptors with the aspartic acid variant in $\alpha5$.[37] This finding suggests that decreased nicotinic receptor function is associated with increased risk for nicotine dependence.

In-depth analyses of the region led to the discovery of additional SNPs that form a haplotype with rs16969968 to modify the expression of *CHRNA5*.[32,36,38] The SNP rs588765 was found to be associated with nicotine dependence and to modify expression of *CHRNA5*. In addition, together with rs16969968, it forms a haplotype to alter the risk of nicotine dependence. Although rs588765 can lead to high expression and low expression of *CHRNA5*, and rs16969968 can lead to high risk and low risk for nicotine dependence, only 3 haplotypes exist in the population (**Table 1**): high risk (rs16969968) and low expression (rs588765), low risk (rs16969968) and low expression (rs588765), and low risk (rs16969968) and high expression (rs588765). The lowest risk of nicotine dependence occurs with the low-expression allele of

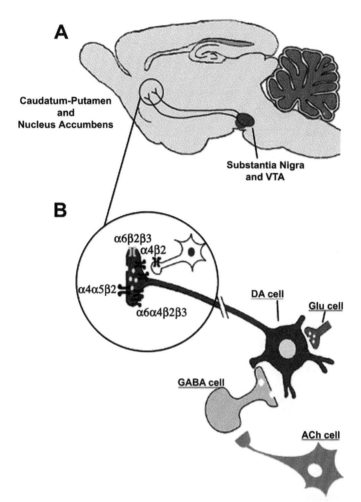

Fig. 3. nAChRs in the striatum of the rodent central nervous system. (*A*) The mesostriatal dopaminergic pathway. (*B*) Subunit composition of the functional nAChRs expressed by dopaminergic nerve terminals ($\alpha6\beta2\beta3$, $\alpha6\alpha4\beta2\beta3$, $\alpha4\beta2$, $\alpha4\alpha5\beta2$). VTA, ventral tegmental area. (*Reproduced from* Gotti C, Clementi F. Neuronal nicotinic receptors: from structure to pathology. Prog Neurobiol 2004;74(6):363–96; with permission.)

rs588765 and the low-risk allele of rs16969968, and the highest risk for nicotine dependence occurs with the low-expression allele of rs588765 and the high-risk allele of rs16969968. A similar association was seen in a population of African Americans with the SNP rs555018, an SNP in high LD with rs588765 in European Americans and African Americans, suggesting that rs555018 is associated with variable expression of *CHRNA5*.[32]

The GWAS results and corresponding biologic experiments suggest that *CHRNA5* is involved in the development of nicotine dependence, but the relationship between changes in structure and expression of *CHRNA5* and the development of smoking behavior remains unknown. Various research groups are evaluating the relationship between these genes and smoking initiation, the pleasurable responses associated with smoking, and the age of onset of smoking.[39–41]

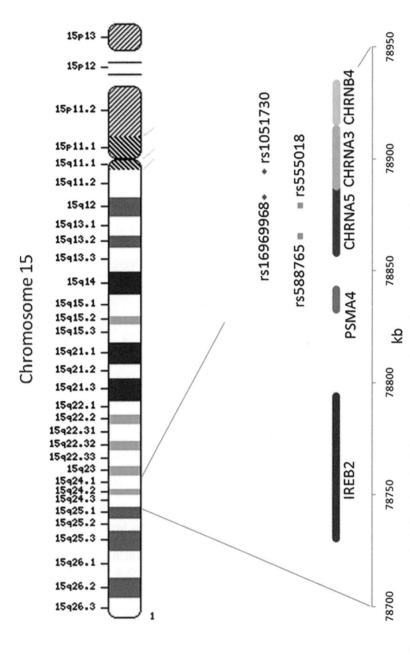

Fig. 4. Chromosome 15q25, including the nicotinic receptor gene cluster. The SNPs associated with nicotine dependence are highlighted.

Table 1
Risk of nicotine dependence based on haplotypes constructed from rs16969968 and rs588765

	Haplotype Risk of Nicotine Dependence		
	High	**Intermediate**	**Low**
rs16969968	High-risk allele	Low-risk allele	Low-risk allele
rs588765	Low-expression allele	High-expression allele	Low-expression allele

Alleles of rs16969968 are represented as high-risk allele for nicotine dependence and low-risk allele for nicotine dependence. Alleles for rs588765 are represented as high expression of *CHRNA5* and low expression of *CHRNA5*. The haplotype of high-risk allele (rs16969968) and high-expression allele (rs588765) is not listed because it is rare in the population.

The purpose of understanding the genetics of nicotine dependence is, ultimately, to change behavior and effectively treat the disorder. Therefore, research has been conducted on the genetics of smoking cessation. Because the greatest predictor of smoking cessation is nicotine dependence, a negative correlation would be expected between smoking cessation and the major SNP associated with nicotine dependence, rs16969968. The initial population-based study to assess genetic associations with smoking cessation did not find an association with rs16969968.[42] However, 2 recent studies selected participants specifically targeted for smoking cessation, and both found the minor allele of rs16969968 to be significantly associated with inability to quit smoking or high likelihood of relapse.[43,44] This finding suggests that rs16969968 increases the risk of nicotine dependence, and decreases the ability to quit.

The *CHRNA5/CHRNA3/CHRNB4* region has also been associated with lung cancer and chronic obstructive pulmonary disease (COPD). Because lung cancer and COPD are nearly completely attributable to smoking it is difficult to determine whether the observed association is independent of nicotine dependence. The difficulty with interpretation has been emphasized in multiple studies.

Associations have been found between lung cancer and an SNP in LD with rs16969968, rs1051730.[33,34,45,46] Various methodologies have been used to try to separate the environmental contribution of nicotine dependence from a direct genetic contribution to lung cancer of rs1051730 or a related SNP. Several researchers found increased risk for lung cancer after adjusting for smoking, supporting the hypothesis that rs1051730 contributes to lung cancer independent of nicotine dependence.[33,45,46] Amos and colleagues[46] found an association between lung cancer and rs1051730 in 3 independent samples, robust to adjustment for pack-years of cigarette exposure. However, the association between rs1051730 and lung cancer was absent in nonsmokers. If rs1051730 were related to lung cancer independent of smoking exposure the effect would be present in nonsmokers. Despite this, the repeated evidence of association of this variant with lung cancer independent of degree of smoking exposure among those who have smoked argues that there is an association between rs1051730 (and related SNPs) and lung cancer beyond the impact on risk of nicotine dependence itself.

The relationship between rs1051730, nicotine dependence, and lung cancer was more specifically explored by Spitz and colleagues.[43] This was accomplished by using 3 samples: (1) patients with lung cancer and controls with a history of smoking, (2) patients with lung cancer and controls who were lifetime nonsmokers, and (3) patients with bladder cancer and controls with a history of smoking. The investigators found a statistically significant association of rs1051730 with lung cancer in subjects with a history of smoking. When stratified for number of cigarettes smoked per day, the highest risk was seen in the lightest smokers, subjects smoking less than 20 cigarettes per day. There was no association between lung cancer and rs1051730 in subjects who had never smoked and no association between rs1051730 and bladder and renal cancers. The investigators concluded that because the highest risk group was in the subjects who smoked the least, rs1051730 mediated risk to lung cancer beyond the cigarette exposure from nicotine dependence.

A recent GWAS for COPD also found association of rs1051730 with COPD.[47] This association remained significant after adjusting for pack-years ($P = 5.7 \times 10^{-10}$). Although this finding suggests that this is a true association with COPD, the investigators acknowledged that the lack of further smoking variables makes it difficult to identify the full contribution of nicotine exposure on COPD.

One explanation for the association of rs16969968 with lung disease independent of cigarette quantity is that the quantity of toxin inhaled when smoking is not well explained by the number of cigarettes smoked per day, suggesting that people with the risk allele of rs16969968 may inhale more deeply. To investigate this possibility, Le Marchand and colleagues[48] conducted a study that evaluated the amount of nicotine and carcinogens consumed in a sample of 819 smokers. A positive association was found between the amount of nicotine metabolites seen in urine, a measure of the amount of nicotine consumed, and the minor variant of rs16969968 after adjusting for number of cigarettes smoked per day. This finding indicates that more nicotine and associated carcinogens are absorbed by individuals with the risk allele than individuals without the risk allele. Moreover, the differential absorption is not accounted for by number of cigarettes smoked per day. Because these data argue that number of cigarettes smoked per day is not a complete proxy for nicotine and toxin absorption, the association between lung cancer and rs16969968 may still be confounded by the increased nicotine and toxin intake in nicotine dependence even after adjusting for number of cigarettes smoked per day.

In summary, multiple associations have been found between nicotine dependence and nicotinic receptor subunit genes. The strongest and most robust association is seen with a nonsynonymous SNP in the nicotinic receptor gene *CHRNA5*, rs16969968. This SNP is also associated with lung cancer and COPD, both smoking-related disorders. The current scientific question is whether there is an association between these smoking-related disorders and rs16969968, independent of nicotine dependence.

COCAINE DEPENDENCE

It is estimated that approximately 2.1% of US residents have used cocaine in the past month, the second most prevalent nonmedical drug to marijuana.[49] Similar to nicotine and alcohol dependence, cocaine dependence has a strong component of heritability: siblings of cocaine-dependent probands had an estimated relative risk of 1.8 of developing cocaine dependence compared with probands without cocaine-dependent siblings.[50] Because of the hypothesis that common genetic factors may lead to dependence on various classes of drugs, a study evaluated the relationship between cocaine dependence and rs16969968, the nonsynonymous *CHRNA5* SNP associated with increased risk for nicotine dependence.[51] The minor allele of rs16969968 that is associated with increased risk for nicotine dependence is associated with decreased risk for cocaine dependence. The bidirectional association is hypothesized to be due to the involvement of nAChRs with excitatory and inhibitory modulation of dopamine-mediated reward pathways. A negative association was also seen between the

CHRNA5 SNP rs588765 and alcohol dependence in a sample that was heavily comorbid with cocaine dependence.[52] This association suggests that the *CHRNA5* gene may play a dual role in modulating susceptibility to addiction via the different mechanisms of action of cocaine and nicotine.

GENETIC ASSOCIATION OF SUBSTANCE DEPENDENCE WITH OTHER MENTAL ILLNESS

The tendency of subjects with mental illness to use substances has been extensively discussed. A traditional hypothesis was that substance use is a means of self-medicating and dependence is therefore 'caused' by mental illness. On the contrary, data have been published that smoking precedes the diagnosis of mental illness and may contribute to the disorder. For example, there is an increased risk of first onset major depression in smokers[53–56] and an increase in depressive symptoms in persons who smoked in adolescence.[57–59] Ex-smokers do not differ from current smokers in their risk for mood disorders, although daily smoking may be a causal factor in panic disorder and agoraphobia.[60] One interpretation of these data is that smoking confers additional risk in the development of psychiatric disorders.

An alternative explanation for the comorbidity of substance dependence and other psychiatric illness is a shared cause. The heritability of major psychiatric illness is high, with estimates of 64% in schizophrenia,[61] 59% in bipolar disorder,[61] and 42% in major depressive disorder.[62] The combination of the heritability of substance dependence, the heritability of psychiatric illnesses, and comorbidity of substance dependence with psychiatric illness indicates that specific genes may be pleiotropic (ie, contribute to substance dependence and other psychiatric illness).

Because of the phenotypic complexity of psychiatric illnesses, the search for pleiotropic genes may help clarify psychiatric diagnoses and help understand biologic causes of mental illness. For example, suspicion of shared genetic susceptibilities with bipolar disorder and illegal substance dependence has been the subject of recent research. A bipolar GWAS data set and an illegal substance dependence GWAS data set were compared for overlap of top signals, and evidence was found of shared associations.[63] These studies suggest that advances may be made by understanding genetic pleiotropy and interconnections between addiction and other major psychiatric illnesses.

SUMMARY

Addictions are common heritable disorders with multiple psychiatric and medical comorbidities. Persons with substance abuse are approximately twice as likely to suffer psychiatric morbidities as those without substance abuse, and have an increased risk of using inpatient and emergency facilities. In addition, public mental health clients had a decreased life span of 13 to 30 years; most deaths are caused by heart disease and cancer. Cigarette smoking is therefore the largest modifiable risk factor for morbidity and mortality in the general population and in the psychiatric population.

Alcohol dependence was the first behavioral disorder to have validated genetic findings. The alcohol metabolism gene, *ALDH2*, was initially found in the early 1980s to decrease the risk of alcohol dependence by increasing the levels of acetaldehyde in the blood, leading to uncomfortable physiologic effects including facial flushing, nausea, and tachycardia. A second alcohol-metabolizing gene, *ADH1B*, also decreases the risk for alcohol dependence by increasing ethanol oxidation to acetaldehyde. In addition to associations between alcoholism and alcohol-metabolizing genes, a GABA receptor gene, *GABRA2*, has been associated with alcohol dependence.

The mechanism for this association is believed to be due to GABA mediation of behavioral affects of alcohol.

Recently, strong genetic associations with nicotine dependence have been found in the nicotinic receptor subunit CHRNA5. It seems that there are at least 2 distinct biologic mechanisms that alter the risk of nicotine dependence. The first biologic mechanism is caused by an amino acid change in *CHRNA5*, in the nonsynonymous SNP rs16969968. Functional studies have found that expression of the minor variant leads to reduced response to a nicotinic agonist. The second mechanism altering risk of nicotine dependence is through altered expression of the $\alpha5$ mRNA. A second group of SNPs in the region, including rs588765 and rs555018, is associated with variable expression of *CHRNA5*. The combination of altered protein and variable mRNA expression leads to different levels of addiction risk.

Although there have been major advances in understanding the genetics of addictions, the current evidence accounts for only a small proportion of the genetic variance. As new statistical and genetic tools allow a better understanding of the mechanism by which multiple genes lead to psychiatric and medical illness, new discoveries will inform and challenge understanding of these illnesses.

Medical disorders that occur in the context of substance dependence seem to have genetic associations that are not entirely explained by the contribution of the genetic variant to substance use. Specifically, gene variants in ADH were protective for cancers of the upper aerodigestive tract, even after adjusting for alcohol consumption. Similarly, SNPs correlated with rs16969968 are associated with an increased risk of COPD and lung cancer, after adjusting for cigarette use. Although the interpretation of these studies is difficult because of the confounding between the medical illness and substance exposure, there is evidence of a genetic interaction in both cases.

Substance dependence is strongly heritable and heavily comorbid with other medical illnesses. Therefore, the importance of understanding the genetics of substance dependence in the context of its many related medical and psychiatric disorders cannot be overstated.

REFERENCES

1. American Psychiatric Association. Task Force on DSM-IV. Diagnostic and statistical manual of mental disorders: DSM-IV-TR. 4th edition. Washington, DC: American Psychiatric Association; 2000.
2. Grant BF, Hasin DS, Chou SP, et al. Nicotine dependence and psychiatric disorders in the United States: results from the national epidemiologic survey on alcohol and related conditions. Arch Gen Psychiatry 2004;61(11):1107–15.
3. Regier DA, Farmer ME, Rae DS, et al. Comorbidity of mental disorders with alcohol and other drug abuse. Results from the Epidemiologic Catchment Area (ECA) Study. JAMA 1990;264(19):2511–8.
4. Clark RE, Samnaliev M, McGovern MP. Treatment for co-occurring mental and substance use disorders in five state Medicaid programs. Psychiatr Serv 2007; 58(7):942–8.
5. Lasser K, Boyd JW, Woolhandler S, et al. Smoking and mental illness: a population-based prevalence study. JAMA 2000;284(20):2606–10.
6. Colton CW, Manderscheid RW. Congruencies in increased mortality rates, years of potential life lost, and causes of death among public mental health clients in eight states. Prev Chronic Dis 2006;3(2):A42.

7. Parks J, Svendsen D, Singer P, et al. Morbidity and mortality in people with serious mental illness. Alexandria (VA): National Association of State Mental Health Program Directors; 2006.
8. Ostacher MJ, Nierenberg AA, Perlis RH, et al. The relationship between smoking and suicidal behavior, comorbidity, and course of illness in bipolar disorder. J Clin Psychiatry 2006;67(12):1907–11.
9. Reich T, Edenberg HJ, Goate A, et al. Genome-wide search for genes affecting the risk for alcohol dependence. Am J Med Genet 1998;81(3):207–15.
10. Wolff PH. Ethnic differences in alcohol sensitivity. Science 1972;175(20): 449–50.
11. Goedde HW, Agarwal DP, Harada S. Genetic studies on alcohol-metabolizing enzymes: detection of isozymes in human hair roots. Enzyme 1980;25(4):281–6.
12. Harada S, Agarwal DP, Goedde HW, et al. Possible protective role against alcoholism for aldehyde dehydrogenase isozyme deficiency in Japan. Lancet 1982; 2(8302):827.
13. Edenberg HJ. The genetics of alcohol metabolism: role of alcohol dehydrogenase and aldehyde dehydrogenase variants. Alcohol Res Health 2007;30(1):5–13.
14. Oota H, Pakstis AJ, Bonne-Tamir B, et al. The evolution and population genetics of the ALDH2 locus: random genetic drift, selection, and low levels of recombination. Ann Hum Genet 2004;68(Pt 2):93–109.
15. Chen CC, Lu RB, Chen YC, et al. Interaction between the functional polymorphisms of the alcohol-metabolism genes in protection against alcoholism. Am J Hum Genet 1999;65(3):795–807.
16. Luczak SE, Glatt SJ, Wall TL. Meta-analyses of ALDH2 and ADH1B with alcohol dependence in Asians. Psychol Bull 2006;132(4):607–21.
17. Thomasson HR, Edenberg HJ, Crabb DW, et al. Alcohol and aldehyde dehydrogenase genotypes and alcoholism in Chinese men. Am J Hum Genet 1991;48(4): 677–81.
18. Higuchi S, Matsushita S, Imazeki H, et al. Aldehyde dehydrogenase genotypes in Japanese alcoholics. Lancet 1994;343(8899):741–2.
19. Whitfield JB. Alcohol dehydrogenase and alcohol dependence: variation in genotype-associated risk between populations. Am J Hum Genet 2002;71(5):1247–50 [author reply: 1250–1].
20. Edenberg HJ, Dick DM, Xuei X, et al. Variations in GABRA2, encoding the alpha 2 subunit of the GABA(A) receptor, are associated with alcohol dependence and with brain oscillations. Am J Hum Genet 2004;74(4):705–14.
21. Agrawal A, Edenberg HJ, Foroud T, et al. Association of GABRA2 with drug dependence in the collaborative study of the genetics of alcoholism sample. Behav Genet 2006;36(5):640–50.
22. Covault J, Gelernter J, Hesselbrock V, et al. Allelic and haplotypic association of GABRA2 with alcohol dependence. Am J Med Genet B Neuropsychiatr Genet 2004;129(1):104–9.
23. Fehr C, Sander T, Tadic A, et al. Confirmation of association of the GABRA2 gene with alcohol dependence by subtype-specific analysis. Psychiatr Genet 2006; 16(1):9–17.
24. Soyka M, Preuss UW, Hesselbrock V, et al. GABA-A2 receptor subunit gene (GABRA2) polymorphisms and risk for alcohol dependence. J Psychiatr Res 2008;42(3):184–91.
25. Glowa JR, Crawley J, Suzdak PD, et al. Ethanol and the GABA receptor complex: studies with the partial inverse benzodiazepine receptor agonist Ro 15-4513. Pharmacol Biochem Behav 1988;31(3):767–72.

26. Boyle AE, Segal R, Smith BR, et al. Bidirectional effects of GABAergic agonists and antagonists on maintenance of voluntary ethanol intake in rats. Pharmacol Biochem Behav 1993;46(1):179–82.

27. Treutlein J, Cichon S, Ridinger M, et al. Genome-wide association study of alcohol dependence. Arch Gen Psychiatry 2009;66(7):773–84.

28. Hashibe M, McKay JD, Curado MP, et al. Multiple ADH genes are associated with upper aerodigestive cancers. Nat Genet 2008;40(6):707–9.

29. Vink JM, Willemsen G, Boomsma DI. Heritability of smoking initiation and nicotine dependence. Behav Genet 2005;35(4):397–406.

30. Bierut LJ, Madden PA, Breslau N, et al. Novel genes identified in a high-density genome wide association study for nicotine dependence. Hum Mol Genet 2007; 16(1):24–35.

31. Saccone SF, Hinrichs AL, Saccone NL, et al. Cholinergic nicotinic receptor genes implicated in a nicotine dependence association study targeting 348 candidate genes with 3713 SNPs. Hum Mol Genet 2007;16(1):36–49.

32. Saccone N, Wang JC, Breslau N, et al. The CHRNA5-CHRNA3-CHRNB4 nicotinic receptor subunit gene cluster affects risk for nicotine dependence in African-Americans and in European-Americans. Cancer Res 2009;69(17):6848–56.

33. Spitz MR, Amos CI, Dong Q, et al. The CHRNA5-A3 region on chromosome 15q24-25.1 is a risk factor both for nicotine dependence and for lung cancer. J Natl Cancer Inst 2008;100(21):1552–6.

34. Thorgeirsson TE, Geller F, Sulem P, et al. A variant associated with nicotine dependence, lung cancer and peripheral arterial disease. Nature 2008;452(7187):638–42.

35. Weiss RB, Baker TB, Cannon DS, et al. A candidate gene approach identifies the CHRNA5-A3-B4 region as a risk factor for age-dependent nicotine addiction. PLoS Genet 2008;4(7):e1000125.

36. Berrettini W, Yuan X, Tozzi F, et al. Alpha-5/alpha-3 nicotinic receptor subunit alleles increase risk for heavy smoking. Mol Psychiatry 2008;13(4):368–73.

37. Bierut LJ, Stitzel JA, Wang JC, et al. Variants in nicotinic receptors and risk for nicotine dependence. Am J Psychiatry 2008;165(9):1163–71.

38. Wang JC, Cruchaga C, Saccone N, et al. Risk for nicotine dependence and lung cancer is conferred by mRNA expression levels and amino acid change in CHRNA5. Hum Mol Genet 2009;18(16):3125–35.

39. Ehringer MA, Clegg HV, Collins AC, et al. Association of the neuronal nicotinic receptor beta2 subunit gene (CHRNB2) with subjective responses to alcohol and nicotine. Am J Med Genet B Neuropsychiatr Genet 2007;144(5):596–604.

40. Ehringer MA, McQueen MB, Hoft NR, et al. Association of CHRN genes with "dizziness" to tobacco. Am J Med Genet B Neuropsychiatr Genet 2009. [Epub ahead of print].

41. Sherva R, Wilhelmsen K, Pomerleau CS, et al. Association of a single nucleotide polymorphism in neuronal acetylcholine receptor subunit alpha 5 (CHRNA5) with smoking status and with 'pleasurable buzz' during early experimentation with smoking. Addiction 2008;103(9):1544–52.

42. Breitling LP, Dahmen N, Mittelstrass K, et al. Smoking cessation and variations in nicotinic acetylcholine receptor subunits alpha-5, alpha-3, and beta-4 genes. Biol Psychiatry 2009;65(8):691–5.

43. Baker TB, Weiss RB, Bolt D, et al. Human neuronal acetylcholine receptor A5-A3-B4 haplotypes are associated with multiple nicotine dependence phenotypes. Nicotine Tob Res 2009;11(7):785–96.

44. Freathy RM, Ring SM, Shields B, et al. A common genetic variant in the 15q24 nicotinic acetylcholine receptor gene cluster (CHRNA5-CHRNA3-CHRNB4) is

associated with a reduced ability of women to quit smoking in pregnancy. Hum Mol Genet 2009;18(15):2922–7.

45. Hung RJ, McKay JD, Gaborieau V, et al. A susceptibility locus for lung cancer maps to nicotinic acetylcholine receptor subunit genes on 15q25. Nature 2008; 452(7187):633–7.

46. Amos CI, Wu X, Broderick P, et al. Genome-wide association scan of tag SNPs identifies a susceptibility locus for lung cancer at 15q25.1. Nat Genet 2008; 40(5):616–22.

47. Pillai SG, Ge D, Zhu G, et al. A genome-wide association study in chronic obstructive pulmonary disease (COPD): identification of two major susceptibility loci. PLoS Genet 2009;5(3):e1000421.

48. Le Marchand L, Derby KS, Murphy SE, et al. Smokers with the CHRNA lung cancer-associated variants are exposed to higher levels of nicotine equivalents and a carcinogenic tobacco-specific nitrosamine. Cancer Res 2008;68(22):9137–40.

49. Substance Abuse and Mental Health Services Administration, Office of Applied Studies (2008). Results from the 2007 National Survey on Drug Use and Health: National Findings (NSDUH Series H-34, DHHS Publication No. SMA 08-4343). Rockville, MD. Available at: http://www.oas.samhsa.gov/NSDUH/2k7NSDUH/2k7results.cfm. Accessed October 16, 2009.

50. Bierut LJ, Dinwiddie SH, Begleiter H, et al. Familial transmission of substance dependence: alcohol, marijuana, cocaine, and habitual smoking: a report from the Collaborative Study on the Genetics of Alcoholism. Arch Gen Psychiatry 1998;55(11):982–8.

51. Grucza RA, Wang JC, Stitzel JA, et al. A risk allele for nicotine dependence in CHRNA5 is a protective allele for cocaine dependence. Biol Psychiatry 2008; 64(11):922–9.

52. Wang JC, Grucza R, Cruchaga C, et al. Genetic variation in the CHRNA5 gene affects mRNA levels and is associated with risk for alcohol dependence. Mol Psychiatry 2009;14(5):501–10.

53. Klungsoyr O, Nygard JF, Sorensen T, et al. Cigarette smoking and incidence of first depressive episode: an 11-year, population-based follow-up study. Am J Epidemiol 2006;163(5):421–32.

54. Breslau N, Peterson EL, Schultz LR, et al. Major depression and stages of smoking. A longitudinal investigation. Arch Gen Psychiatry 1998;55(2):161–6.

55. Brown RA, Lewinsohn PM, Seeley JR, et al. Cigarette smoking, major depression, and other psychiatric disorders among adolescents. J Am Acad Child Adolesc Psychiatry 1996;35(12):1602–10.

56. Kendler KS, Neale MC, MacLean CJ, et al. Smoking and major depression. A causal analysis. Arch Gen Psychiatry 1993;50(1):36–43.

57. Goodman E, Capitman J. Depressive symptoms and cigarette smoking among teens. Pediatrics 2000;106(4):748–55.

58. Kandel DB, Davies M, Karus D, et al. The consequences in young adulthood of adolescent drug involvement. An overview. Arch Gen Psychiatry 1986;43(8): 746–54.

59. Wu LT, Anthony JC. Tobacco smoking and depressed mood in late childhood and early adolescence. Am J Public Health 1999;89(12):1837–40.

60. Breslau N, Novak SP, Kessler RC. Daily smoking and the subsequent onset of psychiatric disorders. Psychol Med 2004;34(2):323–33.

61. Lichtenstein P, Yip BH, Bjork C, et al. Common genetic determinants of schizophrenia and bipolar disorder in Swedish families: a population-based study. Lancet 2009;373(9659):234–9.

62. Edvardsen J, Torgersen S, Roysamb E, et al. Unipolar depressive disorders have a common genotype. J Affect Disord 2009;117(1–2):30–41.
63. Johnson C, Drgon T, McMahon FJ, et al. Convergent genome wide association results for bipolar disorder and substance dependence. Am J Med Genet B Neuropsychiatr Genet 2009;150(2):182–90.

The Genetics of Major Depression: Moving Beyond the Monoamine Hypothesis

Stanley I. Shyn, MD, PhD, Steven P. Hamilton, MD, PhD*

KEYWORDS

• Genetics • Major depression • Genome-wide association

Over the course of a lifetime, major depressive disorder (MDD) afflicts 1 in 6 individuals in the general United States population,[1] women twice as often as men,[2] and is the leading cause of disability among adults younger than 45 years.[3] MDD is characterized by dysphoria or anhedonia plus several additional symptoms for diagnosis, which may include changes in sleep/appetite, excessive feelings of guilt or worthlessness, anergia, psychomotor slowing, impaired ability to think and, in more severe cases, suicidality. The *Diagnostic and Statistical Manual of Mental Disorders* (Fourth Edition, Text Revised) (DSM-IV) further defines MDD as the presence of at least one 2-week depressive episode, and excludes cases in which bipolar disorder, substances, or a general medical condition is etiologic.[4]

The pathophysiology of MDD remains a mystery almost half a century since Joseph Schildkraut first proposed the monoamine hypothesis of depression,[5] which followed the twin serendipitous discoveries of the therapeutic benefits of iproniazid (an antimycobacterial with inhibitory effects on monoamine oxidase)[6] and imipramine (a failed antipsychotic that came to represent a new class of drugs known as tricyclic antidepressants).[7] Despite the compelling nature of this disease model, to date no DNA variants in monoamine synthesis or signaling genes have been consistently linked to the etiology of affective disorders.[8] This review explores current efforts in gene discovery and alternative hypothesis generation for unipolar depression.

This work was supported by fellowship support (R25 MH060482-08 and T32 MH19126-19) from the National Institutes of Mental Health.
Department of Psychiatry, Langley Porter Psychiatric Institute, University of California, San Francisco, Box 0984 - NGL, 401 Parnassus Avenue, San Francisco, CA 94143-0984, USA
* Corresponding author.
E-mail address: steveh@lppi.ucsf.edu (S.P. Hamilton).

EPIDEMIOLOGY AND MDD SUBTYPES

Family studies demonstrate that first-degree relatives of MDD probands have a relative risk for MDD of 2.8 over the general population risk.[9] This number is further increased to between 3.0 and 8.0 for recurrent early-onset depression (MDD-REO).[10] Recurrence of depressive episodes and earlier age of onset have been the 2 clinical features that have shown the most consistent ability to predict greater familial aggregation, though it has been observed that the relative risk estimates quoted for MDD-REO are derived from family studies and not large population-based analyses.[11] The most optimal age at which to define a cut-off for "early-onset" is also unclear, but, in the GenRED (Genetics of Recurrent Early-onset Depression) project, the largest MDD-REO genetic study effort to date, Levinson and colleagues used a cut-off of 30 years or less. The argument for a genetic contribution to MDD comes from twin studies, which estimate an overall heritability of 37% to 43%, despite a lack of biological markers and reliance on an imperfect set of syndromal criteria for diagnosis.[9] While less heritable than schizophrenia and bipolar affective disorder, this estimate is similar to that described for type 2 diabetes mellitus,[12] a complex trait for which several risk loci have been successfully identified.[13]

There are multiple DSM-defined specifiers elaborating a range of clinical subtypes of MDD. These specifiers include severe MDD with psychotic features, melancholic depression, atypical depression, and depression with postpartum onset. Dysthymic disorder, a frequently more chronic MDD-spectrum disorder, albeit with a lower symptom burden, is also clinically recognized. Finally, there is a growing awareness of "anxious depression" as an MDD variant, but as yet there is no consistent or formalized definition for this clinical construct.[14]

The need for such varied specifiers and nosological exclusions highlights the extraordinary clinical heterogeneity of depression—a heterogeneity that also represents one of the great stumbling blocks in epidemiological and genetic studies of MDD. Most research efforts have focused on nonpsychotic depression. Meanwhile, subtypes, such as melancholic and atypical depression, though generally not excluded from MDD studies, have received less individual attention than the construct of MDD as a whole.

Melancholic depression seems to represent a more severe variant of MDD as patients' loss of pleasure more closely approaches absolute anhedonia and neurovegetative symptoms take on greater intensity. A twin study of melancholic depression concluded that melancholic and nonmelancholic depression demonstrated quantitative (eg, higher concordance rates of MDD in melancholic cotwins compared with nonmelancholic cotwins) but not qualitative differences, suggesting shared rather than disparate etiological mechanisms.[15]

Atypical depression is characterized by hypersomnia, hyperphagia, and mood reactivity (eg, brightening in response to positive events). Atypical criteria also include "leaden paralysis" in the limbs and long-standing patterns of "interpersonal rejection sensitivity," symptoms that are inherently more difficult to standardize or objectively measure. Despite the possible presence of mood reactivity, it is not necessarily the case that atypical depression represents a "milder" form of MDD: atypical depression shows greater chronicity, has higher comorbidity with anxiety disorders and Cluster B and C personalities, displays an earlier age of onset, and has a greater propensity to include females.[16]

Postpartum depression, or depression occurring in the first 4 weeks after childbirth, is a specialized case of major depression, and may lie on a continuum with postpartum blues (a non-DSM-defined syndrome whereby full criteria for a major depressive episode are not met) as well as with antepartum depression. There are suggestions of a familial component to both perinatal and postpartum depression (stronger for post-partum depression) in an analysis of the GenRED sample,[17] but with the limited number of perinatal depression cases in that study, it was not possible to determine if this was due to genetic factors distinct from those responsible for major depression in women more generally. The GenRED sample was also not specifically collected for the purpose of examining questions about perinatal depression, and the investigators rightly point out that recall bias and cohort effects cannot be ruled out. As we were unable to locate any major genetic studies of postpartum depression, this topic is not further discussed in this review. Postpartum psychosis, believed to be more closely associated with bipolar disorder than MDD,[18] is also not discussed here.

Dysthymic disorder, or the presence of 2 years of depressive symptoms that are subthreshold for an episode, has received comparatively less attention than has MDD. By DSM-IV criteria, dysthymic disorder is not mutually exclusive with MDD if a major depressive episode occurs after the first 2 years of dysthymia or remits 2 months before the onset of dysthymia. These idiosyncratic timing requirements, however, complicate the ability of research groups to collect accurate data and prop-erly classify research participants whose recall of the chronology of past episodes may be imprecise.

The issue of anxious depression raises questions about whether it is more useful to use syndromal or subsyndromal criteria for anxiety and depression, and whether these clinical components have common etiological mechanisms or if it is more appropriate to treat them as separate entities.[14] DSM-IV preliminarily outlines a set of research criteria for "mixed anxiety-depressive disorder" (MADD), which effectively hybridizes symptom checklists for MDD and generalized anxiety disorder (GAD).[4] There are con-flicting reports about the prevalence of MADD, its longitudinal stability, and therefore its diagnostic validity,[19,20] and further revision to clinical criteria for anxious depression will likely be necessary. There does seem to be a difference in treatment outcomes, however; Fava and colleagues[21] found that 53% of the MDD cases in the Sequenced Treatment Alternatives to Relieve Depression (STAR*D) study were anxious-depressed, and that remission was less likely and took longer to be achieved in this subset. Of note, Fava and colleagues did not use DSM-IV-defined research criteria for MADD, but instead defined a cut-off for anxious depression using the anxiety-so-matization factor of the Hamilton Rating Scale for Depression. Whether these poorer outcomes stem from quantitative or qualitative differences between anxious and non-anxious depression is not yet known. At present, there are few published genetic studies on shared genetic risk factors between anxiety and depression. A recent review[22] finds that whereas the evidence for common genetic etiologies is mixed in family studies, that from twin studies is more consistently supportive. Factor analyses demonstrate a particularly strong correlation between MDD and GAD, and suggest this may be mediated by shared personality traits that may represent more optimal phenotypes for identifying relevant genes. One such personality trait, neuroticism, is discussed further later in this article.

ENDOPHENOTYPES

An endophenotype is a trait that is intermediate between genotype and disease, not necessarily beholden to the diagnostic criteria for a single illness, but a construct whose purpose is to help simplify one's understanding of otherwise complex or heterogeneous disorders. As outlined by Gottesman and Gould,[23] an endophenotype can be "[neuro]-physiologic[al], biochemical, endocrinological, [neuro]anatomic, cognitive, or [neuro]psychological." They further propose that an endophenotype should: (1) be "associated with illness in a population"; (2) be heritable; (3) manifest, when inherited, regardless of the presence/absence of the full syndromic condition; (4) cosegregate with illness in families; and (5) be found in affected and unaffected family members or probands "at higher rate[s] than in the general population."

Perhaps one of the best studied endophenotypes related to MDD is neuroticism, a construct first introduced by Eysenck to describe a high-order personality factor associated with "dysphoria, anxiety, tension, and emotional reactivity."[24] Approximately 55% of MDD's genetic risk may be shared with neuroticism,[25] and, indeed, several of the linkage studies summarized in this article used neuroticism as the study phenotype. Hasler and colleagues[26] raise some concerns about insufficient reduction of complexity substituting MDD with neuroticism, and, in an elegant outline of alternative MDD endophenotypes, mention other possibilities such as tryptophan depletion, the dexamethasone suppression test, and neuroimaging—though these run into limitations of their own (typically related to ease of high-throughput administration and cost). Many of these alternatives, unfortunately, also have not yet received sufficient epidemiological examination and validation.

LINKAGE STUDIES

Linkage studies are genetic analyses of pedigrees and are well-suited for studying disorders with a clear pattern of Mendelian inheritance and disorders driven by genes of large effect. Although neither of these conditions is likely to operate in depression, the discovery and definition of a rare familial variant would still accelerate the development of greater insight into etiological mechanisms. There have been few reports of notable pedigrees segregating an identifiably high-penetrance syndrome involving depression,[27,28] and even then, these have typically demonstrated additional psychiatric disorders other than MDD in members of the same family. A comprehensive summary of MDD linkage studies was recently published[24] and will not be repeated here. Summarized in this previous review were 4 linkage studies of 3 MDD samples that used a range of phenotypes from MDD to MDD-REO, with/without anxiety disorders, and including/excluding cases of bipolar I and bipolar II as affected family members. Supportive findings include regions on chromosomes 1, 3, 4, 6, 8, 11, 12, 15, and 18. It has generally been difficult to replicate linkage findings at a level comparable to that reported in any region's initial respective positive report, and power analyses suggest that much larger samples (on the order of approximately 1000 affected sibling pairs) would be necessary to reliably detect a locus with a risk odds ratio (OR) of 1.25.[24]

Since Levinson's review, there have been 3 additional published linkage studies of MDD. These studies include 2 reports from the GenRED group[29,30] and a third article by Middeldorp and colleagues.[31] Holmans and colleagues[30] present the final genome-wide linkage scan report for GenRED, a collection of 656 families, each with at least 2 MDD-REO cases. Included in this group were 1494 informative affected relative pairs and 894 independent affected sibling pairs. The same group had earlier published their first wave of samples (ie, 297 families) and preliminarily identified a region on chromosome 15q25-26 as genome-wide significant.[10] This same region again emerged as their most significant linkage peak, though with a reduced logarithm of odds (LOD) score of 2.06 (down from the original score of 3.73). Holmans and colleagues were unable to identify a clinical feature that distinguished their first and second waves of family samples, and, therefore, to explain why their second wave did not further bolster their linkage signal at 15q. The proposed (and most likely) scenario is that upward bias in the first half of their sample overestimated the magnitude of linkage. In a companion article, a follow-up fine-mapping effort focused on 88 single nucleotide polymorphisms (SNPs) in a 22.5 megabase (Mb) window (from 77.6 to 100.1 Mb) centered on the 15q linkage peak.[29] Of note, only families of European ancestry (631 of the original 656 families) were retained for this second analysis because there were insufficient numbers in the non-European families for a meaningful linkage study. A maximum LOD score of 4.78 (exact P value of 1.4×10^{-6}) was detected at 92.6 Mb, and, somewhat reassuringly, there was nominal significance even for the second wave of the GenRED sample (P<.04). These investigators then tested 781 SNPs in a subset of their pedigrees involving 1195 individuals in 300 families across a 9 Mb segment of the linkage region. The investigators noted nominally significant family-based association results near NTRK3, a gene encoding a receptor for neurotrophin 3. Based on a prevailing hypothesis linking depression and neuronal growth factors, the investigators resequenced the coding regions of NTRK3 in 176 cases and 176 controls to examine association for novel DNA variants. Although they did not discover any plausible functional variants at appreciable allele frequencies (eg, 2 predicted nonsynonymous SNPs were each seen in single individuals), they found several common variants showing continuing support for association to MDD (including rs4887379, one-tailed $P = .008$, allelic OR 1.61, 95% confidence interval 1.11–2.32).[32] None of these SNP results were considered significant after correcting for multiple tests, but the study does generate interest in NTRK3 as a potential MDD risk locus.

Middeldorp and colleagues[31] examined 110 Australian and 23 Dutch MDD pedigrees (1943 subjects genotyped) with at least 2 affected siblings. Both samples were drawn from twin registries, but the Australian group was preselected for either highly discordant or highly concordant normalized scores for neuroticism and the Dutch group was screened with a factor score reflecting genetic predisposition to "anxious depression." Neither of these traits served as proxies for MDD, however, as blinded interviewers subsequently conducted a telephone-administered Composite International Diagnostic Interview (CIDI) to screen for MDD. Individuals with a history of hypomanic episodes or bipolar disorder were excluded. The ensuing linkage scan identified a maximum LOD score of 2.11 on chromosome 17 (52.6 cM), an interval that includes SLC6A4, the serotonin transporter. Of note, however, their follow-up analysis did not identify the promoter length polymorphism in SLC6A4 to be associated with MDD or any related proxy phenotype, strongly suggesting that another SLC6A4 polymorphism or a polymorphism in a different gene within this linkage region drove their signal. Middeldorp and colleagues[31] suggested that their most promising finding was on chromosome 8 (2.7 cM), where they obtained a smaller LOD score of 1.87, but which had also been implicated in 2 previous linkage studies of personality traits—one, at a significant level, examining harm avoidance (another potential endophenotype)[33] and a second, at a suggestive level, examining neuroticism.[34]

Although linkage efforts in the study of MDD have yet to yield confirmed gene candidates, the studies performed to date represent an important effort that may yet have further use in correlating data from other types of genetic studies (such as those detailed here). A summary of MDD linkage results is provided in **Table 1**.

CANDIDATE GENE STUDIES

An alternative to linkage studies is the association study, in which the frequencies of specific polymorphic alleles are measured for enrichment in one group versus another.

Table 1
Summary of published MDD linkage results

Chr	Region (cM)[a]	LOD	Phenotype	Analysis Model	Sample Size	Authors
1	43–70	2.2	Neuroticism	Nonparametric	297 sib-pairs	Nash et al[35]
1	126	4.0[b]	Neuroticism	Nonparametric	561 sib-pairs	Fullerton et al[34]
2	237	~2	MDD-R	Nonparametric	81 families	Zubenko et al[36]
3	105	3.8	MDD-REO or anxiety	Parametric, dominant	611 individuals, 112 pedigrees	Camp et al[37]
4	176	3.8[b]	Neuroticism	Nonparametric	561 sib-pairs	Fullerton et al[34]
5	108	~2	MDD-REO	Nonparametric	81 families	Zubenko et al[36]
5	130	~2	MDD-R	Nonparametric	81 families	Zubenko et al[36]
6	34–63	2.7	Neuroticism	Nonparametric	297 sib-pairs	Nash et al[35]
7	0.1	2.9	MDD-REO or anxiety	Parametric, dominant	718 individuals, 78 pedigrees	Camp et al[37]
7	42	3.9[b]	Neuroticism	Nonparametric	561 sib-pairs	Fullerton et al[34]
8	8	2.9[b]	Neuroticism	Nonparametric	561 sib-pairs	Fullerton et al[34]
8	17	3.2	Harm avoidance	Nonparametric	758 sib-pairs	Cloninger et al[33]
11	2	4.2	MDD-R	Nonparametric	81 families	Zubenko et al[36]
11	85	2.5	MDD-REO	Nonparametric	81 families	Zubenko et al[36]
11	99	3.7[b]	Neuroticism	Nonparametric	561 sib-pairs	Fullerton et al[34]
12	105	4.7[b]	Neuroticism	Nonparametric	561 sib-pairs	Fullerton et al[34]
13	64	3.8[b]	Neuroticism	Nonparametric	561 sib-pairs	Fullerton et al[34]
15	36	2.0	MDD-R	Nonparametric	81 families	Zubenko et al[36]
15	105	2.1	MDD-REO	Nonparametric	1494 affected relative pairs	Holmans et al[30]
18	73	3.8	MDD-REO and anxiety	Parametric, dominant	96 individuals, 21 pedigrees	Camp et al[37]

Several of the studies shown here included secondary analyses that used covariates, sex-specific linkage, or alternative phenotypic definitions. For simplicity, only the primary analysis results of these studies are shown.

Camp et al used an a priori pedigree-splitting algorithm to address potential intrafamilial heterogeneity in large, multigenerational pedigrees; this accounts for the varied sample sizes at different loci.

Abbreviations: MDD-R, recurrent MDD; MDD-REO, recurrent, early-onset MDD.

[a] Centimorgan (cM) map distances given in Marshfield units.

[b] Denotes −logP instead of LOD score.

Abkevich et al is not tabulated because Camp et al used the same Utah pedigree resource. (*Data from* Abkevich V, Camp NJ, Hensel CH, et al. Predisposition locus for major depression at chromosome 12q22-12q23.2. Am J Hum Genet 2003;73(6):1271–81.)

Typically a group of unrelated individuals comprising the case group is compared at one or many loci with a group of similarly unrelated individuals comprising the control group, although family-based designs are also available. A gene traditionally was chosen for its location within a linkage peak. At present, the choice of candidate loci typically constitutes part of an investigator's best guess or hypothesis about etiological mechanisms, and is informed by biological plausibility based on the limited knowledge gleaned from sources such as animal models, disease-correlated changes in clinical indices, or existing treatments for a disorder. There have been hundreds of candidate gene studies of MDD (most frequently examining candidates related to monoamine signaling, neurotrophins, neuroendocrinology, or immunology/inflammation), and it would be beyond the scope of this review to completely catalog each of these efforts. Instead, the focus here is on several recently published meta-analyses of candidate gene studies.

Lopez-Leon and colleagues[38] recently published the most comprehensive of these meta-analyses and, after surveying 183 articles covering 393 polymorphisms in 102 genes, found that only 22 polymorphisms (5.6%) were examined in at least 3 independent primary studies. The strongest evidence for association (meta-analysis $P \leq .001$) was found for a polymorphism in *APOE* (apolipoprotein E), with lower levels of significance ($P \leq .01$) for variants in *GNB3* (guanine nucleotide-binding protein, beta 3), *MTHFR* (methylene tetrahydrafolate reductase), and *SLC6A4* (serotonin transporter).

In the case of *APOE*, there were a total of 827 cases and 1616 controls (over 7 studies), and a pooled per-allele OR of 0.51, suggesting decreased risk of MDD with the ε2 allele v. the ε3 allele. *APOE*, one may recall, is also the locus that was found to be a major susceptibility factor for late-onset Alzheimer disease (AD) when an individual carries 1 or 2 copies of a third allele, ε4.[39] A more recent study investigated the *APOE*-MDD question stratifying by AD (because cognitive status is a potential confounder), and found that, although MDD was overrepresented in ε4 carriers ($P<.001$), this association did not survive stratification in either the AD(+) or AD(−) groups. The dataset here was underpowered to examine the ε2 allele but, importantly, did not demonstrate a trend toward an effect on MDD by ε2.[40]

The short/long (s/l) polymorphism in the promoter region of *SLC6A4* has been the subject of the most studies to date (n = 24), for a total count of 3752 cases and 5707 controls in the Lopez-Leon and colleagues meta-analysis. The s-allele demonstrated a per-allele OR of 1.11 over the l-allele, suggesting a modest increase in risk for MDD with the s-allele.

For *MTHFR*, Lopez-Leon and colleagues examined the C677T (rs1801133) polymorphism in a pool of 875 cases and 3859 controls, and obtained a pooled per-allele OR of 1.20 (ie, greater risk with the minor allele, T). A subsequent meta-analysis by Gaysina and colleagues[41] (1443 cases and 1123 controls), however, found no statistically significant association with MDD.

Of note, Lopez-Leon and colleagues did not find a robust association with the often-studied Val66Met (rs6265) polymorphism in *BDNF* (brain-derived neurotrophic factor). A more recent meta-analysis of *BDNF* and MDD employing 3879 cases also obtained a negative result at rs6265.[42]

TPH1 encodes tryptophan hydroxylase-1, which is the rate-limiting enzyme in serotonin (5HT) synthesis. The most extensively studied *TPH1* polymorphism, A218C (rs1800532), was recently examined in a meta-analysis by Chen and colleagues.[43] Across 8 MDD samples (1812 cases and 2223 controls), no association was found for any rs1800532 genotype and MDD. Of note, within the same article, a separate meta-analysis across a different set of study samples did find an association with bipolar disorder. Several years ago, a group studying *TPH2* (a separate tryptophan hydroxylase locus with greater central nervous system expression) identified what appeared to be a variant overrepresented in MDD cases.[44] This locus, G1463A (rs7305115), initially generated a great deal of enthusiasm because it was found to functionally reduce 5HT synthesis by up to 80%. At least 3 groups subsequently communicated, however, that the A allele could not be detected in either cases or controls in multiple additional large samples.[45–47]

While candidate gene studies of MDD have allowed investigators to test favored hypotheses about the neurobiological origins of the disorder, they have yielded few solidly replicated findings. Indeed, those candidate genes best supported in meta-analysis have often been those with the least obvious mechanistic connection to depression, such as *APOE*, *GNB3*, and *MTHFR*. Moreover, the available replicated genes confer very small amounts of risk, suggesting that many as-yet unidentified loci may contribute to predisposition to MDD.

GENOME-WIDE ASSOCIATION STUDIES

Linkage studies, as previously discussed, are best suited for detecting genetic variants (including rare variants) of strong effect and with a clear pattern of Mendelian transmission. Association studies, in contrast, are better suited to detecting multiple variants of modest effect, and perform best when the variants being studied are relatively common in the general population. When association studies are focused on particular candidate genes, they are constrained by the limits of investigator imagination and the body of previously accumulated evidence (which may not be sizeable). With the advent of multicenter genomics initiatives such as the International HapMap Project[48] and of improved genotyping technologies for higher throughput analysis, a new type of association study, the genome-wide association study (GWAS), exploded onto the scene. GWAS, presaged in an exposition by Risch and Merikangas,[49] typically interrogate hundreds of thousands to upwards of 1 million biallelic SNPs located throughout the genome. GWAS represent an advance in human genetics because they are more comprehensive and less biased than candidate studies. Because of the unprecedented amount of hypothesis testing (and the resultant inflation of type I error), the standard in the field has been to set "genome-wide significance" at $P \le 5.0 \times 10^{-8}$ (or 0.05 divided by 1 million, the predicted number of independent common DNA variants in the human genome). This calibration raises interesting theoretical questions about how to evaluate single candidate gene association articles achieving P values on the order of 10^{-2} or 10^{-3} even if the history of a sample or a given locus does not include the execution of a GWAS.

GWAS have already advanced the understanding of mechanisms underlying general medical illnesses such as diabetes, Crohn disease, and rheumatoid arthritis, as exemplified by a seminal article published by the Wellcome Trust.[50] For MDD, there are now 4 published GWAS.

The first of these, by Sullivan and colleagues,[51] was facilitated by the Genetic Association Information Network (GAIN) and used a semi-community-based sample of 1738 cases and 1802 controls from the Netherlands. The study examined 435,291 SNPs and found their top signal to be at rs1558477 (trend-test P value of 1×10^{-6}), 12.4 kb downstream of *ADCYAP1R1*, or adenylate cyclase-activating polypeptide 1 (pituitary) receptor type I. The investigators focused their subsequent efforts, however, on a set of 11 clustered association signals (within their top 200 findings) localized to the region of *PCLO* (or Piccolo), a presynpatic protein also known as Aczonin. The investigators pursued this finding with an expanded collection of close to 12,000 independent subjects, but were unable to replicate their *PCLO* findings. A retrospective analysis suggested that the *PCLO*-MDD association may only be optimally detected in population-based (as opposed to clinically obtained) case samples such as the original GAIN MDD sample and only one of their replication samples. Although this hypothesis has not yet been tested, *PCLO* remains an intriguing candidate. Beyond a possible role in facilitating dopamine transporter internalization,[52] PCLO seems to more generally negatively regulate synaptic vesicle exocytosis by decreasing transport of vesicles from reserve pools to readily-releasable pools through an action on synapsin.[53] *PCLO* is also expressed outside the CNS at such diverse locations as the neuromuscular junction[54] and in pancreatic beta cells (where it helps regulate insulin release),[55] though these are less likely to have relevance to MDD.

The second published GWAS of MDD, by Muglia and colleagues,[56] used a German clinic-based sample of 1022 recurrent depression (MDD-R) cases and 1000 controls, and interrogated 494,678 SNPs. As in the Sullivan and colleagues study, there were no genome-wide significant findings. Muglia and colleagues performed a meta-analysis combining the first sample with a second population-based sample of Swiss origin (494 cases and 1052 controls), and found their best signal at rs4238010 ($P = 5.8 \times 10^{-6}$), 260 kb from the closest gene (*CCND2*, or cyclin D2). A gene-based analysis obtained results generally similar to those of their original SNP-based analysis. These investigators then performed a more focused examination of SNPs in the vicinity of several previously published MDD and bipolar disorder candidate loci, where they found that their most significant association lay in *GRM7* (metabotropic glutamate receptor 7) at rs162209, though this is not in linkage disequilibrium with rs1485171, the SNP previously identified by the Wellcome Trust as moderately associated with bipolar disorder at a P value of 9.7×10^{-5}.

Additional GWAS of MDD, one derived from GenRED[57] and another from STAR*D,[58] have followed. For simplification, the authors focus on the results of a meta-analysis by Shyn and colleagues,[58] which combined results from GenRED, STAR*D, and the GAIN MDD study. The GenRED GWAS consisted of 1020 MDD-REO cases whereas the STAR*D GWAS consisted of 1221 MDD cases. Both were sampled from North American individuals of European ancestry and both shared a common set of 1636 controls. By including subjects contributed from the publicly available GAIN MDD GWAS, there were a total of 3956 cases and 3428 controls in this 3-sample meta-analysis. Using imputation (a method that takes known correlations between individual markers to probabilistically "fill-in" genotypes missing in one, 2, or all 3 studies), a total of 2,339,408 autosomal and 51,795 x chromosome SNPs were analyzed. The model was a broadly inclusive one, and treated as cases all patients with DSM-IV-defined MDD. Additional exploratory analyses, however, were also examined and included a "narrow" analysis (MDD-REO only) and sex-specific analyses. There were no genome-wide significant findings in either the primary analysis or any of the secondary analyses. Intronic markers from 3 genes, however, achieved meta-analysis P values of better than 10^{-6}: *ATP6V1B2*, *GRM7*, and *SP4*. *ATP6V1B2* encodes a vacuolar protein pump ATPase subunit, and has a potentially related finding in bipolar disorder: Sklar and colleagues[59] obtained a P value of approximately 10^{-5} in an SNP in *ATP6V1G1*, a gene that contributes a distinct subunit to the same molecular complex. In addition, it remains possible that the implicated *ATP6V1B2* SNP in the MDD GWAS meta-analysis may affect the adjacent gene *VMAT1* (or vesicular monoamine transporter 1). *GRM7*, which was additionally highlighted in Muglia and colleagues (and also mentioned briefly in Sullivan and colleagues), is perhaps the most promising finding because there is a significant body of literature linking GRM7 to the mechanistic action of mood stabilizers and antidepressants.[60–62] As a cell surface receptor, GRM7 would represent a highly tractable target for novel therapeutic agents, should subsequent studies continue to suggest a prominent role for this receptor in mood regulation. Finally, *SP4* encodes a brain-specific zinc-finger transcription factor. Most notable for *SP4*, so far, are studies demonstrating an association between bipolar disorder and *SP4*[63] and an Sp4-binding site in *GRK3* (G-protein receptor kinase 3),[64] as well as a series of murine studies demonstrating that mice with *SP4* deleted have deficits in hippocampal granule cell density in the dentate gyrus[65] and in hippocampal integrity (with resultant phenotypes in contextual memory).[66] Adult neurogenesis of hippocampal granule cells has been linked to depression and to antidepressant action,[67] and so the locus of these *SP4* mutant phenotypes is intriguing. **Table 2** gives a summary of published MDD GWAS to date.

Although the results of each individual GWAS and the 3-study GAIN/GenRED/STAR*D meta-analysis did not reach the desired level of statistical significance, these studies do support interesting candidate genes and genomic regions for further study. In addition, pooled analysis of multiple GWAS samples has yielded findings for other complex traits that were not apparent in any single GWAS.[13,68,69] With this in mind, a meta-analysis of MDD using over 12,000 cases and nearly 10,000 controls is underway.[70]

ENVIRONMENT

One possible explanation for poor replication of psychiatric genetic findings is insufficient consideration of gene-environment (or "G × E") interactions. An elegant demonstration of a possible G × E effect was reported by Caspi and colleagues[71] in an examination of the s/l polymorphism in *SLC6A4* (abbreviated 5HTTLPR) in 847 prospectively studied Caucasians from age 3 to 26 years. Alone, genotypic data for this locus had little predictive value for whether an individual developed adult MDD, but, using multiple regression methodology, Caspi and colleagues found that the number of stressful life events was significantly correlated with probability of developing MDD when 1 or 2 copies of the "s" allele were present (at a significance level of approximately $P \sim 10^{-2}$–10^{-3}). These findings were also robust to an examination of sequence of events (ie, stressful life events predating adult diagnosis with MDD).

Subsequent research employing similar approaches to the study of MDD or dimensional measures of depressive or anxious symptomatology in adults ± a history of childhood abuse and *CRHR1* (corticotropin-releasing hormone receptor 1) SNPs[72]—and in healthy adults ± early life stress and the *BDNF* SNP, rs6265.[73] "G × E" interaction studies are still relatively few in number, however, and this is likely due, in part, to difficulties inherent in standardizing or quantifying disparate life experiences as well as the challenges posed by extra instances of multiple-hypothesis testing. Finally, a recent systematic review and meta-analysis suggests that the original Caspi and colleagues[71] finding, when extended to the subsequent "5HTTLPR and stressful life events" literature, has only equivocal support at best.[74] A similar meta-analysis of this literature, comprising more than 14,000 individuals, with 1769 having MDD, showed that serotonin transporter genotype was not associated with depression, or depression when measured in interaction with stressful life events.[75]

FUTURE DIRECTIONS

Despite its unmatched impact on public health among psychiatric disorders, MDD has received only comparatively recent attention in human genetic studies because of its lower heritability, likely propensity for phenocopies, and significant clinical heterogeneity. This review summarizes possible approaches to deconstructing this

Table 2
Summary of published MDD GWAS results

GWAS	Authors	Sample	Cases	Controls	Platform	Markers	Top Findings
GAIN	Sullivan et al	Semi-community-based	1738	1820	Perlegen	435,291	PCLO
GSK	Muglia et al	Mix of clinic- & community-based	[a]1516	[a]2052	Illumina 550 (first sample), Affymetrix 5.0 (second sample)	[b]494,678	CCND2; [c]GRM7
GAIN, GenRED, STAR*D meta-analysis	Shyn et al	—	[d]3956	[d]3428	—	2,391,203	ATP6V1B2, GRM7, & SP4
GenRED-MGS[e]	Shi et al	Clinical	1020	1636	Affymetrix 6.0	662,206	[f]BC053410
STAR*D-MGS[e]	Shyn et al	Clinical	1221	1636	Affymetrix 500K, Affymetrix 5.0, Affymetrix 6.0	260,474	Intergenic regions in 19q12, 2q23.3

None of the studies achieved genome-wide significant findings (ie, P value $\leq 5 \times 10^{-8}$).

Abbreviations: GAIN, Genetic Association Information Network; GenRED, Genetics of Recurrent Early-onset Depression; GSK, GlaxoSmithKline; GWAS, genome-wide association study; STAR*D, Sequenced Treatment Alternatives to Relieve Depression.

[a] The Muglia et al study was a 2-stage study; case and control tallies represent the sum across their 2 samples.

[b] This figure represents the total number of markers analyzed across both platforms, after quality control and imputation.

[c] This was the top finding among a panel of mood disorder-related candidate genes suggested by previous literature.

[d] These figures are the sum totals for cases and controls across the 3 MDD GWAS studies; of note, because Sullivan et al was not yet published at the time of this meta-analysis, the exact numbers of cases and controls retained for analysis from GAIN diverged modestly.

[e] MGS refers to the Molecular Genetics of Schizophrenia control sample. A portion of these controls were retained (after screening-out MDD) for the GenRED and STAR*D MDD GWAS.

[f] Putative mRNA identified from pooled brain samples; no annotated gene.

heterogeneity and identifying subpopulations within MDD cohorts who are likely to have enriched heritability. In addition, key highlights from linkage analysis, candidate and genome-wide association studies, the use of endophenotypes, and "G × E" interaction analyses are discussed, which are beginning to move the understanding of the biology of MDD from beyond the shadow of the monoamine hypothesis of depression. In the near future, efforts will likely be extended to larger collaborations and pooled analyses, to integration of disease genetics with results generated from pharmacogenomics and, also, to the use of newer approaches such as analysis of copy-number variations and other types of genomic rearrangements. As the cost of large-scale sequencing continues to come down, next-generation sequencing approaches will undoubtedly also grow in importance and allow investigators access to rarer sequence variants, perhaps allowing for a more complete accounting of "missing heritability." These technologies may additionally allow efficient identification of epigenetic variation, such as cytosine methylation and histone modification, which could impact MDD risk. Finally, growing sophistication not only with "G × E" interaction analyses, but "G × G" (or gene × gene) interaction studies, must necessarily complement these future steps.

REFERENCES

1. Kessler RC, Berglund P, Demler O, et al. Lifetime prevalence and age-of-onset distributions of DSM-IV disorders in the National Comorbidity Survey Replication. Arch Gen Psychiatry 2005;62(6):593–602.
2. Weissman MM, Bland R, Joyce PR, et al. Sex differences in rates of depression: cross-national perspectives. J Affect Disord 1993;29(2–3):77–84.
3. World Health Organization. The global burden of disease: a comprehensive assessment of mortality and disability from diseases, injuries, and risk factors in 1990 and projected to 2020; summary. Published by the Harvard School of Public Health on behalf of the World Health Organization and the World Bank. Cambridge (MA): Harvard University Press; 1996. p. 43.
4. American Psychiatric Association. Diagnostic and statistical manual of mental disorders: DSM-IV-TR. 4th edition. Washington, DC: American Psychiatric Association; 2000.
5. Schildkraut JJ, Kety SS. Biogenic amines and emotion. Science 1967;156(771): 21–37.
6. Deverteuil RL, Lehmann HE. Therapeutic trial of iproniazid (marsilid) in depressed and apathetic patients. Can Med Assoc J 1958;78(2):131–3.
7. Kuhn R. The treatment of depressive states with G 22355 (imipramine hydrochloride). Am J Psychiatry 1958;115(5):459–64.
8. Stahl SM. Blue genes and the monoamine hypothesis of depression. J Clin Psychiatry 2000;61(2):77–8.
9. Sullivan PF, Neale MC, Kendler KS. Genetic epidemiology of major depression: review and meta-analysis. Am J Psychiatry 2000;157(10):1552–62.
10. Holmans P, Zubenko GS, Crowe RR, et al. Genomewide significant linkage to recurrent, early-onset major depressive disorder on chromosome 15q. Am J Hum Genet 2004;74(6):1154–67.
11. Levinson DF, Zubenko GS, Crowe RR, et al. Genetics of recurrent early-onset depression (GenRED): design and preliminary clinical characteristics of a repository sample for genetic linkage studies. Am J Med Genet B Neuropsychiatr Genet 2003;119B(1):118–30.

12. Krishnan V, Nestler EJ. The molecular neurobiology of depression. Nature 2008; 455(7215):894–902.
13. Zeggini E, Scott LJ, Saxena R, et al. Meta-analysis of genome-wide association data and large-scale replication identifies additional susceptibility loci for type 2 diabetes. Nat Genet 2008;40(5):638–45.
14. McGrath PJ, Miller JM. Anxious depression: concepts, significance, and treatment implications. In: Simpson HB, Neria Y, Lewis-Fernandez R, et al, editors. Understanding anxiety; in press.
15. Kendler KS. The diagnostic validity of melancholic major depression in a population-based sample of female twins. Arch Gen Psychiatry 1997;54(4):299–304.
16. Thase ME. Recognition and diagnosis of atypical depression. J Clin Psychiatry 2007;68(Suppl 8):11–6.
17. Murphy-Eberenz K, Zandi PP, March D, et al. Is perinatal depression familial? J Affect Disord 2006;90(1):49–55.
18. Jones I, Hamshere M, Nangle JM, et al. Bipolar affective puerperal psychosis: genome-wide significant evidence for linkage to chromosome 16. Am J Psychiatry 2007;164(7):1099–104.
19. Zinbarg RE, Barlow DH, Liebowitz M, et al. The DSM-IV field trial for mixed anxiety-depression. Am J Psychiatry 1994;151(8):1153–62.
20. Weisberg RB, Maki KM, Culpepper L, et al. Is anyone really M.A.D.?: the occurrence and course of mixed anxiety-depressive disorder in a sample of primary care patients. J Nerv Ment Dis 2005;193(4):223–30.
21. Fava M, Rush AJ, Alpert JE, et al. Difference in treatment outcome in outpatients with anxious versus nonanxious depression: a STAR*D report. Am J Psychiatry 2008;165(3):342–51.
22. Hettema JM. What is the genetic relationship between anxiety and depression? Am J Med Genet C Semin Med Genet 2008;148C(2):140–6.
23. Gottesman II, Gould TD. The endophenotype concept in psychiatry: etymology and strategic intentions. Am J Psychiatry 2003;160(4):636–45.
24. Levinson DF. The genetics of depression: a review. Biol Psychiatry 2006;60(2): 84–92.
25. Kendler KS, Neale MC, Kessler RC, et al. A longitudinal twin study of personality and major depression in women. Arch Gen Psychiatry 1993;50(11):853–62.
26. Hasler G, Drevets WC, Manji HK, et al. Discovering endophenotypes for major depression. Neuropsychopharmacology 2004;29(10):1765–81.
27. Mercuro G, Carpiniello B, Ruscazio M, et al. Association between psychiatric disorders and Marfan's syndrome in a large Sardinian family with a high prevalence of cardiac abnormalities. Clin Cardiol 1997;20(3):243–5.
28. St Clair D, Blackwood D, Muir W, et al. Association within a family of a balanced autosomal translocation with major mental illness. Lancet 1990; 336(8706):13–6.
29. Levinson DF, Evgrafov OV, Knowles JA, et al. Genetics of recurrent early-onset major depression (GenRED): significant linkage on chromosome 15q25-q26 after fine mapping with single nucleotide polymorphism markers. Am J Psychiatry 2007;164(2):259–64.
30. Holmans P, Weissman MM, Zubenko GS, et al. Genetics of recurrent early-onset major depression (GenRED): final genome scan report. Am J Psychiatry 2007; 164(2):248–58.
31. Middeldorp CM, Sullivan PF, Wray NR, et al. Suggestive linkage on chromosome 2, 8, and 17 for lifetime major depression. Am J Med Genet B Neuropsychiatr Genet 2009;150B(3):352–8.

32. Verma R, Holmans P, Knowles JA, et al. Linkage disequilibrium mapping of a chromosome 15q25-26 major depression linkage region and sequencing of NTRK3. Biol Psychiatry 2008;63(12):1185–9.

33. Cloninger CR, Van Eerdewegh P, Goate A, et al. Anxiety proneness linked to epistatic loci in genome scan of human personality traits. Am J Med Genet 1998;81(4):313–7.

34. Fullerton J, Cubin M, Tiwari H, et al. Linkage analysis of extremely discordant and concordant sibling pairs identifies quantitative-trait loci that influence variation in the human personality trait neuroticism. Am J Hum Genet 2003;72(4):879–90.

35. Nash MW, Huezo-Diaz P, Williamson RJ, et al. Genome-wide linkage analysis of a composite index of neuroticism and mood-related scales in extreme selected sibships. Hum Mol Genet 2004;13(19):2173–82.

36. Zubenko GS, Maher B, Hughes HB 3rd, et al. Genome-wide linkage survey for genetic loci that influence the development of depressive disorders in families with recurrent, early-onset, major depression. Am J Med Genet B Neuropsychiatr Genet 2003;123B(1):1–18.

37. Camp NJ, Lowry MR, Richards RL, et al. Genome-wide linkage analyses of extended Utah pedigrees identifies loci that influence recurrent, early-onset major depression and anxiety disorders. Am J Med Genet B Neuropsychiatr Genet 2005;135B(1):85–93.

38. Lopez-Leon S, Janssens AC, Gonzalez-Zuloeta Ladd AM, et al. Meta-analyses of genetic studies on major depressive disorder. Mol Psychiatry 2008;13(8): 772–85.

39. Corder EH, Saunders AM, Strittmatter WJ, et al. Gene dose of apolipoprotein E type 4 allele and the risk of Alzheimer's disease in late onset families. Science 1993;261(5123):921–3.

40. Slifer MA, Martin ER, Gilbert JR, et al. Resolving the relationship between Apolipoprotein E and depression. Neurosci Lett 2009;455(2):116–9.

41. Gaysina D, Cohen S, Craddock N, et al. No association with the 5,10-methylene-tetrahydrofolate reductase gene and major depressive disorder: results of the depression case control (DeCC) study and a meta-analysis. Am J Med Genet B Neuropsychiatr Genet 2008;147B(6):699–706.

42. Chen L, Lawlor DA, Lewis SJ, et al. Genetic association study of BDNF in depression: finding from two cohort studies and a meta-analysis. Am J Med Genet B Neuropsychiatr Genet 2008;147B(6):814–21.

43. Chen C, Glatt SJ, Tsuang MT. The tryptophan hydroxylase gene influences risk for bipolar disorder but not major depressive disorder: results of meta-analyses. Bipolar Disord 2008;10(7):816–21.

44. Zhang X, Gainetdinov RR, Beaulieu JM, et al. Loss-of-function mutation in tryptophan hydroxylase-2 identified in unipolar major depression. Neuron 2005;45(1): 11–6.

45. Glatt CE, Carlson E, Taylor TR, et al. Response to Zhang et al. (2005): loss-of-function mutation in tryptophan hydroxylase-2 identified in unipolar major depression. Neuron 45, 11–16. Neuron 2005;48(5):704–5 [author reply: 705–6].

46. Van Den Bogaert A, De Zutter S, Heyrman L, et al. Response to Zhang, et al (2005): loss-of-function mutation in tryptophan hydroxylase-2 identified in unipolar major depression. Neuron 45, 11–16. Neuron 2005;48(5):704 [author reply: 705–6].

47. Zhou Z, Peters EJ, Hamilton SP, et al. Response to Zhang, et al. (2005): loss-of-function mutation in tryptophan hydroxylase-2 identified in unipolar major depression. Neuron 45, 11–16. Neuron 2005;48(5):702–3 [author reply: 705–6].

48. International HapMap Consortium. The International HapMap Project. Nature 2003;426(6968):789–96.
49. Risch N, Merikangas K. The future of genetic studies of complex human diseases. Science 1996;273(5281):1516–7.
50. Wellcome Trust Case Control Consortium. Genome-wide association study of 14,000 cases of seven common diseases and 3,000 shared controls. Nature 2007;447(7145):661–78.
51. Sullivan PF, de Geus EJ, Willemsen G, et al. Genome-wide association for major depressive disorder: a possible role for the presynaptic protein piccolo. Mol Psychiatry 2009;14(4):359–75.
52. Cen X, Nitta A, Ibi D, et al. Identification of Piccolo as a regulator of behavioral plasticity and dopamine transporter internalization. Mol Psychiatry 2008;13(4): 349, 451–63.
53. Leal-Ortiz S, Waites CL, Terry-Lorenzo R, et al. Piccolo modulation of Synapsin1a dynamics regulates synaptic vesicle exocytosis. J Cell Biol 2008;181(5):831–46.
54. Tokoro T, Higa S, Deguchi-Tawarada M, et al. Localization of the active zone proteins CAST, ELKS, and Piccolo at neuromuscular junctions. Neuroreport 2007;18(4):313–6.
55. Shibasaki T, Sunaga Y, Fujimoto K, et al. Interaction of ATP sensor, cAMP sensor, Ca2+ sensor, and voltage-dependent Ca2+ channel in insulin granule exocytosis. J Biol Chem 2004;279(9):7956–61.
56. Muglia P, Tozzi F, Galwey NW, et al. Genome-wide association study of recurrent major depressive disorder in two European case-control cohorts. Mol Psychiatry 2008 [Epub ahead of print].
57. Shi J, Potash JB, Knowles JA, et al. Genomewide association study of recurrent early-onset major depressive disorder. Mol Psychiatry, in press.
58. Shyn SI, Shi J, Potash JB, et al. Novel loci for major depression identified by genome-wide association study of STAR*D and meta-analysis of three studies. Mol Psychiatry 2009 [Epub ahead of print].
59. Sklar P, Smoller JW, Fan J, et al. Whole-genome association study of bipolar disorder. Mol Psychiatry 2008;13(6):558–69.
60. Zhou R, Yuan P, Wang Y, et al. Evidence for selective microRNAs and their effectors as common long-term targets for the actions of mood stabilizers. Neuropsychopharmacology 2009;34(6):1395–405.
61. Palucha A, Klak K, Branski P, et al. Activation of the mGlu7 receptor elicits antidepressant-like effects in mice. Psychopharmacology (Berl) 2007;194(4):555–62.
62. Wieronska JM, Klak K, Palucha A, et al. Citalopram influences mGlu7, but not mGlu4 receptors' expression in the rat brain hippocampus and cortex. Brain Res 2007;1184:88–95.
63. Zhou X, Tang W, Greenwood TA, et al. Transcription factor SP4 is a susceptibility gene for bipolar disorder. PLoS One 2009;4(4):e5196.
64. Zhou X, Barrett TB, Kelsoe JR. Promoter variant in the GRK3 gene associated with bipolar disorder alters gene expression. Biol Psychiatry 2008;64(2):104–10.
65. Zhou X, Qyang Y, Kelsoe JR, et al. Impaired postnatal development of hippocampal dentate gyrus in Sp4 null mutant mice. Genes Brain Behav 2007;6(3):269–76.
66. Zhou X, Long JM, Geyer MA, et al. Reduced expression of the Sp4 gene in mice causes deficits in sensorimotor gating and memory associated with hippocampal vacuolization. Mol Psychiatry 2005;10(4):393–406.
67. Jacobs BL, Praag H, Gage FH. Adult brain neurogenesis and psychiatry: a novel theory of depression. Mol Psychiatry 2000;5(3):262–9.

68. Barrett JC, Hansoul S, Nicolae DL, et al. Genome-wide association defines more than 30 distinct susceptibility loci for Crohn's disease. Nat Genet 2008;40(8): 955–62.

69. Ferreira MA, O'Donovan MC, Meng YA, et al. Collaborative genome-wide association analysis supports a role for ANK3 and CACNA1C in bipolar disorder. Nat Genet 2008;40(9):1056–8.

70. Psychiatric GWAS Consortium Coordinating Committee, Cichon S, Craddock N, et al. Genomewide association studies: history, rationale, and prospects for psychiatric disorders. Am J Psychiatry 2009;166(5):540–56.

71. Caspi A, Sugden K, Moffitt TE, et al. Influence of life stress on depression: moderation by a polymorphism in the 5-HTT gene. Science 2003;301(5631):386–9.

72. Bradley RG, Binder EB, Epstein MP, et al. Influence of child abuse on adult depression: moderation by the corticotropin-releasing hormone receptor gene. Arch Gen Psychiatry 2008;65(2):190–200.

73. Gatt JM, Nemeroff CB, Dobson-Stone C, et al. Interactions between BDNF Val66-Met polymorphism and early life stress predict brain and arousal pathways to syndromal depression and anxiety. Mol Psychiatry 2009;14(7):681–95.

74. Munafo MR, Durrant C, Lewis G, et al. Gene × environment interactions at the serotonin transporter locus. Biol Psychiatry 2009;65(3):211–9.

75. Risch N, Herrell R, Lehner T, et al. Interaction between the serotonin transporter gene (5-HTTLPR), stressful life events, and risk of depression: a meta-analysis. JAMA 2009;301(23):2462–71.

Genetics of Obsessive-Compulsive Disorder

Gerald Nestadt, MD, MPH*, Marco Grados, MD, MSc,
Jack F. Samuels, PhD

KEYWORDS

• Obsessive-compulsive disorder • Genetics • Psychiatry

Obsessive-compulsive disorder (OCD) is a psychiatric condition first described 100 years ago.[1] The pathognomic features of the disorder are persistent, intrusive, senseless thoughts and impulses (obsessions) and repetitive, intentional behaviors (compulsions). Patients with the disorder recognize that their thoughts and behaviors are excessive and unreasonable, and they struggle to resist them. The lifetime prevalence of OCD is estimated to be 1% to 3%, based on population-based surveys conducted in many communities nationally and internationally.[2,3] Although the disorder affects individuals of all ages, the period of greatest risk is from childhood to early adulthood.[4,5] Patients experience a chronic or episodic course with exacerbations that can substantially impair social, occupational, and academic functioning; according to the World Health Organization, OCD is among the 10 most disabling medical conditions worldwide.[6] Moreover, the burden placed on, and stresses experienced by, family members are considerable.[7] Medications and behavioral therapy can partially control symptoms, but the course is chronic or relapsing in most cases, and cure is rare.

There is compelling evidence for a biological basis of OCD. First, obsessions and compulsions are common in several medical conditions, including Huntington chorea; encephalitis lethargica (von Economo encephalitis); Parkinson disease; Tourette syndrome; schizophrenia; Sydenham chorea; certain epilepsies; and insults to specific brain regions caused by trauma, ischemia, and tumors.[8] Second, serotonin reuptake inhibitors (clomipramine) and selective serotonin reuptake inhibitors (eg, fluoxetine, fluvoxamine, and sertraline) have demonstrated efficacy in controlling obsessions and compulsions.[9,10] Third, functional imaging studies have revealed increased metabolic activity in specific brain regions of patients with OCD, at rest and when challenged with stimuli that provoke obsessions and compulsions.[11]

Supported by National Institutes of Health grants R01-MH-50214, R01-MH-071507, and NCRR/OPD-GERCRR00052.

Department of Psychiatry and Behavioral Sciences, Johns Hopkins School of Medicine, Johns Hopkins Hospital, Meyer 113, 600 North Wolfe Street, Baltimore, MD 21287, USA

* Corresponding author.

E-mail address: gnestadt@jhmi.edu (G. Nestadt).

Psychiatr Clin N Am 33 (2010) 141–158
doi:10.1016/j.psc.2009.11.001
0193-953X/10/$ – see front matter © 2010 Elsevier Inc. All rights reserved.

Evidence implicating cortico-striatal-thalamic-cortico (CSTC) pathways in the manifestation of the disorder is accumulating,[12,13] and the neurocircuitry models of OCD are the most developed of any neuropsychiatric disorder. There has been a considerable body of neuroimaging,[14] and to a lesser extent cognitive neuroscience research in this area.[15] Although a primary pathological process underlying core OCD symptoms has not yet been definitively identified, functional imaging studies have established that metabolism or perfusion in CSTC circuits is affected. Further, MRI and MR spectroscopy studies in OCD also suggest striatal pathology. Influential theories suggest that these patterns of activity arise from failed striatothalamic inhibition.[13] Genes affecting development, connectivity, and neurotransmission and signal transduction in CSTC circuits are natural foci of interest.

Neuropharmacological hypotheses of OCD pathophysiology have been greatly influenced by strong evidence that serotonergic systems modulate OCD symptomatology. Interestingly, both the serotonin transporter and the serotonin receptor subtypes implicated in OCD are at their highest levels in the brain in the ventral striatum[16] where they could influence the functioning of the CSTC circuits. In theory, other neurotransmitter systems within CSTC circuits, individually or by their interactions, may play a role in susceptibility, course, or response to OCD treatment. For example, dopaminergic mechanisms have been implicated by controlled studies demonstrating that neuroleptics are beneficial when added to ongoing serotonin reuptake inhibitor treatment.[17,18] Other CSTC neurotransmitter systems that are candidates for involvement in OCD on the basis of their anatomical localization or functional roles in CSTC circuits include glutamate, γ-aminobutyric acid, substance P, cholinergic, and endogenous opioid systems.[13,19,20]

The discovery of the genetic etiology of OCD is the best hope at present of unraveling the pathophysiology of this condition. There is compelling evidence that the disorder has a genetic basis. In contrast, other than the reported relationship of streptococcal infection in a subset of OCD[21] cases, there are no current environmental hypotheses with strong empirical support. The discovery of genes is crucial for elucidation of pathogenic mechanisms and for developing rational treatments.

GENETIC EPIDEMIOLOGY

Since the early years of the twentieth century, clinicians have suspected that heredity plays an important role in the development of OCD. One of the first reports in the English literature was based on 50 cases of "obsessional neurosis" treated at the Maudsley Hospital in London. A total of 37% of parents and 21% of siblings of cases were diagnosed with this disorder.[22] The findings from the Hopkins OCD Family Study are remarkably similar.[23] There have been over 15 family studies of OCD, and most support the familial transmission of OCD.[24–32] Black and colleagues[33] found that the age-corrected morbid risk of "broadly defined OCD" (ie, OCD plus subsyndromal obsessive-compulsive symptoms) was substantially greater in the parents of OCD probands as compared with those of controls (16% vs 3%). Pauls and colleagues[34] found that the morbid risk of OCD was significantly greater in first-degree relatives of OCD subjects as compared with relatives of psychiatrically normal controls (10% vs 1.9%); they found similar results for the morbid risks of OCD plus subthreshold OCD (18% vs 4%). The Hopkins OCD Family Study[23] found that the prevalence of OCD in the first-degree relatives of case probands was 11.7%, compared with 2.7% in the relatives of controls; the prevalence of OCD in the siblings of early onset probands was 17.9% (λsib = 7.8), within the range of other psychiatric disorders, such as bipolar disorder and panic disorder.

Family studies report prevalence rates of 7% to 15% in first-degree relatives of child and adolescent probands with OCD.[28,29,31,35] These findings are consistent with reports of an increased familial loading in probands with early age at onset (AAO). Pauls and colleagues[34] reported a significantly higher morbid risk of OCD in the relatives of probands with an onset age less than 19 years. In the Hopkins OCD Family Study, there were no secondary cases of OCD in the families of probands with an AAO greater than 17 years: the prevalence of OCD in all relatives of probands with an onset before 18 was 13.8%, compared with 0% in probands with older AAO ($P = .006$). Hanna[36] reported a risk ratio (λsib = 8.7) in a family study of early onset OCD probands, similar to the authors' finding (λsib = 7.8) in that subgroup. Finally, results from a recent study of families ascertained through children and adolescents with OCD are consistent with these findings; the estimated odd ratios for OCD in first-degree relatives was 32.5 (95% confidence interval, 4.5–230.8).[37] Early AAO differentiates a strongly inherited subtype in other conditions[35,38] and has been fruitfully used in the subclassification of disorders, such as schizophrenia,[39] breast cancer,[40,41] and Alzheimer's disease.[42]

Since Lewis'[22] first report in 1936, there have been several reports of monozygotic twins concordant for obsessive-compulsive symptoms.[43–46] One series reported a concordance of 80% in monozygotic twin pairs, as compared with 50% in dizygotic pairs.[47] Carey and Gottesman[48] reported concordance rates in monozygotic and dizygotic twin pairs of 87% and 47%, respectively, giving a heritability estimate of 80%. Overall, in the twin studies published to date, 54 (68%) of 80 monozygotic twin pairs were reported as concordant, as compared with 9 (31%) of 29 dizygotic twin pairs. In larger studies, in which diagnoses were questionnaire-derived, moderate heritabilities were found.[49–51] There have been no adoption studies in OCD.

Published segregation analyses of OCD implicate a gene of major effect in the etiology of OCD. Nicolini and colleagues[52] concluded that their family data are most consistent with a highly penetrant dominant major gene. In a more recent study, based on a much larger sample, the data best fit a dominant model of transmission.[53] Alsobrook and colleagues[54] reported statistical evidence for transmission consistent with genetic models; no specific model fit the data better than any other. When they analyzed a subset of 52 families in which at least two individuals were affected with OCD, however, they found that models of no inheritance, polygenic inheritance, and single locus inheritance could all be statistically rejected and that the most parsimonious explanation for the inheritance patterns in these families was a mixed model of inheritance. Segregation analyses of the Hopkins OCD Family Study data strongly rejected sporadic and environmental models, whereas mendelian dominant and codominant models could not be rejected.[55]

CANDIDATE GENE STUDIES

Candidate genes for association studies have been selected based on knowledge of the pathophysiology and pharmacology of the condition. The serotonergic system has been a primary focus. The 5-HTTLPR serotonin transporter,[56–62] 5HT1-D beta serotonin receptor gene,[63,64] 5HT2A serotonin receptor,[65–67] and the serotonin 5HT2C receptor[68] have all been investigated with several positive studies. Ozaki and colleagues[69] have recently shown, in two independent families, that a novel, uncommon gain-of-function missense variant in the serotonin transporter coding region (SLC6A4-Ile425Val) was associated with OCD plus comorbid disorders (anorexia nervosa, Asperger syndrome and autism). This finding is intriguing because the probands and their siblings who had the coding region variant and the more highly transcribed allele of the serotonin transporter promoter polymorphism had OCD of unusual severity and treatment resistance, suggesting a possible "double-hit" effect of two variants that increase transporter function.[69] This finding has been supported in two more recent studies of OCD families.[70,71] This particular variant, however, may play a role in only a small number of affected families. Hu and colleagues[72] have observed the overtransmission of the L(a) allele to individuals with OCD. These findings have not been consistently replicated, however, and recent family-based and case-control association studies have not found associations with serotonin transporter, trypophan hydroxylase, or serotonin *1B*, *2A*, or *1D-beta* receptor polymorphisms.[63,66,73]

An association between OCD and a repeat in the dopamine receptor type 4 (*DRD4*) gene has been found by some,[74,75] whereas others have reported suggestive evidence (not quite statistically significant). Associations have not been found between OCD and the dopamine *D2* receptor,[61,76,77] except in individuals with OCD and tics.[78] Associations were not found for the DRD3 dopamine receptor[76,77] or the dopamine transporter.[61,63]

Karayiorgou and colleagues[79] reported that OCD is associated with a low-activity allele of an enzyme involved in the degradation of dopamine, catechol-O-methyltrans-ferase (*COMT*), particularly in male probands. Niehaus and colleagues[80] found that the heterozygous genotype was more frequent in OCD patients, but these results have not been confirmed.[81–83] In contrast to Karyiorgou and colleagues[79] Alsobrook and colleagues[84] found an association between *COMT* and OCD in females but not males. Similarly, OCD was found to be associated with monoamine oxidase A (*MAO-A*) in male subjects in one study[85] but female subjects in another.[58] Recently, there have been reported associations between OCD and the *BDNF* locus,[86] glutamate (*NMDA*) subunit receptor gene,[87] γ-aminobutyric acid type B receptor 1 (*GABBR1*) gene has been observed to be overtransmitted at the A-7265G polymorphism,[88] *OLIG2*[89] and myelin oligodendrocyte glycoprotein (*MOG*) gene.[69,90]

The limited state of knowledge about pathophysiological pathways and networks of interacting genes in OCD, and conflicting results from association studies, makes it premature to restrict the focus to associations of OCD with specific candidate genes.

A productive research approach has been to identify and study animal models rele-vant to OCD. Welch and colleagues[91] showed that mice with a genetic deletion of *Sa-pap3* (a postsynaptic scaffolding protein at excitatory synapses) exhibited compulsive grooming behavior leading to facial hair loss and skin lesions. These behaviors were alleviated by a selective serotonin reuptake inhibitor. Electrophysiological, structural, and biochemical studies of *Sapap3*-mutant mice revealed defects in cortico-striatal synapses. Sequencing exons and exon-intron junctions of the *SAPAP3* gene in 165 OCD and trichotillomania samples revealed six nonsynonymous changes.[92] Further-more, Bienvenu and colleagues[93] showed evidence for association for a single nucle-otide polymorphism (SNP) in the *Sapap3* gene in a sample of "grooming disordered" patients with OCD.

LINKAGE STUDIES

There have been only three genome-wide linkage studies of OCD. In 56 relatives in seven families ascertained through pediatric probands, Hanna[36] found suggestive linkage to a region near the telomere of chromosome 9 (9p24;LOD 1.97). The Johns Hopkins University group replicated this finding in 50 families, finding linkage peaks within 0.5 cM (<350 kb) of the original 9p24 linkage signal.[94] Subsequently, five inde-pendent groups have replicated evidence for association within *SLC1A1*,

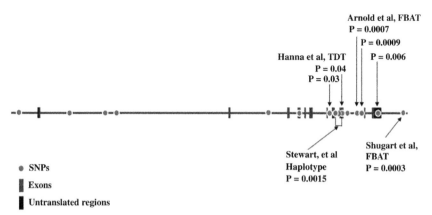

Fig. 1. Results of association studies of *SLC1A1* in OCD. FBAT, family based association test; SNP, single nucleotide polymorphism; TDT, transmission disequilibrium test.

a glutamatergic transporter gene in that region (**Fig. 1**).[95–99] In a sequencing experiment of this gene, Wang and colleagues[100] identified one nonsynonymous coding SNP in a single family (c.490A>G, T164A).

The largest linkage scan for OCD was conducted by the OCD Collaborative Genetics Study group ([OCGS] including Johns Hopkins, UCLA, Columbia, Brown, and Harvard Universities, and the National Institute of Mental Health). Genotyping for the OCGS was performed at the Center for Inherited Disease Research using 386 microsatellite markers spaced at an average of 9 cM across the genome. For the whole genome scan, 1008 subjects in 219 families were genotyped. The analysis was conducted using a nonparametric linkage method[101,102] implemented in the analysis program Merlin. Both Kong and Cox LODall and Kong and Cox LODpairs statistics were computed, and empirical *P* values for all "significant signals" were computed with Merlin using 10,000 replicates. The genome-scan results for multiple point analysis are presented in **Fig. 2**. The locations of the chromosomal regions are shown on the X axis, and the statistical significance of the linkage signals (in units of −log of the *P* values) is shown on the Y axis.

The multipoint nonparametric analyses showed suggestive linkage regions on chromosomes 1 (*P* = .003) and 3 (*P* = .0002). The highest Kong and Cox LOD score of 2.67 (asymptotic *P* value of .0002) was obtained at marker D3S2398. Also computed was an empirical *P* value for a marker situated at this location using the same allele frequencies and 10,000 replicates. The chance of observing a Kong and Cox LOD score of 2.67 was 4 in 10,000, making it unlikely that this is a chance finding.

More recently, Hanna and colleagues[103] conducted a genome-wide linkage scan in 121 individuals from 26 families ascertained through probands with early onset OCD. They found suggestive evidence for linkage on chromosome 10p15. They also found association with three SNPs in a gene in this linkage region, *ADAR3*.

USING OCD SUBTYPES

The limited success identifying genetic determinants for OCD may be related to the etiological heterogeneity of OCD. Multiple approaches have been proposed to delineate more etiologically homogeneous groups within the broader definition of the disorder. Addressed next are some of the possible subtypes that may usefully be used to identify genetic etiologies.

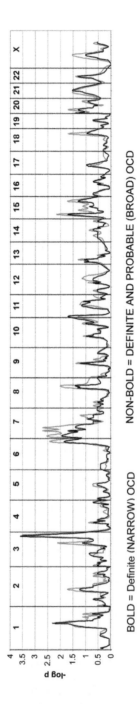

Fig. 2. Linkage results from the OCD Collaborative Genetics Study. Bold, definite (narrow) OCD; nonbold, definite and probable (broad) OCD.

AAO has proved useful in the clinical categorization of patients with respect to their genetic risk. Results from the Hopkins OCD Family Study and the Childhood OCD Family Study suggest an inverse relationship between AAO of OCD in probands and the risk of OCD in relatives. This is consistent with findings from other family studies.[34,36] The authors found a significant inverse relationship between the proband's AAO and the prevalence of OCD in their first-degree relatives (odds per year = 0.92 [0.85–0.99]; P = .02). Interestingly, this relationship was found for relatives of female, but not male, probands.

In addition to the increased familial risk, early onset OCD has been distinguished from later-onset OCD based on the nature of the OCD symptoms,[104] patterns of co-morbidity,[105,106] course and treatment response,[107] and regional cerebral blood flow in frontal-subcortical circuits.[108] Unfortunately, no twin study has compared AAO concordance patterns. To date, there is no clinical or other type of variable with stronger support in OCD.

Family studies found that AAO of OCD before 18 years indicates a substantially more familial subgroup.[23,33,34] Using familiality as the outcome measure, the Hopkins group found evidence that an AAO earlier than 18 years was more useful than the standard phenotype.[23,33,34] In the linkage study described previously, AAO was used as a covariate in covariate-based linkage analysis. The LOD score was 2.94 at D1S1679 (empirical P = .001). After stratifying the sample by AAO it was determined that it was younger AAO that increased the linkage estimate.[109]

Given previous work of differential penetrance by gender (segregation analysis), the authors stratified the sample based on proband gender (78 male proband families, 141 female proband families), with a subsequent substantial increase in the linkage signal at 11p15.[110] After genotyping additional microsatellite markers, at approximately a 1- to 2-cM density, from 2.8 to 15 cM, the stratified analyses showed a LOD = 5.66 (P<.00001) in the male group. This first stage fine-mapping reduced the 1-LOD support interval from 25.9 to 4 Mb. This region contains plausible candidate genes, such as dopamine D4 receptor (*DRD4*), tyrosine hydroxylase (*TH*), neuronal nicotinic, alpha polypeptide 10 (*CHRNA10*), and the cholecystokinin B receptor (*CCKBR*).

In addition to AAO and gender, several clinical features potentially may be useful for categorizing OCD into homogeneous phenotypes for etiologic investigation. Clinical characteristics that may distinguish a familial subtype of OCD include tic disorders,[34,111,112] affective and anxiety disorders,[33,113,114] obsessive-compulsive personality disorder,[115] and specific obsessive-compulsive symptom classes.[116–119]

In a large sample of multiply affected families, the authors identified three OCD classes: (1) OCD simplex, (2) comorbid OCD tic-related, and (3) comorbid OCD affective-related. These classes suggest that the co-occurrence of other psychiatric disorders (eg, tics, anxiety, and affective disorders) with OCD may be indicative of different phenotypic subgroups.[120] It is possible that one or more of these OCD subtypes represents a more homogenous genetic group yielding greater ability to detect genetic variation relevant to the disorder. The tic-related group points to the widely investigated relationship between Tourette syndrome and OCD. There is compelling evidence that OCD is a familially related phenotype in families with Tourette syndrome.[121] It has not been established, however, whether those individuals with OCD in Tourette syndrome families share, or do not share, a genetic etiology with other cases of OCD.

Several groups have reported that OCD subjects with hoarding behaviors are clinically distinct from other individuals with OCD.[122–125] The Hopkins OCD Family Study also found that relatives of hoarding OCD probands had a higher prevalence of hoarding behaviors.[126]

In addition to subtyping by individual clinical features, it may be fruitful to subtype based on symptom clusters. Consistent with several prior studies,[127] the authors' research group found four or five OCD symptom dimensions using different statistical approaches on data collected with the YBOCS symptom checklist. In 221 OCD-affected individuals examined during the Johns Hopkins University OCD Family Study, Cullen and colleagues[128] using dichotomous factor analysis of 16 YBOCS symptom categories found four symptom factors: (1) aggressive-sexual-religious obsessions, (2) contamination-cleaning, (3) symmetry-order, and (4) hoarding. These dimensions were differentially associated with onset of symptoms, treatment responsiveness, and comorbid diagnoses, and magnitude of sib-sib correlation.[128] Similar dimensions were evident using principal components factor analysis of YBOCS symptom checklist categories in 418 OCD-affected individuals (251 affected sibling pairs) ascertained during the OCD Collaborative Genetics Study. These factors had significant sib-sib correlations, with the hoarding dimension being the most familial.[129] More recently, using exploratory dichotomous factor analysis on individual YBOCS symptom checklist items in 485 adults ascertained in the OCGS, the authors found similar dimensions (and a taboo factor) and strong sib-sib correlations, especially for the hoarding factor.[130] This structure has been replicated in children and adolescents.[131]

It has been reported that OCD subjects with hoarding behaviors were clinically different from other OCD subjects, and that hoarding was more frequent in their first-degree relatives.[126] When families were stratified based on the presence of two or more relatives with compulsive hoarding (74 hoarding families, 145 nonhoarding families), suggestive linkage for the stratum with hoarding was found (LOD = 2.99; $P = .0001$).[132] The 1-LOD support region at 14q31-32 is 10.9 Mb. This region contains the positional candidate genes potassium channel, voltage-gated, subfamily H, member 5 (KCNH5), subfamily K, member 10 (KCNK10), estrogen receptor 2 (ESR2), neurexin 3 (NRXN3), and others. These analyses were repeated using OCD hoarding as the phenotypic outcome (ie, only subjects with OCD hoarding, regardless of the presence of any other OCD symptoms, were the affected phenotype). This reduced the number of informative families to 60 but still there was a signal (LOD = 1.6; $P = .003$), albeit the peak was marginally proximal to the one using the stratified sample. The linkage signal on the X chromosome, when stratified for compulsive hoarding, was strengthened considerably (LOD = 2.81; $P = .0002$) suggesting that these two chromosomal regions are likely to harbor susceptibility genes for compulsive hoarding.

INTERMEDIATE PHENOTYPES

Another phenotypic approach to OCD genetics is through the use of intermediate phenotypes. Recently, measures of specific cognitive domains have been found to be associated with OCD; moreover, several studies have shown the familial nature of the measures in OCD such that unaffected relatives of probands with OCD also have abnormalities on these measures.[133–135] Cognitive measures investigated in OCD have addressed both the clinical characteristics of the phenomena (obsessions and compulsions) and the brain regions implicated in OCD. This is illustrated by the executive task "set shifting," which is intended to measure the apparent inability of the OCD patient to stop repetitive behaviors. Tests of this process (eg, the Wisconsin Card Sort) have been found to be impaired in OCD patients and their unaffected first-degree relatives.[136] Other tasks involve impaired decision making, also considered a hallmark of OCD. The Iowa Gambling Task aims to simulate real-life decision making and is known to be sensitive to frontal lobe dysfunction. OCD patients are impaired in completing this task; however, there are some negative findings.[137–139] Response inhibition deficits have been reported in OCD patients when performing the Stop Signal Reaction Time, which measures the time taken to internally suppress prepotent motor responses.[140] Unaffected first-degree relatives of OCD patients are also impaired on this task compared with unrelated healthy controls, suggesting that response inhibition may be an endophenotype for OCD. Menzies and colleagues[135] showed that two anatomical brain systems, a parieto-cingulo-striatal system (increased gray matter) and a predominantly fronto-temporal system including OFC and inferior frontal gyri (decreased gray matter), were associated with impairment on the Stop Signal Reaction Time in both OCD patients and their unaffected first-degree relatives compared with healthy controls. Recently, Chamberlain and colleagues[134] found that a reversal learning paradigm, the facilitation of behavioral flexibility after negative feedback, distinguished both OCD patients and their unaffected relatives from controls and was associated with abnormally reduced activation of several cortical regions, including the lateral orbitofrontal cortex, suggesting another potential OCD endophenotype.

It seems plausible that, like other neuropsychiatric conditions, OCD is an etiologically heterogeneous condition, and that in addition to genetic causes (involving one or more major genes and several genes of smaller effect) there are environmental causes (eg, trauma and infection) and gene-by-environmental interaction that are all involved in the emergence of the disorder.

FUTURE DIRECTIONS

With advances in analytic and molecular genetic technology today, investigators are faced with several options to identify the genetic causes of diseases. The field has been enormously successful identifying genes responsible for mendelian disorders; however, complex genetic conditions have been less tractable to study. Linkage studies remain the design of choice for rare, highly penetrant conditions with genes of major effect. For disorders accounted for by genes of modest effect, linkage studies have been less rewarding. The sample size required for detecting genes of small effect by linkage is prohibitively large. In contrast, association studies are promising for detecting genetic variants of modest effect.[122] Genome-wide association studies are now feasible and, as Carlson and colleagues[141] state, "the technical, informatic, and statistical foundations have been laid for whole genome analyses." Indeed, there are several recent examples of the success of the genome-wide association approach. For example, although Hirschsprung disease is a well-studied condition with eight identified mutations, a genome-wide association study identified a chromosomal region not previously known to be related to the disorder, and epistasis between two known genes was detected and confirmed in an animal model.[142] More recently, investigators compared 96 cases with age-related macular degeneration with 50 control subjects at 116,204 SNPs[143] and found a highly significant association with the CFH gene, which was located within a region of previously reported linkage to age-related macular degeneration. Two Whole Genome Association studies for OCD are in progress, and it is hoped that findings from these studies will inform the understanding of the etiology of OCD.

There are limitations to the association approach. A negative linkage-disequilibrium result in a particular genomic region does not exclude a significant gene effect in that region. It may be that the SNPs used through the region are too widely spaced to detect the extent of linkage-disequilibrium in the region. In a genome-wide random SNP approach, even at high density, disease-causing genes might be missed.[144]

Moreover, although linkage-disequilibrium is useful in identifying common variants affecting disease susceptibility, if there are many rare susceptibility variants at a disease locus, linkage-disequilibrium is unlikely to be useful to identify the locus.[145]

OCD is a complex genetic disorder with unknown genetic and environmental bases. There are likely common genetic influences of modest effect (possibly in addition to other less common genetic factors), and many of these genetic determinants have probably not been detected using traditional linkage methodologies. Moreover, the biological basis of OCD is largely unknown, preventing a more focused genetic search in particular metabolic pathways. The authors recognize the merits of gene-based association studies,[146] but this is premature in OCD. There are biological hypotheses regarding the pathophysiology of OCD, and a few studies have found associations with candidate genes; however, these studies have had limited power, results have not been replicated, and the available evidence does not support a sustainable biological hypothesis. Awaited are the results of genome-wide association studies using dense genome-wide SNP panels to identify SNPs and ultimately genes associated with OCD in biologically plausible pathways. The optimal approach in determining genetic variants relevant to OCD requires a variety of strategies, some of which are in progress and others of which have yet to be applied to this condition. These strategies involve improved understanding of the phenotype from both clinical and cognitive perspectives, approaching investigations from an epigenetic perspective, searching for copy number variations in the genome, and using deep genetic sequencing techniques.

The identification of genetic and environmental causes of OCD should ultimately be of substantial benefit to those who suffer from this debilitating condition. The expectation is that rational treatments will become available and preventive measures will be possible.

REFERENCES

1. Janet P. Les obsessions and psychasthenie. Paris: Bailliere; 1903.
2. Karno M, Golding JM. Obsessive compulsive disorder. In: Robins LN, Regier DA, editors. Psychiatric disorders in America. New York: Free Press; 1991. p. 204–19.
3. Weissman MM, Bland RC, Canino GJ, et al. The cross national epidemiology of obsessive compulsive disorder. The Cross National Collaborative Group. J Clin Psychiatry 1994;55(Suppl):5–10.
4. Nestadt G, Samuels JF, Romanoski AJ, et al. Obsessions and compulsions in the community. Acta Psychiatr Scand 1994;89:219–24.
5. Nestadt G, Bienvenu OJ, Cai G, et al. Incidence of obsessive-compulsive disorder in adults. J Nerv Ment Dis 1998;186:401–6.
6. Murray CL, Lopez AD. The global burden of disease. Cambridge: Harvard University Press; 1996.
7. Steketee G. Disability and family burden in obsessive-compulsive disorder. Can J Philos 1997;42:919–28.
8. Stein DJ. Advances in the neurobiology of obsessive-compulsive disorder: implications for conceptualizing putative obsessive-compulsive and spectrum disorders. Psychiatr Clin North Am 2000;23:545–62.
9. Clomipramine Collaborative Study Group. Clomipramine in the treatment of patients with obsessive-compulsive disorder. The Clomipramine Collaborative Study Group. Arch Gen Psychiatry 1991;48:730–8.

10. Goodman WK, Price LH, Rasmussen SA, et al. Efficacy of fluvoxamine in obsessive-compulsive disorder: a double-blind comparison with placebo. Arch Gen Psychiatry 1989;46:36–44.
11. Hoehn-Saric RGB. Psychobiology of obsessive-compulsive disorder: anatomical and physiological considerations. Int Rev Psychiatry 1997;9:15–29.
12. Rauch SL, Savage CR, Alpert NM, et al. Probing striatal function in obsessive-compulsive disorder: a PET study of implicit sequence learning. J Neuropsychiatry Clin Neurosci 1997;9:568–73.
13. Saxena S, Rauch SL. Functional neuroimaging and the neuroanatomy of obsessive-compulsive disorder. Psychiatr Clin North Am 2000;23:563–86.
14. Saxena S, Brody AL, Schwartz JM, et al. Neuroimaging and frontal-subcortical circuitry in obsessive-compulsive disorder. Br J Psychol Suppl 1998;35:26–37.
15. Rauch SL. Neuroimaging and neurocircuitry models pertaining to the neurosurgical treatment of psychiatric disorders. Neurosurg Clin N Am 2003;14(2):213–23.
16. Hoyer D, Pazos A, Probst A, et al. Serotonin receptors in the human brain. I. Characterization and autoradiographic localization of 5-HT1A recognition sites. Apparent absence of 5-HT1B recognition sites. Brain Res 1986;376:85–96.
17. McDougle CJ, Goodman WK, Leckman JF, et al. Haloperidol addition in fluvoxamine-refractory obsessive-compulsive disorder: a double-blind, placebo-controlled study in patients with and without tics. Arch Gen Psychiatry 1994;51:302–8.
18. McDougle CJ, Epperson CN, Pelton GH, et al. A double-blind, placebo-controlled study of risperidone addition in serotonin reuptake inhibitor-refractory obsessive-compulsive disorder. Arch Gen Psychiatry 2000;57:794–801.
19. Carlsson ML. On the role of cortical glutamate in obsessive-compulsive disorder and attention-deficit hyperactivity disorder, two phenomenologically antithetical conditions. Acta Psychiatr Scand 2000;102:401–13.
20. Haber SN, McFarland NR. The concept of the ventral striatum in nonhuman primates. Ann N Y Acad Sci 1999;877:33–48.
21. Leonard HL, Swedo SE. Paediatric autoimmune neuropsychiatric disorders associated with streptococcal infection (PANDAS). Int J Neuropsychopharmacol 2001;4:191–8.
22. Lewis A. Problems of obsessional illness. Proc R Soc Med 1936;29:325–36.
23. Nestadt G, Samuels J, Riddle M, et al. A family study of obsessive-compulsive disorder. Arch Gen Psychiatry 2000;57:358–63.
24. Bellodi L, Sciuto G, Diaferia G, et al. Psychiatric disorders in the families of patients with obsessive-compulsive disorder. Psychiatry Res 1992;42:111–20.
25. Brown FW. Heredity in the psychoneuroses. Proceedings of the Royal Society of Medicine 1942;35:785–90.
26. Hoover CF, Insel TR. Families of origin in obsessive-compulsive disorder. J Nerv Ment Dis 1984;172:207–15.
27. Insel TR, Hoover C, Murphy DL. Parents of patients with obsessive-compulsive disorder. Psychol Methods 1983;13:807–11.
28. Lenane MC, Swedo SE, Leonard H, et al. Psychiatric disorders in first degree relatives of children and adolescents with obsessive compulsive disorder. J Am Acad Child Adolesc Psychiatry 1990;29:407–12.
29. Leonard HL, Lenane MC, Swedo SE, et al. Tics and Tourette's disorder: a 2- to 7-year follow-up of 54 obsessive-compulsive children. Am J Psychiatry 1992;149:1244–51.
30. Rasmussen SA, Tsuang MT. Clinical characteristics and family history in DSM-III obsessive-compulsive disorder. Am J Psychiatry 1986;143:317–22.

31. Riddle MA, Scahill L, King R, et al. Obsessive compulsive disorder in children and adolescents: phenomenology and family history. J Am Acad Child Adolesc Psychiatry 1990;29:766–72.
32. Rosenberg CM. Familial aspects of obsessional neurosis. Br J Psychol 1967; 113:405–13.
33. Black DW, Noyes R Jr, Goldstein RB, et al. A family study of obsessive-compulsive disorder. Arch Gen Psychiatry 1992;49:362–8.
34. Pauls DL, Alsobrook JP, Goodman W, et al. A family study of obsessive-compulsive disorder. Am J Psychiatry 1995;152:76–84.
35. Swedo SE, Rapoport JL, Leonard H, et al. Obsessive-compulsive disorder in children and adolescents: clinical phenomenology of 70 consecutive cases. Arch Gen Psychiatry 1989;46:335–41.
36. Hanna G. Abstract. Biological Psychiatry Conference, 2000 2004.
37. do Rosario-Campos MC, Leckman JF, Curi M, et al. A family study of early-onset obsessive-compulsive disorder. Am J Med Genet B Neuropsychiatr Genet 2005; 136B(1):92–7.
38. Childs B, Scriver CR. Age at onset and causes of disease. Perspect Biol Med 1986;29:437–60.
39. Pulver AE, Liang KY. Estimating effects of proband characteristics on familial risk: II. The association between age at onset and familial risk in the Maryland schizophrenia sample. Genet Epidemiol 1991;8:339–50.
40. Claus EB. Genetic epidemiology of breast cancer in younger women. J Natl Cancer Inst Monogr 1994;16:49–53.
41. Hall JM, Lee MK, Newman B, et al. Linkage of early-onset familial breast cancer to chromosome 17q21. Science 1990;250:1684–9.
42. Roses AD. Alzheimer diseases: a model of gene mutations and susceptibility polymorphisms for complex psychiatric diseases. Am J Med Genet 1998;81:49–57.
43. Cryan EM, Butcher GJ, Webb MG. Obsessive-compulsive disorder and paraphilia in a monozygotic twin pair. Br J Psychol 1992;161:694–8.
44. Marks IM, Crowe M, Drewe E, et al. Obsessive compulsive neurosis in identical twins. Br J Psychol 1969;115:991–8.
45. McGuffin P, Mawson D. Obsessive-compulsive neurosis: two identical twin pairs. Br J Psychol 1980;137:285–7.
46. Woodruff R, Pitts FM. Monozygotic twins with obsessional illness. Am J Psychiatry 1964;120:1075–80.
47. Inyoue E. Similar and dissimilar manifestations of obsessive-compulsive neurosis in monozygotic twins. Am J Psychiatry 1965;121:1171–5.
48. Carey G, Gottesman I. Twin and family studies of anxiety, phobic, and obsessive disorders anxiety: new research and changing concepts. In: Klein DF, Rabkin JG, editors. Anxiety: new research and changing concepts. New York: Raven Press; 1981. p. 117–36.
49. Jonnal AH, Gardner CO, Prescott CA, et al. Obsessive and compulsive symptoms in a general population sample of female twins. Am J Med Genet 2000;96:791–6.
50. Bolton D, Rijsdijk F, O'Connor TG, et al. Obsessive-compulsive disorder, tics and anxiety in 6-year-old twins. Psychol Methods 2007;37:39–48.
51. Hudziak JJ, Van Beijsterveldt CE, Althoff RR, et al. Genetic and environmental contributions to the child behavior checklist obsessive-compulsive scale: a cross-cultural twin study. Arch Gen Psychiatry 2004;61(6):608–16.
52. Nicolini H, Hanna G, Baxter L, et al. Segregation analysis of obsessive compulsive and associated disorders: preliminary results. Ursus Medicus 1991;1:25–8.

53. Cavallini MC, Pasquale L, Bellodi L, et al. Complex segregation analysis for obsessive compulsive disorder and related disorders. Am J Med Genet 1999; 88:38–43.
54. Alsobrook JP II, Leckman JF, Goodman WK, et al. Segregation analysis of obsessive-compulsive disorder using symptom-based factor scores. Am J Med Genet 1999;88:669–75.
55. Nestadt G, Lan T, Samuels J, et al. Complex segregation analysis provides compelling evidence for a major gene underlying obsessive-compulsive disorder and for heterogeneity by sex. Am J Hum Genet 2000;67:1611–6.
56. Bengel D, Greenberg BD, Cora-Locatelli G, et al. Association of the serotonin transporter promoter regulatory region polymorphism and obsessive-compulsive disorder. Mol Psychiatry 1999;4:463–6.
57. Billett EA, Richter MA, King N, et al. Obsessive compulsive disorder, response to serotonin reuptake inhibitors and the serotonin transporter gene. Mol Psychiatry 1997;2:403–6.
58. Camarena B, Rinetti G, Cruz C, et al. Additional evidence that genetic variation of MAO-A gene supports a gender subtype in obsessive-compulsive disorder. Am J Med Genet 2001;105:279–82.
59. Camarena B, Rinetti G, Cruz C, et al. Association study of the serotonin transporter gene polymorphism in obsessive-compulsive disorder. Int J Neuropsychopharmacol 2001;4:269–72.
60. Di Bella D, Erzegovesi S, Cavallini MC, et al. Obsessive-compulsive disorder, 5-HTTLPR polymorphism and treatment response. Pharmacogenomics J 2002;2:176–81.
61. Frisch A, Michaelovsky E, Rockah R, et al. Association between obsessive-compulsive disorder and polymorphisms of genes encoding components of the serotonergic and dopaminergic pathways. Eur Neurol 2000;10:205–9.
62. McDougle CJ, Epperson CN, Price LH, et al. Evidence for linkage disequilibrium between serotonin transporter protein gene (SLC6A4) and obsessive compulsive disorder. Mol Psychiatry 1998;3:270–3.
63. Hemmings SM, Kinnear CJ, Niehaus DJ, et al. Investigating the role of dopaminergic and serotonergic candidate genes in obsessive-compulsive disorder. Eur Neurol 2003;13:93–8.
64. Mundo E, Richter MA, Zai G, et al. 5HT1Dbeta Receptor gene implicated in the pathogenesis of obsessive-compulsive disorder: further evidence from a family-based association study. Mol Psychiatry 2002;7:805–9.
65. Enoch MA, Greenberg BD, Murphy DL, et al. Sexually dimorphic relationship of a 5-HT2A promoter polymorphism with obsessive-compulsive disorder. Biol Psychiatry 2001;49:385–8.
66. Walitza S, Wewetzer C, Warnke A, et al. 5-HT2A promoter polymorphism -1438G/A in children and adolescents with obsessive-compulsive disorders. Mol Psychiatry 2002;7:1054–7.
67. Meira-Lima I, Shavitt RG, Miguita K, et al. Association analysis of the catechol-o-methyltransferase (COMT), serotonin transporter (5-HTT) and serotonin 2A receptor (5HT2A) gene polymorphisms with obsessive-compulsive disorder. Genes Brain Behav 2004;3:75–9.
68. Cavallini MC, Di Bella D, Pasquale L, et al. 5HT2C CYS23/SER23 polymorphism is not associated with obsessive-compulsive disorder. Psychiatry Res 1998;77:97–104.
69. Ozaki N, Goldman D, Kaye WH, et al. Serotonin transporter missense mutation associated with a complex neuropsychiatric phenotype. Mol Psychiatry 2003;8: 933–6.

70. Delorme R, Betancur C, Wagner M, et al. Support for the association between the rare functional variant I425V of the serotonin transporter gene and susceptibility to obsessive compulsive disorder. Mol Psychiatry 2005;10:1059–61.
71. Wendland JR, DeGuzman TB, Rudnick G, et al. SERT Ileu425Val and other uncommon SERT variants in Asperger syndrome, autism and obsessive-compulsive disorder. Psychiatr Genet 2008;18(1):31–9.
72. Hu XZ, Lipsky RH, Zhu G, et al. Serotonin transporter promoter gain-of-function genotypes are linked to obsessive-compulsive disorder. Am J Hum Genet 2006; 78:815–26.
73. Chabane N, Millet B, Delorme R, et al. Lack of evidence for association between serotonin transporter gene (5-HTTLPR) and obsessive-compulsive disorder by case control and family association study in humans. Neurosci Lett 2004;363: 154–6.
74. Cruz C, Camarena B, King N, et al. Increased prevalence of the seven-repeat variant of the dopamine D4 receptor gene in patients with obsessive-compulsive disorder with tics. Neurosci Lett 1997;231:1–4.
75. Millet B, Chabane N, Delorme R, et al. Association between the dopamine receptor D4 (DRD4) gene and obsessive-compulsive disorder. Am J Med Genet 2003;116B:55–9.
76. Billett EA, Richter MA, Sam F, et al. Investigation of dopamine system genes in obsessive-compulsive disorder. Psychiatr Genet 1998;8:163–9.
77. Catalano M, Sciuto G, Di Bella D, et al. Lack of association between obsessive-compulsive disorder and the dopamine D3 receptor gene: some preliminary considerations. Am J Med Genet 1994;54:253–5.
78. Nicolini H, Cruz C, Camarena B, et al. DRD2, DRD3 and 5HT2A receptor genes polymorphisms in obsessive-compulsive disorder. Mol Psychiatry 1996;1:461–5.
79. Karayiorgou M, Altemus M, Galke BL, et al. Genotype determining low catechol-O-methyltransferase activity as a risk factor for obsessive-compulsive disorder. Proc Natl Acad Sci U S A 1997;94:4572–5.
80. Niehaus DJ, Kinnear CJ, Corfield VA, et al. Association between a catechol-o-methyltransferase polymorphism and obsessive-compulsive disorder in the Afrikaner population. J Atten Disord 2001;65:61–5.
81. Schindler KM, Richter MA, Kennedy JL, et al. Association between homozygosity at the COMT gene locus and obsessive compulsive disorder. Am J Med Genet 2000;96:721–4.
82. Azzam A, Mathews CA. Meta-analysis of the association between the catecholamine-O-methyl-transferase gene and obsessive-compulsive disorder. Am J Med Genet 2003;123B:64–9.
83. Erdal ME, Tot S, Yazici K, et al. Lack of association of catechol-O-methyltransferase gene polymorphism in obsessive-compulsive disorder. Depress Anxiety 2003;18:41–5.
84. Alsobrook JP, Zohar AH, Leboyer M, et al. Association between the COMT locus and obsessive-compulsive disorder in females but not males. Am J Med Genet 2002;114:116–20.
85. Karayiorgou M, Sobin C, Blundell ML, et al. Family-based association studies support a sexually dimorphic effect of COMT and MAOA on genetic susceptibility to obsessive-compulsive disorder. Biol Psychiatry 1999;45:1178–89.
86. Hall D, Dhilla A, Charalambous A, et al. Sequence variants of the brain-derived neurotrophic factor (BDNF) gene are strongly associated with obsessive-compulsive disorder. Am J Hum Genet 2003;73:370–6.

87. Arnold PD, Rosenberg DR, Mundo E, et al. Association of a glutamate (NMDA) subunit receptor gene (GRIN2B) with obsessive-compulsive disorder: a preliminary study. Psychopharmacology (Berl) 2004;174:530–8.

88. Zai G, Arnold P, Burroughs E, et al. Evidence for the gamma-amino-butyric acid type B receptor 1 (GABBR1) gene as a susceptibility factor in obsessive-compulsive disorder. Am J Med Genet B Neuropsychiatr Genet 2005;134B(1):25–9.

89. Stewart SE, Platko J, Fagerness J, et al. A genetic family-based association study of OLIG2 in obsessive-compulsive disorder. Arch Gen Psychiatry 2007; 64:209–14.

90. Zai G, Bezchlibnyk YB, Richter MA, et al. Myelin oligodendrocyte glycoprotein (MOG) gene is associated with obsessive-compulsive disorder. Am J Med Genet 2004;129B:64–8.

91. Welch JM, Lu J, Rodriguiz RM, et al. Cortico-striatal synaptic defects and OCD-like behaviours in Sapap3-mutant mice. Nature 2007;448:894–900.

92. Zuchner S, Wendland JR, Ashley-Koch AE, et al. Multiple rare SAPAP3 missense variants in trichotillomania and OCD. Mol Psychiatry 2009;14:6–9.

93. Bienvenu OJ, Wang Y, Shugart YY, et al. Sapap3 and pathological grooming in humans: Results from the OCD collaborative genetics study. Am J Med Genet B Neuropsychiatr Genet 2009;150B:710–20.

94. Willour VL, Yao SY, Samuels J, et al. Replication study supports evidence for linkage to 9p24 in obsessive-compulsive disorder. Am J Hum Genet 2004;75:508–13.

95. Arnold PD, Sicard T, Burroughs E, et al. Glutamate transporter gene SLC1A1 associated with obsessive-compulsive disorder. Arch Gen Psychiatry 2006;63:769–76.

96. Dickel DE, Veenstra-VanderWeele J, Cox NJ, et al. Association testing of the positional and functional candidate gene SLC1A1/EAAC1 in early-onset obsessive-compulsive disorder. Arch Gen Psychiatry 2006;63:778–85.

97. Shugart Y, Wang Y, Samuels J, et al. A family-based association study of the glutamate transporter gene SLC1A1 obsessive-compulsive disorder in 378 families. Am J Med Genet B Neuropsychiatr Genet 2009;150B(6):886–92.

98. Stewart SE, Fagerness JA, Platko J, et al. Association of the SLC1A1 glutamate transporter gene and obsessive-compulsive disorder. Am J Med Genet B Neuropsychiatr Genet 2007;144:1027–33.

99. Wendland JR, Moya PR, Timpano KR, et al. A haplotype containing quantitative trait loci for SLC1A1 gene expression and its association with obsessive-compulsive disorder. Arch Gen Psychiatry 2009;66:408–16.

100. Wang Y, Adamczyk A, Shugart Y, et al. A screen of SLC1A1 for OCD-related alleles. Am J Med Genet, 2009 [Epub ahead of print].

101. Kong A, Cox NJ. Allele-sharing models: LOD scores and accurate linkage tests. Am J Hum Genet 1997;61:1179–88.

102. Abecasis GR, Cherny SS, Cookson WO, et al. Merlin: rapid analysis of dense genetic maps using sparse gene flow trees. Nat Genet 2002;30:97–101.

103. Hanna GL, Veenstra-VanderWeele J, Cox NJ, et al. Evidence for a susceptibility locus on chromosome 10p15 in early-onset obsessive-compulsive disorder. Biol Psychiatry 2007;62:856–62.

104. Geller D, Biederman J, Jones J, et al. Is juvenile obsessive-compulsive disorder a developmental subtype of the disorder? A review of the pediatric literature. J Am Acad Child Adolesc Psychiatry 1998;37:420–7.

105. March JS, Leonard HL. Obsessive-compulsive disorder in children and adolescents: a review of the past 10 years. J Am Acad Child Adolesc Psychiatry 1996; 35:1265–73.

106. Rosario-Campos MC, Leckman JF, Mercadante MT, et al. Adults with early-onset obsessive-compulsive disorder. Am J Psychiatry 2001;158: 1899–903.
107. Skoog G, Skoog I. A 40-year follow-up of patients with obsessive-compulsive disorder [see comments]. Arch Gen Psychiatry 1999;56:121–7.
108. Busatto GF, Buchpiguel CA, Zamignani DR, et al. Regional cerebral blood flow abnormalities in early-onset obsessive-compulsive disorder: an exploratory SPECT study. J Am Acad Child Adolesc Psychiatry 2001;40:347–54.
109. Shugart YY, Samuels J, Willour VL, et al. Genomewide linkage scan for obsessive-compulsive disorder: evidence for susceptibility loci on chromosomes 3q, 7p, 1q, 15q, and 6q. Mol Psychiatry 2006;11:763–70.
110. Wang Y, Samuels JF, Chang YC, et al. Gender differences in genetic linkage and association on 11p15 in obsessive-compulsive disorder families. Am J Med Genet B Neuropsychiatr Genet 2009;150(B):33–40.
111. Grados MA, Riddle MA, Samuels JF, et al. The familial phenotype of obsessive-compulsive disorder in relation to tic disorders: the Hopkins OCD Family Study. Biol Psychiatry 2001;50(8):559–65.
112. Pauls DL, Leckman JF. The inheritance of Gilles de la Tourette's syndrome and associated behaviors: evidence for autosomal dominant transmission. N Engl J Med 1986;315:993–7.
113. Nestadt G, Samuels J, Riddle MA, et al. The relationship between obsessive-compulsive disorder and anxiety and affective disorders: results from the Johns Hopkins OCD Family Study. Psychol Methods 2001;31(3):481–7.
114. Nestadt G, Addington A, Samuels J, et al. The identification of OCD-related subgroups based on comorbidity. Biol Psychiatry 2003;53:914–20.
115. Samuels J, Nestadt G, Bienvenu OJ, et al. Personality disorders and normal personality dimensions in obsessive-compulsive disorder. Br J Psychol 2000; 177:457–62.
116. Baer L. Factor analysis of symptom subtypes of obsessive compulsive disorder and their relation to personality and tic disorders. J Clin Psychiatry 1994; 55(Suppl):18–23.
117. Leckman JF, Grice DE, Boardman J, et al. Symptoms of obsessive-compulsive disorder. Am J Psychiatry 1997;154:911–7.
118. Mataix-Cols D, Rauch SL, Manzo PA, et al. Use of factor-analyzed symptom dimensions to predict outcome with serotonin reuptake inhibitors and placebo in the treatment of obsessive-compulsive disorder. Am J Psychiatry 1999;156: 1409–16.
119. Rasmussen SA, Eisen JL. The epidemiology and clinical features of obsessive compulsive disorder. Psychiatr Clin North Am 1992;15:743–58.
120. Nestadt G, Di CZ, Riddle MA, et al. Obsessive-compulsive disorder: subclassification based on co-morbidity. Psychol Med 2009;39(9):1491–501.
121. Pauls DL, Towbin KE, Leckman JF, et al. Gilles de la Tourette's syndrome and obsessive-compulsive disorder: evidence supporting a genetic relationship. Arch Gen Psychiatry 1986;43:1180–2.
122. Frost RO, Steketee G, Williams LF, et al. Mood, personality disorder symptoms and disability in obsessive compulsive hoarders: a comparison with clinical and nonclinical controls. Behav Res Ther 2000;38:1071–81.
123. Winsberg ME, Cassic KS, Koran LM. Hoarding in obsessive-compulsive disorder: a report of 20 cases. J Clin Psychiatry 1999;60:591–7.
124. Saxena S, Brody AL, Maidment KM, et al. Cerebral glucose metabolism in obsessive-compulsive hoarding. Am J Psychiatry 2004;161:1038–48.

125. Mataix-Cols D, Wooderson S, Lawrence N, et al. Distinct neural correlates of washing, checking, and hoarding symptom dimensions in obsessive-compulsive disorder. Arch Gen Psychiatry 2004;61:564–76.

126. Samuels J, Bienvenu OJ III, Riddle MA, et al. Hoarding in obsessive compulsive disorder: results from a case-control study. Behav Res Ther 2002;40:517–28.

127. Mataix-Cols D, Rosario-Campos MC, Leckman JF. A multidimensional model of obsessive-compulsive disorder. Am J Psychiatry 2005;162:228–38.

128. Cullen B, Brown CH, Riddle MA, et al. Factor analysis of the Yale-brown obsessive compulsive scale in a family study of obsessive-compulsive disorder. Depress Anxiety 2007;24:130–8.

129. Hasler G, Pinto A, Greenberg BD, et al. Familiality of factor analysis-derived YBOCS dimensions in OCD-affected sibling pairs from the OCD Collaborative Genetics Study. Biol Psychiatry 2007;61:617–25.

130. Pinto A, Greenberg B, Grados M, et al. OCD Collaborative Genetics Study: further development of YBOCS dimensions in the OCD Collaborative Genetics Study: symptoms vs. categories. Psychiatry Res 2008;160:83–93.

131. Stewart SE, Rosario MC, Brown TA, et al. Principal components analysis of obsessive-compulsive disorder symptoms in children and adolescents. Biol Psychiatry 2007;61:285–91.

132. Samuels J, Shugart Y, Grados M, et al. Significant linkage to compulsive hoarding on chromosome 14 in families with obsessive-compulsive disorder: results from the OCD Collaborative Genetics Study. Am J Psychiatry 2007; 164:493–9.

133. Tolin DF, Kiehl KA, Worhunsky P, et al. An exploratory study of the neural mechanisms of decision making in compulsive hoarding. Psychol Methods 2009;39:325–36.

134. Chamberlain SR, Menzies L, Hampshire A, et al. Orbitofrontal dysfunction in patients with obsessive-compulsive disorder and their unaffected relatives. Science 2008;321:421–2.

135. Menzies L, Achard S, Chamberlain SR, et al. Neurocognitive endophenotypes of obsessive-compulsive disorder. Brain 2007;130:3223–36.

136. Chamberlain SR, Fineberg NA, Menzies LA, et al. Impaired cognitive flexibility and motor inhibition in unaffected first-degree relatives of patients with obsessive-compulsive disorder. Am J Psychiatry 2007;164:335–8.

137. Bechara A, Damasio AR, Damasio H, et al. Insensitivity to future consequences following damage to human prefrontal cortex. Cognition 1994;50:7–15.

138. Cavedini P, Riboldi G, D'Annucci A, et al. Decision-making heterogeneity in obsessive-compulsive disorder: ventromedial prefrontal cortex function predicts different treatment outcomes. Neuropsychologia 2002;40:205–11.

139. Nielen MM, Veltman DJ, de Jong R, et al. Decision making performance in obsessive compulsive disorder. J Affect Disord 2002;69:257–60.

140. Chamberlain SR, Fineberg NA, Blackwell AD, et al. Motor inhibition and cognitive flexibility in obsessive-compulsive disorder and trichotillomania. Am J Psychiatry 2006;163:1282–4.

141. Carlson CS, Eberle MA, Kruglyak L, et al. Mapping complex disease loci in whole-genome association studies. Nature 2004;429:446–52.

142. Carrasquillo MM, McCallion AS, Puffenberger EG, et al. Genome-wide association study and mouse model identify interaction between RET and EDNRB pathways in Hirschsprung disease. Nat Genet 2002;32:237–44.

143. Klein RJ, Zeiss C, Chew EY, et al. Complement factor H polymorphism in age-related macular degeneration. Science 2005;308:385–9.

144. Botstein D, Risch N. Discovering genotypes underlying human phenotypes: past successes for mendelian disease, future approaches for complex disease. Nat Genet 2003;33(Suppl):228–37.

145. Ohashi J, Tokunaga K. The expected power of genome-wide linkage disequilibrium testing using single nucleotide polymorphism markers for detecting a low-frequency disease variant. Ann Hum Genet 2002;66:297–306.

146. Neale BM, Sham PC. The future of association studies: gene-based analysis and replication. Am J Hum Genet 2004;75:353–62.

Molecular Genetics of Attention Deficit Hyperactivity Disorder

Stephen V. Faraone, PhD[a,b,]*, Eric Mick, ScD[c]

KEYWORDS

- Attention deficit/hyperactivity disorder • ADHD • Genetics

Attention deficit/hyperactivity disorder (ADHD) is among the most common childhood-onset psychiatric disorders. The worldwide prevalence of ADHD in children is 8% to 12%,[1] and estimated to be 4% in adults in the United States by the National Comorbidity Survey.[2] Early studies found the risk for ADHD among parents of children who had ADHD to be increased by between two- and eightfold, with similarly elevated risk among siblings.[3] Faraone and colleagues[4] extended these findings to families ascertained through adult probands meeting Diagnostic and Statistical Manual of Mental Disorders, Fourth Edition (DSM-IV) criteria for either full ADHD or late-onset ADHD.

However, adoption and twin studies are necessary to disentangle genetic from environmental sources of transmission observed in family studies. Three studies found that biologic relatives of ADHD[5] or hyperactive children[6,7] were more likely to have hyperactivity than adoptive relatives. A more direct method of examining the heritability of ADHD is to study twins. The extent to which monozygotic twins are more concordant for ADHD than dizygotic twins can be used to compute the degree to which variability in ADHD in the population can be accounted for by genes (ie, heritability). Faraone and colleagues[8] reviewed 20 twin studies from the United States, Australia, Scandinavia, and the European Union and reported a mean heritability estimate of 76%, showing that ADHD is among the most heritable of psychiatric disorders.

[a] Department of Psychiatry and Behavioral Sciences, SUNY Upstate Medical University, 750 East Adams Street, Syracuse, NY 13210-2375, USA
[b] Department of Neuroscience & Physiology, SUNY Upstate Medical University, 750 East Adams Street, Syracuse, NY 13210-2375, USA
[c] Department of Psychiatry, Massachusetts General Hospital and Harvard Medical School, 55 Fruit Street–Warren 705, Boston, MA 02114, USA
* Corresponding author. Department of Psychiatry and Behavioral Sciences, SUNY Upstate Medical University, 750 East Adams Street, Syracuse, NY 13210-2375.
E-mail address: faraones@upstate.edu (S.V. Faraone).

Psychiatr Clin N Am 33 (2010) 159–180
doi:10.1016/j.psc.2009.12.004
0193-953X/10/$ – see front matter © 2010 Elsevier Inc. All rights reserved.

GENETIC LINKAGE STUDIES

To find regions of chromosomes that might harbor genes for ADHD, several groups have conducted genome-wide linkage scans.[9–14] This approach examines many DNA markers across the genome to determine if any chromosomal regions are shared more often than expected among family members who have ADHD.

A study of 126 American affected sibling pairs found four regions that showed some evidence of linkage (LOD scores >1.5): 5p12, 10q26, 12q23, and 16p13.[9] An expanded sample of 203 families found stronger evidence for the 16p13 region, previously implicated in autism, with a maximum LOD score of 4.[10] A study of 164 Dutch affected sibling pairs also identified a peak previously noted in autism, at 15q15, with a peak LOD score of 3.5.[11] Two other peaks at 7p13 and 9q33 yielded LOD scores of 3.0 and 2.1, respectively. A genome-wide scan of families from a genetically isolated community in Columbia implicated 8q12, 11q23, 4q13, 17p11, 12q23, and 8p23.[12] Pooled analyses[10,11] suggest that the genetic background in the differing populations is distinct and that the lack of consistent findings is a reflection of this between-population heterogeneity,[13] but did identify an area of linkage in these pooled analyses (5p13) that may reflect a common risk locus.

A study of 155 sibling pairs from Germany reported a maximum LOD score of 2.59 for chromosome 5p at 17cM. They also reported nominal evidence for linkage to chromosomes 6q, 7p, 9q, 11q, 12q, and 17p, which had also been identified in previous scans.[14] Faraone and colleagues[15] found no regions of significant or suggestive linkage in an affected sibling pair linkage analysis on 217 families with 601 siblings diagnosed with ADHD.

Although some overlap is present in nominally significant linkage peaks, no evidence exists for the replication of a genome-wide significant finding using strict criteria.[16] To determine if any common linkage signals were present among these studies, Zhou and colleagues[17] conducted a Genome Scan Meta Analysis of these data. They reported genome-wide significant linkage ($P_{Statistical\ Ratio}$ = .00034; $P_{Odds\ Ratio}$ = .04) for a region on chromosome 16 between 64 Mb and 83 Mb. Although this finding is intriguing and worthy of follow-up, the lack of significant findings for other loci suggests that many genes of moderately large effect are unlikely to exist and that the method of association will be more fruitful in the search for ADHD susceptibility genes.

Genetic Association Studies

In contrast to the scarcity of linkage studies, many candidate gene association studies have been conducted. Several meta-analyses suggest strong association with ADHD and the dopamine D4 receptor gene (DRD4, 48-bp VNTR),[18,19] the dopamine D5 receptor gene (DRD5, 148-bp microsatellite marker),[18,20] the dopamine β-hydroxylase gene (DBH, 5' taq1 A allele),[8] the synaptosomal-associated protein 25 gene (SNAP-25, T1065G single-nucleotide polymorphism [SNP]),[8] the serotonin transporter gene (SLC6A4, 44-bp insertion/deletion in the promoter region [5-HTTLPR]),[8] and the serotonin 1B receptor gene (HTR1B, G861C SNP).[8] Meta-analysis has also suggested a weak association with ADHD and the dopamine transporter gene (SLC6A3, 480-bp VNTR in the 3' untranslated region [UTR]),[18,21,22] but no association with the catechol-O-methyltransferase gene (COMT, Val108Met polymorphism).[23]

A major advance in the molecular genetics of ADHD was the publication of the International Multisite ADHD Gene (IMAGE) project in which 51 genes were analyzed for association with ADHD. Families were recruited through an ADHD combined-type child proband (N = 674) who had at least one full sibling (n = 808) and one biologic parent (N = 1227 parents) available for study. A high density SNP map was constructed for genes involved in the regulation of neurotransmitter pathways implicated in ADHD (dopamine, norepinephrine, and serotonin) based on tagging SNPs and SNPs within known functional regions. This study is the most in-depth genetic association study performed in the largest set of ADHD patients to date and found evidence of association with ADHD and 18 genes.

Taken together this literature strongly suggests a contribution of genetic factors in the etiology of ADHD. In this review, we provide an update on the progress of molecular genetic studies published since the completion of these meta-analyses. Results from the IMAGE project will be discussed separately for each gene.

ASSOCIATION STUDIES OF CATECHOLAMINERGIC GENES
The Dopamine D4 Receptor (DRD4)

Both noradrenaline and dopamine are potent agonists of DRD4,[24] and the D4 receptor is prevalent in frontal-subcortical networks implicated in the pathophysiology of ADHD by neuroimaging and neuropsychological studies.[25] Researchers have predominantly focused on a tandem repeat polymorphism in exon III of DRD4 because in vitro studies have shown that one variant (the 7-repeat allele) produces a blunted response to dopamine.[26,27] Faraone and colleagues[8] conducted a meta analysis of the 7-repeat allele of the exon III polymorphism and found statistically significant association with ADHD in both case-control (odds ratio = 1.45 (95% CI 1.27–1.65)) and family based OR = 1.16 (95% CI 1.03–1.31) studies. Li and colleagues[18] reported a pooled OR of 1.34 (1.23–1.45) in 33 studies.

Not included in these meta-analyses of the exon III DRD4 48-bp VNTR were a prospective follow-up study of German children in which the 7-repeat DRD4 allele was associated with increased incidence and persistence of ADHD in boys up to 11 years of age,[28] a positive association with the 6 and 7 repeat alleles in a sample of 44 Indian ADHD trios (RR = 1.81; P = .03),[29] and a negative association in 126 Korean ADHD families (P = .67).[30] Carrasco and colleagues[31] also failed to document an association with the 7 repeat allele in a small case-control study of 26 Chilean children with ADHD, but found a significant interaction with this DRD4 marker and the dopamine transporter gene suggesting that children with the risk alleles at both loci are at greater risk of ADHD. In the large and comprehensive IMAGE project, the association with this VNTR and ADHD was not statistically significant (P<.09) but the odds ratio (1.18) was very close to that observed in meta-analyses.

A small number of studies have assessed other DRD4 polymorphisms; however, these data have not been conclusive. McCracken and colleagues[32,33] found an association between ADHD and a 5' 120-bp repeat 1.2 kb upstream of the initiation codon. However, Barr and colleagues,[34] Todd and colleagues,[35] Brookes and colleagues,[36] and Bhaduri and colleagues[37] found no association between ADHD and this marker. Significant evidence of association was found by Arcos-Burgos and colleagues,[12] but only with the 5' 120-bp marker included with the exon III 48-bp 7-repeat allele in haplotype analysis.

Barr and colleagues[34] found no association between ADHD and two SNPs in the promoter region (rs747302 and rs1800955), but Lowe and colleagues[38] observed a significant over transmission of the rs1800955-A allele and a trend toward association with the rs747302-C allele. Brookes and colleagues[39] did not genotype these SNPS in the IMAGE project, but observed nominal association with a SNP (rs9195457) for which the LD structure with previously associated SNPs could not be determined.

Although it has been suggested that the DRD4 gene may be particularly relevant to symptoms of inattention, the literature suggests that this may not be so. Rowe and colleagues[40] found that fathers of ADHD children with the 7-repeat allele had higher levels of retrospectively reported inattention symptoms, and Levitan and colleagues[41] found an association between this allele and greater self-reported childhood inattention in women with seasonal affective disorder. However, Todd and colleagues[42] found no association with the exon III 48-bp VNTR and any ADHD symptom profiles or DSM-IV subtypes in pooled analysis of 2,090 children. Similarly, Mill and colleagues[43] found no association with the 7-repeat allele and a quantitative measure of ADHD symptom profiles in 329 pairs of male twins ascertained in England and Wales. Although the 7-repeat allele was not present in a sample of Korean ADHD children, Kim and colleagues[30] reported no variation of inattentive symptoms with the number of repeats but rather observed a greater severity of hyperactive/impulsive symptoms in subjects with a 5-repeat allele.

Furthermore, on neuropsychological measures of attention, subjects possessing the 7-repeat allele have demonstrated significantly better attention than subjects with fewer repeats[44–46] or demonstrated no difference on similar measures of attention.[47] However, Bellgrove and colleagues[46] found that the rs747302-A allele was associated with sustained attention deficits while the 7-repeat allele of the exon III VNTR was associated with improved performance. Thus, they conclude that such risk alleles have dissociable effects on cognition in ADHD children.[46]

Two studies have provided evidence documenting strength of a DRD4-ADHD relationship relative to other phenotypes hypothesized to also be associated with DRD4: autism[48] and a novelty seeking temperament.[49] Grady and colleagues[48] found no evidence of an over-representation of rare DRD4 variants in a sample of children with autism relative to geographically matched controls, while a sample of ADHD children had a fourfold increase in novel alleles compare with geographically matched controls. Furthermore, Lynn and colleagues[49] examined the relationship between ADHD, novelty seeking and the exon III DRD4 48-bp VNTR and found independent associations with ADHD/novelty seeking, and ADHD/DRD4, but not with DRD4/novelty seeking. Although not conclusive these studies suggest that the association between ADHD and DRD4 is relatively specific (ie, relative to autism) and not confounded by common comorbid behaviors (ie, increased novelty seeking).

The Dopamine 5 Receptor (DRD5)

The most widely studied polymorphism for DRD5 has been a dinucleotide repeat that maps approximately 18.5 kb 5′ to the transcription start site.[50] Meta-analysis of 14 independent family-based studies suggested a significant association of the 148-bp allele with ADHD (OR = 1.2; 95% CI 1.1–1.4)[20] that was confirmed in updated analyses conducted by Li and colleagues[18] (OR = 1.3; 95% CI 1.2–1.5). Not included in these meta-analyses is a study by Mill and colleagues[43] examining quantitative measures of ADHD symptoms in 329 pairs of male twins ascertained in England and Wales. Again, the 148-bp allele was statistically significantly associated with ADHD, but unfortunately the direction of effect was in the opposite direction: the risk allele was associated with lower hyperactivity scores.[43]

Other markers within DRD5 have also been found to be associated with ADHD. Hawi and colleagues[50] studied two additional 5′ microsatellite markers and a SNP in the 3′ UTR. The 3′ SNP was associated with ADHD (relative risk = 1.6) and haplotype analyses showed an association with ADHD and a two-marker haplotype of one of the 5′ microsatellite markers (D4S1582) and the dinucleotide repeat (DRD5-PCR1) (P = .000107), a two-marker haplotype comprising DRD5-PCR1 and the 3′ SNP (P = .0099), and a haplotype comprised of all three of these markers (P = .0013).

The Dopamine Transporter Gene (DAT, SLC6A3)

There are several reasons that SLC6A3 has been considered a suitable candidate for ADHD. Stimulant medications, which are efficacious in treating ADHD, block the dopamine transporter as one mechanism of action for achieving their therapeutic effects.[51] In mice, eliminating SLC6A3 gene function leads to two features suggestive of ADHD: hyperactivity and deficits in inhibitory behavior. Treating these "knockout" mice with stimulants reduces their hyperactivity.[52,53]

Using a family-based association study, Cook and colleagues[54] first reported an association between ADHD and the 10-repeat allele of the 3'UTR VNTR. Our previous meta-analysis of family-based studies resulted in a small but significant odds ratio (1.13, 95% CI 1.03–1.24), however Li and colleagues[18] updated this work and found no evidence of association with ADHD and the 10-repeat allele in family-based studies (OR = 1.04, 95% CI = 0.99–1.14), as well as considerable evidence of heterogeneity between studies (p(Q) = 0.000001). A subsequent meta-analysis of this gene found small but significant association with ADHD for family-based TDT studies (OR = 1.17, 95% CI = 1.05–1.30).[21] The odd ratio for seven family-based HHRR studies was 1.5, but it was not significant. Although there were only six case-control studies, their combined odds ratio of 0.95 would seem to disconfirm the family-based studies.[21]

Thus, the lack of consistent association with the 3' UTR VNTR suggests that this marker itself is not directly involved in the etiology of ADHD, but it may be tagging a proximate functional polymorphism in partial linkage disequilibrium (LD) with the 10-repeat allele. In an attempt to further refine the SLC6A3 risk variant for ADHD, Brookes and colleagues[55] reported association with a haplotype comprised the 10-repeat allele in the 3'UTR and the 6-repeat allele of a 30-bp VNTR in intron 8. Of the four possible haplotype combinations of the two markers, only the 10-6 haplotype was associated with increased risk for ADHD in both populations. This finding was replicated by Brookes and colleagues[39] (OR = 1.19, P<.06) and Asherson and colleagues[56] in the second set of 383 ADHD probands from the IMAGE sample (OR = 1.27, P = .002). Bakker and colleagues[57] failed to identify an overall association with this haplotype (P = .2) or preferential over transmission of the 10-6 variant in 198 Dutch probands with ADHD.

However, evidence is emerging that environmental risk factors for ADHD might be important mediators of the risk for ADHD associated with SLC6A3. Brookes and colleagues[55] also reported a gene-environment interaction suggesting that the risk for ADHD was increased only in the presence of the 10-6 SLC6A3 haplotype when there was also exposesure to maternal alcohol use during pregnancy. Although the 9-repeat allele was significantly over transmitted in the sample[58] used by Neuman and colleagues,[59] they documented an increased risk for the severe combined ADHD profile with both SLC6A3 and the DRD4 7-repeat allele only in children who were exposed to maternal cigarette smoking during pregnancy. Similarly, Laucht and colleagues[60] found that the 3'UTR 10-repeat allele, the intron 8 6-repeat allele, and the 10-6 haplotype were associated with ADHD symptoms only in families exposed to higher psychosocial adversity.

Dopamine Beta-Hydroxylase (DBH)

DBH is the primary enzyme responsible for conversion of dopamine to norepinephrine. Comings and colleagues[61,62] examined a Taq1 restriction site polymorphism in intron 5 and found a significant association with the A1 allele and ADHD symptom scores in children with Tourette's Syndrome (TS).[62] Smith and colleagues[63] subsequently replicated this association (OR = 1.96; 95% CI: 1.01-3.79) in ADHD subjects but Daly and colleagues[64] and Roman and colleagues[65] found over-transmission of the A2 allele. Both also found that the association was stronger in combined-type ADHD cases but Daly and colleagues[64] found that parental history of ADHD strengthened the association while Roman and colleagues[65] found stronger evidence of association in those with no parental history of ADHD. In a Canadian study of 117 families with children with ADHD, Wigg and colleagues[66] reported a non-significant excess transmission of the A2 allele. Subsequently, a case-control study of Indian ADHD children[67] and both case-control and family-based analyses of persistent ADHD cases in Canada[68] have failed to document a significant association with this marker of DBH.

Other markers of DBH have also shown a lack of significant association with ADHD. Wigg and colleagues[66] observed no evidence of linkage or association for the dinucleotide repeat polymorphism and an insertion/deletion polymorphism in the region 5' to the transcription start site (both of which had been associated with serum DBH levels). A G/T SNP in exon 5 of DBH was examined in 104 trios from the UK (Payton and colleagues[69]) and in 86 trios from Ireland[50] and showed no evidence of association. Hawi and colleagues[70] also examined an EcoN1 restriction site polymorphism in exon 2 and an MspI polymorphism in intron 9 and found association for only a haplotype comprised of allele 1 of the exon 2 polymorphism and A2 of the Taq1 polymorphism. A -1021C>T polymorphism in the 5' flanking region of DBH has been shown to account for as much as 50% of plasma DBH activity and was associated with ADHD in the Han Chinese,[71] but not in a sample of Indian ADHD children.[67] Finally, 33 SNPs were tagged for this gene in the IMAGE project, but there were no nominally significant associations with ADHD found.[39]

Monoamine Oxidase A (MAO-A)

The MAO-A enzyme moderates levels of norepinephrine, dopamine, and serotonin, and MAO-A knockout mice display numerous abnormalities in these neurotransmitter systems.[72] A case-control study of a 30-bp pair tandem repeat in the promoter region in 129 Israeli ADHD subjects suggested association with ADHD and noted a particularly large effect in the subset of female cases (n = 19).[73] The 4 and 5 repeat alleles of this promoter-region VNTR were also significantly associated with ADHD in a sample of 133 Israeli families,[73] but not in a similarly-sized family-based study by Lawson and colleagues[74] A CA-repeat microsatellite in intron 2 was associated with ADHD[75] in 82 Chinese, but this was not replicated in Caucasian samples.[69,76]

Domschke and colleagues[76] also examined a SNP in exon 8 (941G>T) and found association with the high activity G941T allele and with a haplotype containing the G941T allele, the 3-repeat allele of 30-bp VNTR and the 6-repeat of the CA microsatellite described above. Xu and colleagues[77] replicated the association with G941T allele and the over-transmission of a haplotype contain the G941T allele and the shorter 3-repeat allele of the promoter VNTR in a Taiwanese sample. Five tagged SNPs for MAO-A were statistically significantly associated with ADHD in the IMAGE sample.[39] The 941G>T SNP was not included in that analysis but the region covered by the widow of significant SNPs incorporated the location of this SNP.

The Dopamine D2 Receptor (DRD2)

The dopamine D2 receptor (DRD2) has been less extensively studied in ADHD than DRD4 and DRD5. Comings[78] compared 104 ADHD subjects (nearly all with comorbid Tourette's syndrome) to controls, and found a significant association with the TaqIA1 allele of DRD2, which they subsequently replicated.[61] This finding was replicated in a case-control sample of Czech boys with ADHD,[79] but not in a sample of Korean alcoholics with and without ADHD.[80]

Family-based studies of DRD2 have been uniformly negative, however. Rowe and colleagues[81] examined 164 ADHD children from 125 families, and found no excess transmission of the Taq1A1 allele. A subsequent study of Taiwanese families likewise found no association.[82] Kirley and colleagues[83] examined two polymorphisms in 118 ADHD children and their families. No significant associations were identified, though they reported a trend toward significance (P = .07) for the Ser311 polymorphism when paternally transmitted. Finally, the IMAGE project examined 23 tag SNPs and found no nominally significant association with ADHD.

The Dopamine D3 Receptor (DRD3)

Barr and colleagues[84] examined a Ser9Gly exon 1 polymorphism and an intron 5 MspI restriction site polymorphism in 100 Canadian families but neither the individual loci nor haplotypes of the two were associated with ADHD. Negative results for the Ser9Gly polymorphism were also reported in a UK family-based study of 105 families[69] and a study of 39 families of ADHD adults.[85] Comings and colleagues[86] also found no evidence for association with ADHD and comorbid Tourette Syndrome. In a sample of 146 German patients referred for forensic evaluation,[87] heterozygosity at this polymorphism was associated with higher impulsivity scores although this effect was only seen among those with a history of violence. Similarly, none of the 28 DRD3 SNPs tagged for the IMAGE project were nominally significant.[39]

Catechol-O-methyltransferase (COMT)

COMT catalyzes a major step in the degradation of dopamine, norepinephrine, and epinephrine. The most extensively studied marker for the COMT gene is the Val108Met polymorphism, which yields either a high- or low- activity form of COMT.[88] Cheuk and colleagues[23] conducted a meta-analysis of this marker and found no evidence of association with ADHD in case-control studies (OR = 0.95 [0.75–1.2], P = .7) or family-based studies using the TDT (OR = 0.95 [0.84–1.09], P = .5) or the HHRR (OR = 1.02 [0.78–1.34], P = .9). Reuter and colleagues[89] found that higher symptom scores were associated with the MET/MET genotype in German adults who were healthy or diagnosed with eating or substance use disorders and Gothelf[90] documented a 5-fold increased risk for the MET allele in 55 subjects with velocardiofacial syndrome and comorbid ADHD relative to those without comorbid ADHD. The lack of significant results from the IMAGE project[91] is consistent with the negative meta-analysis conducted by Cheuk and colleagues[23] Although these association studies rule out a simple role for the Val108Met polymorphism in the etiology of ADHD, it is of note that COMT hass been found to be highly up-regulated in a rat model of ADHD caused by prenatal exposure to polychlorinated biphenyls.[92]

Noradrenergic Receptors: ADRA2A, 2C and 1C

Three adrenergic receptors have been examined in ADHD. The alpha-2A adrenergic receptor (ADRA2A) has a promoter-region SNP (-1291 C>G) which has been examined in both case-control and family-based studies. Comings and colleagues[93] reported an association between genotypes at this SNP and ADHD symptom scores and that the G-1291C allele was associated with ADHD and oppositional defiant or conduct disorder symptoms while the C-1291G allele was associated with a spectrum of other conditions including panic attacks, obsessive compulsive disorder (OCD), addictions, affective, and schizoid symptoms.

However, family-based studies failed to detect association with -1291C>G polymorphism and the diagnosis of ADHD.[94–100] The G-1291C allele of this marker has been shown to be associated with ADHD symptom scores, but the direction of effect has been inconsistent: some studies found association with only inattentive symptoms[101] while others found association with both inattentive and hyperactive symptoms.[95,96] In contrast, Wang and colleagues[99] found no association with ADHD in a sample of Han Chinese but a trend toward lower ADHD symptom score in subjects homozygous for the G-1291C allele. Examination of other markers have been similarly inconsistent with the G-1291C allele being included in a significantly over-transmitted haplotype in a sample of 51 trios[96] while the C-1291G allele was included in a significant haplotype in sib-pair linkage study of 93 ADHD probands and 50 of their unaffected siblings.[100]

While these results suggest either a weak or no association with ADHD and the1291G>C polymorphism, they do not take heterogeneity in the presentation of ADHD into account. Schmitz and colleagues[97] conducted a unique study of exclusively inattentive-type ADHD children and found a significant association with the G-1291C allele in case-control but not family-based analyses. Waldman and colleagues[102] evaluated the moderating and mediating effects of executive function deficits on the association of ADRA2A and ADHD and found that association with ADHD was more robust in children with poorer cognitive performance. Although Stevenson and colleagues[103] reported no overall association with ADRA2A, there was a significant over-transmission of the G-1291C allele in the sub-sample with a reading disability.

A dinucleotide repeat polymorphism located approximately 6 kb from the gene which codes for the alpha-2C adrenergic receptor (ADRA2C;) has also been examined in both case control and family-based analyses. Comings and colleagues[104] found an association between this polymorphism and ADHD symptom scores, but it was not significant after Bonferroni correction. Two subsequent family-based analyses showed no evidence of association.[105,106] The former study also examined a C-to-T SNP in codon 492 of the 1C receptor (ADRA1C) that changes cysteine to arginine but found no evidence of linkage.[105] In the IMAGE project, there was no nominally significant association with any of SNPs tagged for ADRA2A or ADRA2C.[39]

The Norepinephrine Transporter (NET; SLC6A2)

SLC6A2 has been examined in ADHD because drugs that block the norepinephrine transporter are efficacious in treating ADHD.[107] Comings and colleagues[86] found evidence for association of a SNP in SLC6A2 with ADHD symptoms. Subsequently, Barr and colleagues[108] examined 3 SNPs in SLC6A2 (one in exon 9, intron 9 and intron 13, respectively) in 122 ADHD families and found no evidence of association for these loci or haplotypes comprising them. Others have found no association with SNPs in intron 7 or 9[109] or with a restriction fragment length polymorphism in ADHD adults.[106] However, Xu and colleagues[110] investigated 21 SNPs spanning the NET region in 180 cases and 334 controls and reported nominally significant association with rs3785157 that was later replicated by Bobb and colleagues[111] with an additional significant association with rs998424. Although these SNPs were not found to be associated with ADHD in the IMAGE study,[39] two of the 43 tagged SNPs (rs3785143 and rs11568324) for SLC6A2 did reach nominal statistical significance. Finally, a novel promoter SNP has been shown to be possibly associated with ADHD in a set of 94 ADHD cases and 60 controls.[112]

ASSOCIATION STUDIES OF SEROTONERGIC GENES
Serotonin Receptors: HTR1B and HTR2A

Of the family-based association studies of a silent SNP (861G>C) in the gene coding for the serotonin HTR1B receptor,[111,113–116] only the multi-site study by Hawi and colleagues[113] reached statistical significance suggesting over-transmission of the G861C allele. Smoller and colleagues[115] pooled data from[113–115] and identified statistically significant over-transmission of this allele (OR = 1.35 [1.13–1.62], P = .009) that strongly suggested paternal (P = .00005) rather than maternal transmission (P = .2). There was a weak trend suggesting over-transmission of the G681 allele in Li and colleagues[117] when examining primarily inattentive ADHD subjects separately. Smoller and colleagues[115] also identified association with this ADHD subtype and a 6-SNP haplotype including the G681C allele and two promoter SNPs with functional effects on HTR1B expression. Heiser and colleagues[116] identified no association with the G681C allele but examined only the combined ADHD subtype and did not assess for paternal transmission separately. The analysis of combined-type ADHD in the IMAGE project did not identify association with any of the tag SNPs selected.[39]

The T102C, G1438A, and His452Tyr polymorphisms of the serotonin HTR2A receptor gene have also been examined for association with ADHD.[113,116,118–122] No association has been reported for the T102C and the G1438A SNPS for ADHD in.[116,119–122] Likewise Bobb and colleagues[111] found no evidence of association with ADHD and any of the SNPs of the HTR2A gene examined in either case-control or family-based analyses. However, Levitan and colleagues[123] found an association with C102T allele and greater scores on a self-report measure of childhood ADHD in a sample of women with seasonal affective disorder and Li and colleagues[121] found that the A1438G allele was associated with functional remission from ADHD in Han Chinese adolescents. A coding polymorphism in the HTR2A receptor gene (His452Tyr) was associated with ADHD in,[118,122] but not in.[113,116]

Li and colleagues[124] found significant over-transmission of the C-759T/G-697C haplotype within the HTR2C gene, but no association was observed in Bobb and colleagues[111] or in the IMAGE project.[39] Li and colleagues[125] have also reported significant under transmission of the C83097T/G83198A haplotype in the HTR4 gene, but no association with markers in HTR5A and HTR6[120] or HTR1D.[126] Genes for additional serotonin receptors (HTR1E and HTR3B) evaluated in the IMAGE project[39] have also failed to yield any significant association with ADHD.

Serotonin Transporter (HTT, SLC6A4)

A 44-base pair insertion/deletion polymorphism (HTTLPR) in the promoter region of SLC6A4 may be the most studied genetic marker in psychiatric genetics, with associations reported for a broad range of diagnoses and traits.[127,128] When the HTTLPR studies published by 2005 were combined,[8] the pooled odds ratio for the long (L) allele was 1.31 (95% CI 1.09–1.59). Curran and colleagues[129] found nominal evidence of over transmission of the L allele and strong evidence of association with a 4 SNP haplotype upstream that included the 5-HTTPR ins/del polymorphism. However, subsequent studies of this marker in 126 Korean ADHD families,[130] 197 ADHD families from the UK,[131] 196 Taiwanese ADHD familes,[131,132] 56 Indian ADHD families,[133] 209 Canadian ADHD families,[134] and 102 German ADHD families[116] have failed to identify an association with the HTTLPR. Li and colleagues[135] found statistically significant over-transmission of the S (rather than the L) allele in 279 Han Chinese ADHD families.

A 17-bp VNTR in intron 2 of SLC6A4 (STint2) was first associated with ADHD in a case-control study conducted by[119] with the 12-12 genotype being under-represented in cases than controls. Banerjee and colleagues[133] found significant over-transmission of the 12 allele, but Heiser,[116] Xu[131] and Kim and colleagues[130] found no association and Li and colleagues[135] found evidence of under-transmission of a haplotype with the HTTLPR L allele and the STint2 12 allele. The IMAGE project found no association for the tag SNPs examined[39] and Wigg and colleagues[134] found no association with 2 functional SLC6A4 polymorphisms (rs3813034 (T/G) and Ile425Val (A/G)) and ADHD.

Tryptophan Hydroxylase (TPH and TPH-2)

TPH is the rate-limiting enzyme in the synthesis of serotonin, and TPH polymorphisms have been associated with aggression and impulsivity.[136] Two family-based studies examined the TPH gene in ADHD. One study of 69 Han Chinese trios found no association with a SNP (A218C) in intron 7.[137] A second study examined two SNPs among more than 350 Han Chinese youth with ADHD, with and without learning disability, and their families.[138,139] Although neither SNP showed biased transmission individually, a haplotype composed of the A218 and G-6526 alleles appeared to be under-transmitted (P = .03).

The gene for a second form of TPH (TPH2) located on chromosome 12q15 has also been studied. Walitza and colleagues examined two SNPs located in the transcriptional control region of TPH-2 (rs4570625 and rs11178997) a third located in intron 2 (rs4565946). Tests of the transcriptional SNPs individually and in a 2-SNP haplotype were modestly associated with ADHD in the 225 affected children (103 families), but the intron 2 SNP was not associated. Sheehan and colleagues[140] studied 8 additional SNPs in 179 ADHD families and found statistically significant evidence of association with the rs1843809-T allele (P = .0006), the rs1386497-A allele (P = .048), and a trend suggesting association with the rs1386493-C allele (P = .09). In the IMAGE project rs1843809 and rs1386497 were also significantly associated with ADHD, but the alleles implicateded in Sheehan and colleagues[140] were not.[39] Brookes and colleagues also reported an association with rs1007023 which was in perfect LD with rs1386497 from Sheehan and colleagues[39] However, Brookes and colleagues did not replicate the finding reported by Walitza and colleagues[141] and Sheehan and colleagues was not able to replicate their earlier findings in a smaller sample of 63 ADHD trios.[142]

ASSOCIATION STUDIES OF OTHER CANDIDATE GENES
Synaptosomal Associated Protein of 25kD (SNAP25)

SNAP25 is a 206 amino acid protein found on chromosome 20p12. The gene product is a presynaptic plasma membrane protein involved in the regulation of neurotransmitter release. Its relevance to ADHD was motivated by the coloboma mouse, which has a hemizygous two centimorgan deletion of a segment on chromosome 2q, including the gene encoding SNAP-25. The coloboma mutation leads to spontaneous hyperactivity, delays in achieving complex neonatal motor abilities, deficits in hippocampal physiology, which may contribute to learning deficiencies, and deficits in $Ca2+$-dependent dopamine release in dorsal striatum.[143] Four family-based studies of SNAP25 examined two SNPs (1069T>C and 1065T>G) separated by four base pairs at the 3' end of the gene.[144–148] Meta-analysis of these studies showed significant evidence for an association with ADHD and T1065G (OR = 1.19, 95%CI 1.03-1.38). Feng and colleagues[149] examined 12 SNPS in two independent samples of ADHD families and found significant over-transmission of the rs66039806-C, rs362549-A, rs362987-A, and the rs362998-C alleles in families from Toronto, but not California.

The IMAGE analysis of pooled data did not test these specific markers, but did demonstrate nominally statistically significant association with SNAP-25 and other markers (rs363020 and rs362567)[39] the 5'UTR. Kim and colleagues[150] examined the previously implicated SNPs and five additional SNPs (rs6077699, rs363006, rs362549, rs362987, rs362998) but found no evidence of association with ADHD in tests of individual markers or haplotypes. However, a combined TDT analysis of pooled data was modestly significant for rs3746544-T (P = .048) and rs6077690-T (P = .031). Stratification by psychiatric comorbidity further suggested that subjects with ADHD and comorbid depression may demonstrate stronger association with SNPs in SNAP-25.[150]

Acetylcholine Receptors: CHRNA4

The nicotinic acetylcholine receptors are ligand-gated ion channels composed of five subunits, one of which is the alpha-4 subunit (CHRNA4), which has been examined in several studies in ADHD. Comings and colleagues[151] found evidence of association with an intron 1 dinucleotide repeat polymorphism of the CHRNA4 gene and ADHD symptoms in a case-control study of children with Tourette Syndrome, but Kent and colleagues[152] found no significant evidence of association with a Cfo1 restriction site polymorphism in exon 5 in a study of 68 trios. Todd and colleagues[153] examined seven SNPs encompassing exons 2 and 5 as well as haplotypes of these markers and found significant association for inattentive ADHD with an intronic SNP (G/A) near the exon/intron boundary at the 3' end of exon 2. Subsequent examination of CHRNA4 in samples of combined-type ADHD cases have not replicated this association[39,111] although the IMAGE project did report association with a SNP in the 5' flanking region. Lee and colleagues[154] failed to replicate the association with SNPs from Todd and colleagues[153] or the IMAGE study[39] for either categorical ADHD diagnosis or symptom profile scores. In contrast to Todd and colleagues,[153] Lee and colleagues[154] found over-transmission of the rs2273505-G and rs3787141-T alleles with the combined ADHD subtype and hyperactivity–impulsivity scores.

Glutamate Receptors

The GRIN2A gene, which encodes a subunit of the N-methyl D-aspartate receptor has been examined in family-based studies of ADHD. Glutamate and the NMDA receptor have been implicated in cognition in both animal and human studies; the GRIN2A gene is an appealing positional candidate gene as well, located under a linkage peak at 16p13 previously associated with ADHD.[10] In a family-based analysis of 238 families, a SNP in exon 5 (Grin2a_5) was significantly associated with ADHD (P = .01); haplotypes including additional SNPs were more weakly associated[155] However, among 183 families, no evidence for association was identified for this SNP (P = .74) or three others.[156]

Brain-derived Neurotrophic Factor (BDNF)

BDNF is a protein that supports survival of central nervous system neurons and stimulates growth and differentiation of developing neurons. A polymorphism producing an amino acid substitution (valine to methionine) at codon 66 of the BDNF may impact intracellular trafficking and activity-dependent secretion of BDNF.[157] Kent and colleagues[158] found over transmission of the Val66 allele and that this was accounted for by paternal (P = .0005) rather than maternal (P = 1.0) transmission in 341 Caucasian ADHD probands and their family members. However, Xu and colleagues[159] failed to replicate these associations with Val66 in samples from the UK or Taiwan. Xu and colleagues also examined the 270C>T SNP in the 5'-noncoding region of intron1 and found significant over transmission of the C720T allele in Taiwanese, but not UK, ADHD families.[159] Twenty SNPs in the BDNF gene were tagged for the IMAGE project, but none were statistically significantly associated with ADHD.[39]

GENOME-WIDE ASSOCIATION STUDIES

To date, there have been two genome-wide association studies (GWAS) of ADHD. The International ADHD Genetics (IMAGE) project examined 909 trio families (two parents and one ADHD child) using 438,784 tagging SNPs designed to be in high linkage disequilibrium with all untyped SNPs in the genome. No finding achieved genome-wide significance (ie, a P-value of $<5x10^{-8}$) in the primary analysis of the ADHD diagnosis[160] but this analysis and several exploratory analyses implicated some novel genes that require further study.[161,162] Of interest, one of the exploratory analyses implicated the CDH13 gene, which was also implicated in a second GWAS of 343 ADHD adults and 250 controls.[163] CDH 13 lies under the linkage peak implicated in the meta-analysis of ADHD linkage studies discussed.

The IMAGE study also explored the existing candidate genes from the ADHD literature, to place the potential effects in context. They examined two sets of candidates. The first set comprised genes that showed significant association with ADHD in meta-analyses performed by Faraone and colleagues[8] These are SNAP25, DRD4, SLC6A3, HTR1B, SLC6A4, and DBH. The second set consisted of genes that had been nominated by the study investigators as good candidates for ADHD.[39] These were: NR4A2, PER2, SLC6A1, DRD3, SLC9A9, HES1, ADRA2C, ADRB2, ADRA1B, DRD1, HTR1E, DDC, STX1A, ADRA1A, NFIL3, ADRA2A, ADRB1, SLC18A2, TPH1, BDNF, FADS1, FADS2, ADRBK1, ARRB1, DRD2, HTR3B, TPH2, SYT1, HTR2A, SLC6A2, ARRB2, PER1, PNMT, CHRNA4, COMT, ADRBK2, CSNK1E, MAOA, MAOB, and HTR2C. Although none of the SNPs in these achieved genomewide significance, when the SNPs in these genes were analyzed as a group, the results suggested that they were weakly associated with ADHD.[160]

DISCUSSION

Although twin studies demonstrate that ADHD is a highly heritable condition, molecular genetic studies suggest that the genetic architecture of ADHD is complex. The handful of genome-wide scans that have been conducted thus far show divergent findings and are, therefore, not conclusive. Similarly, many of the candidate genes reviewed here (ie, DBH, MAOA, SLC6A2, TPH-2, SLC6A4, CHRNA4, GRIN2A) are theoretically compelling from a neurobiological systems perspective, but available data are sparse and inconsistent. However, candidate gene studies of ADHD have produced substantial evidence implicating several genes in the etiology of the disorder. The literature published since recent meta-analyses is particularly supportive for a role of the genes coding for DRD4, DRD5, SLC6A3, SNAP-25, and HTR1B in the etiology of ADHD.

Yet, even these associations are small and consistent with the idea that the genetic vulnerability to ADHD is mediated by many genes of small effect. These small effects emphasize the need for future candidate gene studies to implement strategies that will provide enough statistical power to detect such small effects. One such strategy, examination of refined phenotypes that may reduce heterogeneity, is beginning to bear fruit but more research is needed to extend the work focused on ADHD subtypes (eg, inattentive subtype and HTR1B); comorbid psychopathology or cognitive impairment (eg, depression and SNAP-25, reading disability and ADRA2A), and gene-environment interactions (eg, prenatal or psychosocial risk factors for ADHD and SLC6A3). It is also possible that ADHD genetics research will benefit from the study of endophenotypes such as neuropsychological functioning or brain imaging.[164–166] The ongoing efforts to develop larger collaborative studies with adequate sizes for genome-wide association studies will also be critical in understanding the molecular genetics of ADHD.

ACKNOWLEDGMENTS

The article was adapted from: Mick, E. & Faraone, S. V. (2008). Genetics of attention deficit hyperactivity disorder. Child Adolesc Psychiatr Clin N Am 17, 261–84, vii–viii.

REFERENCES

1. Faraone SV, Sergeant J, Gillberg C, et al. The worldwide prevalence of ADHD: is it an american condition? World Psychiatry 2003;2(2):104–13.
2. Kessler RC, Adler L, Barkley R, et al. The prevalence and correlates of adult ADHD in the United States: results from the national comorbidity survey replication. Am J Psychiatry 2006;163(4):716–23.
3. Faraone SV, Biederman J. Nature, nurture, and attention deficit hyperactivity disorder. Dev Rev 2000;20:568–81.
4. Faraone SV, Biederman J, Spencer TJ, et al. Diagnosing adult attention deficit hyperactivity disorder: are late onset and subthreshold diagnoses valid? Am J Psychiatry 2006;163(10):1720–9.
5. Sprich S, Biederman J, Crawford MH, et al. Adoptive and biological families of children and adolescents with ADHD. J Am Acad Child Adolesc Psychiatry 2000;39(11):1432–7.
6. Cantwell DP. Genetics of hyperactivity. J Child Psychol Psychiatry 1975;16:261–4.
7. Morrison JR, Stewart MA. The psychiatric status of the legal families of adopted hyperactive children. Arch Gen Psychiatry 1973;28(6):888–91.
8. Faraone SV, Perlis RH, Doyle AE, et al. Molecular genetics of attention-deficit/hyperactivity disorder. Biol Psychiatry 2005;57(11):1313–23.
9. Fisher SE, Francks C, McCracken JT, et al. A genomewide scan for loci involved in attention-deficit/hyperactivity disorder. Am J Hum Genet 2002;70(5):1183–96.
10. Smalley SL, Kustanovich V, Minassian SL, et al. Genetic linkage of attention-deficit/hyperactivity disorder on chromosome 16p13, in a region implicated in autism. Am J Hum Genet 2002;71(4):959–63.
11. Bakker SC, van der Meulen EM, Buitelaar JK, et al. A whole-genome scan in 164 Dutch sib pairs with attention-deficit/hyperactivity disorder: suggestive evidence for linkage on chromosomes 7p and 15q. Am J Hum Genet 2003; 72(5):1251–60.
12. Arcos-Burgos M, Castellanos FX, Konecki D, et al. Pedigree disequilibrium test (PDT) replicates association and linkage between DRD4 and ADHD in multigenerational and extended pedigrees from a genetic isolate. Mol Psychiatry 2004; 9(3):252–9.
13. Ogdie MN, Bakker SC, Fisher SE, et al. Pooled genome-wide linkage data on 424 ADHD ASPs suggests genetic heterogeneity and a common risk locus at 5p13. Mol Psychiatry 2006;11(1):5–8.
14. Hebebrand J, Dempfle A, Saar K, et al. A genome-wide scan for attention-deficit/hyperactivity disorder in 155 german sib-pairs. Mol Psychiatry 2006; 11(2):196–205.
15. Faraone SV, Doyle AE, Lasky-Su J, et al. Linkage analysis of attention deficit hyperactivity disorder. Am J Med Genet B Neuropsychiatr Genet 2007; 147B(8):1387–91.

16. Lander E, Kruglyak L. Genetic dissection of complex traits: guidelines for interpreting and reporting linkage results. Nat Genet 1995;11:241–7.

17. Zhou K, Dempfle A, Arcos-Burgos M, et al. Meta-analysis of genome-wide linkage scans of attention deficit hyperactivity disorder. Am J Med Genet B Neuropsychiatr Genet 2008;147(8):1392–8.

18. Li D, Sham PC, Owen MJ, et al. Meta-analysis shows significant association between dopamine system genes and attention deficit hyperactivity disorder (ADHD). Hum Mol Genet 2006;15(14):2276–84.

19. Faraone SV, Doyle AE, Mick E, et al. Meta-analysis of the association between the 7-repeat allele of the dopamine D (4) receptor gene and attention deficit hyperactivity disorder. Am J Psychiatry 2001;158(7):1052–7.

20. Lowe N, Kirley A, Hawi Z, et al. Joint analysis of DRD5 marker concludes association with ADHD confined to the predominantly inattentive and combined subtypes. Am J Hum Genet 2004;74(2):348–56.

21. Yang B, Chan RC, Jing J, et al. A meta-analysis of association studies between the 10-repeat allele of a VNTR polymorphism in the 3'-UTR of dopamine transporter gene and attention deficit hyperactivity disorder. Am J Med Genet B Neuropsychiatr Genet 2007;144B(4):541–50.

22. Purper-Ouakil D, Wohl M, Mouren MC, et al. Meta-analysis of family-based association studies between the dopamine transporter gene and attention deficit hyperactivity disorder. Psychiatr Genet 2005;15(1):53–9.

23. Cheuk DK, Wong V. Meta-analysis of association between a catechol-o-methyltransferase gene polymorphism and attention deficit hyperactivity disorder. Behav Genet 2006;36(5):651–9.

24. Lanau F, Zenner M, Civelli O, et al. Epinephrine and norepinephrine act as potent agonists at the recombinant human dopamine D4 receptor. J Neurochem 1997;68(2):804–12.

25. Faraone SV, Biederman J. Neurobiology of attention-deficit hyperactivity disorder. Biol Psychiatry 1998;44(10):951–8.

26. Van Tol HH, Wu CM, Guan HC, et al. Multiple dopamine D4 receptor variants in the human population. Nature 1992;358(6382):149–52.

27. Asghari V, Sanyal S, Buchwaldt S, et al. Modulation of intracellular cyclic AMP levels by different human dopamine D4 receptor variants. J Neurochem 1995;65(3):1157–65.

28. El-Faddagh M, Laucht M, Maras A, et al. Association of dopamine D4 receptor (DRD4) gene with attention-deficit/hyperactivity disorder (ADHD) in a high-risk community sample: a longitudinal study from birth to 11 years of age. J Neural Transm 2004;111(7):883–9.

29. Bhaduri N, Sinha S, Chattopadhyay A, et al. Analysis of polymorphisms in the dopamine Beta hydroxylase gene: association with attention deficit hyperactivity disorder in Indian children. Indian Pediatr 2005;42(2):123–9.

30. Kim YS, Leventhal BL, Kim SJ, et al. Family-based association study of DAT1 and DRD4 polymorphism in Korean children with ADHD. Neurosci Lett 2005;390(3):176–81.

31. Carrasco X, Rothhammer P, Moraga M, et al. Genotypic interaction between DRD4 and DAT1 loci is a high risk factor for attention-deficit/hyperactivity disorder in Chilean families. Am J Med Genet B Neuropsychiatr Genet 2006;141(1):51–4.

32. McCracken JT, Smalley SL, McGough JJ, et al. Evidence for linkage of a tandem duplication polymorphism upstream of the dopamine D4 receptor gene (DRD4) with attention deficit hyperactivity disorder (ADHD). Mol Psychiatry 2000;5(5):531–6.

33. Kustanovich V, Ishii J, Crawford L, et al. Transmission disequilibrium testing of dopamine-related candidate gene polymorphisms in ADHD: confirmation of association of ADHD with DRD4 and DRD5. Mol Psychiatry 2004;9(7):711–7.

34. Barr CL, Feng Y, Wigg KG, et al. 5'-untranslated region of the dopamine D4 receptor gene and attention-deficit hyperactivity disorder. Am J Med Genet 2001;105(1):84–90.

35. Todd RD, Neuman RJ, Lobos EA, et al. Lack of association of dopamine D4 receptor gene polymorphisms with ADHD subtypes in a population sample of twins. Am J Med Genet 2001;105(5):432–8.

36. Brookes KJ, Xu X, Chen CK, et al. No evidence for the association of DRD4 with ADHD in a Taiwanese population within-family study. BMC Med Genet 2005;6:31.

37. Bhaduri N, Das M, Sinha S, et al. Association of dopamine D4 receptor (DRD4) polymorphisms with attention deficit hyperactivity disorder in Indian population. Am J Med Genet B Neuropsychiatr Genet 2006;141(1):61–6.

38. Lowe N, Kirley A, Mullins C, et al. Multiple marker analysis at the promoter region of the DRD4 gene and ADHD: evidence of linkage and association with the SNP -616. Am J Med Genet 2004;131(1):33–7.

39. Brookes K, Xu X, Chen W, et al. The analysis of 51 genes in DSM-IV combined type attention deficit hyperactivity disorder: association signals in DRD4, DAT1 and 16 other genes. Mol Psychiatry 2006;11(10):934–54.

40. Rowe DC, Stever C, Chase D, et al. Two dopamine genes related to reports of childhood retrospective inattention and conduct disorder symptoms. Mol Psychiatry 2001;6(4):429–33.

41. Levitan RD, Masellis M, Lam RW, et al. Childhood inattention and dysphoria and adult obesity associated with the dopamine D4 receptor gene in overeating women with seasonal affective disorder. Neuropsychopharmacology 2004; 29(1):179–86.

42. Todd RD, Huang H, Smalley SL, et al. Collaborative analysis of DRD4 and DAT genotypes in population-defined ADHD subtypes. J Child Psychol Psychiatry 2005;46(10):1067–73.

43. Mill J, Xu X, Ronald A, et al. Quantitative trait locus analysis of candidate gene alleles associated with attention deficit hyperactivity disorder (ADHD) in five genes: DRD4, DAT1, DRD5, SNAP-25, and 5HT1B. Am J Med Genet B Neuropsychiatr Genet 2005;133B(1):68–73.

44. Swanson J, Oosterlaan J, Murias M, et al. Attention deficit/hyperactivity disorder children with a 7-repeat allele of the dopamine receptor D4 gene have extreme behavior but normal performance on critical neuropsychological tests of attention. Proc Natl Acad Sci U S A 2000;97(9):4754–9.

45. Manor I, Tyano S, Eisenberg J, et al. The short DRD4 repeats confer risk to attention deficit hyperactivity disorder in a family-based design and impair performance on a continuous performance test (TOVA). Mol Psychiatry 2002;7(7):790–4.

46. Bellgrove MA, Hawi Z, Lowe N, et al. DRD4 gene variants and sustained attention in attention deficit hyperactivity disorder (ADHD): effects of associated alleles at the VNTR and -521 SNP. Am J Med Genet B Neuropsychiatr Genet 2005;136(1):81–6.

47. Langley K, Marshall L, van den Bree M, et al. Association of the dopamine D4 receptor gene 7-repeat allele with neuropsychological test performance of children with ADHD. Am J Psychiatry 2004;161(1):133–8.

48. Grady DL, Harxhi A, Smith M, et al. Sequence variants of the DRD4 gene in autism: further evidence that rare DRD4 7R haplotypes are ADHD specific. Am J Med Genet B Neuropsychiatr Genet 2005;136(1):33–5.

49. Lynn DE, Lubke G, Yang M, et al. Temperament and character profiles and the dopamine d4 receptor gene in ADHD. Am J Psychiatry 2005;162(5):906–13.

50. Hawi Z, Lowe N, Kirley A, et al. Linkage disequilibrium mapping at DAT1, DRD5 and DBH narrows the search for ADHD susceptibility alleles at these loci. Mol Psychiatry 2003;8(3):299–308.

51. Spencer T, Biederman J, Wilens T. Pharmacotherapy of attention deficit hyperactivity disorder. Child Adolesc Psychiatr Clin N Am 2000;9(1):77–97.

52. Giros B, Jaber M, Jones SR, et al. Hyperlocomotion and indifference to cocaine and amphetamine in mice lacking the dopamine transporter. Nature 1996; 379(6566):606–12.

53. Gainetdinov RR, Wetsel WC, Jones SR, et al. Role of serotonin in the paradoxical calming effect of psychostimulants on hyperactivity. Science 1999;283: 397–402.

54. Cook EH, Stein MA, Krasowski MD, et al. Association of attention deficit disorder and the dopamine transporter gene. Am J Med Genet 1995;56:993–8.

55. Brookes KJ, Mill J, Guindalini C, et al. A common haplotype of the dopamine transporter gene associated with attention-deficit/hyperactivity disorder and interacting with maternal use of alcohol during pregnancy. Arch Gen Psychiatry 2006;63(1):74–81.

56. Asherson P, Brookes K, Franke B, et al. Confirmation that a specific haplotype of the dopamine transporter gene is associated with combined-type ADHD. Am J Psychiatry 2007;164(4):674–7.

57. Bakker SC, van der Meulen EM, Oteman N, et al. DAT1, DRD4, and DRD5 polymorphisms are not associated with ADHD in Dutch families. Am J Med Genet B Neuropsychiatr Genet 2005;132(1):50–2.

58. Todd RD. Neural development is regulated by classical neurotransmitters: Dopamine D2 receptor stimulation enhances neurite outgrowth. Biol Psychiatry 1992;31:794–807.

59. Neuman RJ, Lobos E, Reich W, et al. Prenatal smoking exposure and dopaminergic genotypes interact to cause a severe ADHD subtype. Biol Psychiatry 2007;61(12):1320–8.

60. Laucht M, Skowronek MH, Becker K, et al. Interacting effects of the dopamine transporter gene and psychosocial adversity on attention-deficit/hyperactivity disorder symptoms among 15-year-olds from a high-risk community sample. Arch Gen Psychiatry 2007;64(5):585–90.

61. Comings DE, Muhleman D, Gysin R. Dopamine D2 receptors (DRD2) gene and susceptibility to posttraumatic stress disorder: a study and replication. Biol Psychiatry 1996;40:368–72.

62. Comings DE, Wu H, Chiu C, et al. Polygenic inheritance of Tourette syndrome, stuttering, attention deficit hyperactivity, conduct and oppositional defiant disorder: the additive and subtractive effect of the three dopaminergic genes - DRD2, DβH and DAT1. Am J Med B Genet Neuropsychiatr Genet 1996;67:264–88.

63. Smith KM, Daly M, Fischer M, et al. Association of the dopamine beta hydroxylase gene with attention deficit hyperactivity disorder: Genetic analysis of the Milwaukee longitudinal study. Am J Med Genet 2003;119(1):77–85.

64. Daly G, Hawi Z, Fitzgerald M, et al. Mapping susceptibility loci in attention deficit hyperactivity disorder: preferential transmission of parental alleles at DAT1, DBH and DRD5 to affected children. Mol Psychiatry 1999;4:192–6.

65. Roman T, Schmitz M, Polanczyk GV, et al. Further evidence for the association between attention- deficit/hyperactivity disorder and the dopamine-beta-hydroxylase gene. Am J Med Genet 2002;114(2):154–8.

66. Wigg K, Zai G, Schachar R, et al. Attention deficit hyperactivity disorder and the gene for dopamine Beta-hydroxylase. Am J Psychiatry 2002;159(6):1046–8.
67. Bhaduri N, Mukhopadhyay K. Lack of significant association between -1021C->T polymorphism in the dopamine beta hydroxylase gene and attention deficit hyperactivity disorder. Neurosci Lett 2006;402(1-2):12–6.
68. Inkster B, Muglia P, Jain U, et al. Linkage disequilibrium analysis of the dopamine beta-hydroxylase gene in persistent attention deficit hyperactivity disorder. Psychiatr Genet 2004;14(2):117–20.
69. Payton A, Holmes J, Barrett JH, et al. Examining for association between candidate gene polymorphisms in the dopamine pathway and attention-deficit hyperactivity disorder: a family- based study. Am J Med Genet 2001;105(5):464–70.
70. Hawi Z, Foley D, Kirley A, et al. Dopa decarboxylase gene polymorphisms and attention deficit hyperactivity disorder (ADHD): no evidence for association in the Irish population. Mol Psychiatry 2001;6(4):420–4.
71. Zhang HB, Wang YF, Li J, et al. [Association between dopamine beta hydroxylase gene and attention deficit hyperactivity disorder complicated with disruptive behavior disorder]. Zhonghua Er Ke Za Zhi 2005;43(1):26–30 [in Chinese].
72. Cases O, Lebrand C, Giros B, et al. Plasma membrane transporters of serotonin, dopamine, and norepinephrine mediate serotonin accumulation in atypical locations in the developing brain of monoamine oxidase A knock-outs. J Neurosci 1998;18(17):6914–27.
73. Manor I, Tyano S, Mel E, et al. Family-based and association studies of monoamine oxidase A and attention deficit hyperactivity disorder (ADHD): preferential transmission of the long promoter-region repeat and its association with impaired performance on a continuous performance test (TOVA). Mol Psychiatry 2002;7(6):626–32.
74. Lawson DC, Turic D, Langley K, et al. Association analysis of monoamine oxidase A and attention deficit hyperactivity disorder. Am J Med Genet 2003;116(1):84–9.
75. Jiang S, Xin R, Lin S, et al. Linkage studies between attention-deficit hyperactivity disorder and the monoamine oxidase genes. Am J Med Genet 2001; 105(8):783–8.
76. Domschke K, Sheehan K, Lowe N, et al. Association analysis of the monoamine oxidase A and B genes with attention deficit hyperactivity disorder (ADHD) in an Irish sample: Preferential transmission of the MAO-A 941G allele to affected children. Am J Med Genet B Neuropsychiatr Genet 2005;134(1):110–4.
77. Xu X, Brookes K, Chen CK, et al. Association study between the monoamine oxidase A gene and attention deficit hyperactivity disorder in Taiwanese samples. BMC Psychiatry 2007;7(1):10.
78. Comings DE, Comings BG, Muhleman D, et al. The dopamine D2 receptor locus as a modifying gene in neuropsychiatric disorders. JAMA 1991;266(13):1793–800.
79. Sery O, Dritilkova I, Theiner P, et al. Polymorphism of DRD2 gene and ADHD. Neuro Endocrinol Lett 2006;27(1-2):236–40.
80. Kim JW, Park CS, Hwang JW, et al. Clinical and genetic characteristics of Korean male alcoholics with and without attention deficit hyperactivity disorder. Alcohol Alcohol 2006;41(4):407–11.
81. Rowe DC, den Oord EJ, Stever C, et al. The DRD2 TaqI polymorphism and symptoms of attention deficit hyperactivity disorder. Mol Psychiatry 1999;4(6):580–6.
82. Huang YS, Lin SK, Wu YY, et al. A family-based association study of attention-deficit hyperactivity disorder and dopamine D2 receptor TaqI A alleles. Chang Gung Med J 2003;26(12):897–903.

83. Kirley A, Hawi Z, Daly G, et al. Dopaminergic system genes in ADHD: toward a biological hypothesis. Neuropsychopharmacology 2002;27(4):607–19.

84. Barr CL, Wigg KG, Wu J, et al. Linkage study of two polymorphisms at the dopamine D3 receptor gene and attention-deficit hyperactivity disorder. Am J Med Genet 2000;96(1):114–7.

85. Muglia P, Jain U, Kennedy JL. A transmission disequilibrium test of the Ser9/Gly dopamine D3 receptor gene polymorphism in adult attention-deficit hyperactivity disorder. Behav Brain Res 2002;130(1-2):91–5.

86. Comings DE, Gade-Andavolu R, Gonzalez N, et al. Comparison of the role of dopamine, serotonin, and noradrenaline genes in ADHD, ODD and conduct disorder: multivariate regression analysis of 20 genes. Clin Genet 2000;57(3):178–96.

87. Retz W, Rosler M, Supprian T, et al. Dopamine D3 receptor gene polymorphism and violent behavior: relation to impulsiveness and ADHD-related psychopathology. J Neural Transm 2003;110(5):561–72.

88. Syvanen AC, Tilgmann C, Rinne J, et al. Genetic polymorphism of catechol-O-methyltransferase (COMT): correlation of genotype with individual variation of S-COMT activity and comparison of the allele frequencies in the normal population and parkinsonian patients in Finland. Pharmacogenetics 1997;7(1):65–71.

89. Reuter M, Kirsch P, Hennig J. Inferring candidate genes for Attention Deficit Hyperactivity Disorder (ADHD) assessed by the World Health Organization Adult ADHD Self-Report Scale (ASRS). J Neural Transm 2006;113(7):929–38.

90. Gothelf D, Michaelovsky E, Frisch A, et al. Association of the low-activity COMT 158 Met allele with ADHD and OCD in subjects with velocardiofacial syndrome. Int J Neuropsychopharmacol 2007;10(3):301–8.

91. Brookes KJ, Knight J, Xu X, et al. DNA pooling analysis of ADHD and genes regulating vesicle release of neurotransmitters. Am J Med Genet B Neuropsychiatr Genet 2005;139B(1):33–7.

92. Dasbanerjee T, Middleton FA, Berger DF, et al. A comparison of molecular alterations in environmental and genetic rat models of ADHD: a pilot study. Am J Med Genet B Neuropsychiatr Genet 2008;147(8):1554–63.

93. Comings DE, Gonzalez NS, Cheng Li SC, et al. A "line item" approach to the identification of genes involved in polygenic behavioral disorders: the adrenergic alpha2A (ADRA2A) gene. Am J Med Genet 2003;118(1):110–4.

94. Xu C, Schachar R, Tannock R, et al. Linkage study of the alpha2A adrenergic receptor in attention-deficit hyperactivity disorder families. Am J Med Genet 2001;105(2):159–62.

95. Roman T, Schmitz M, Polanczyk GV, et al. Is the alpha-2A adrenergic receptor gene (ADRA2A) associated with attention-deficit/hyperactivity disorder? Am J Med Genet 2003;120(1):116–20.

96. Park L, Nigg JT, Waldman ID, et al. Association and linkage of alpha-2A adrenergic receptor gene polymorphisms with childhood ADHD. Mol Psychiatry 2005; 10(6):572–80.

97. Schmitz M, Denardin D, Silva TL, et al. Association between alpha-2a-adrenergic receptor gene and ADHD inattentive type. Biol Psychiatry 2006;60(10):1028–33.

98. Stevenson J, Asherson P, Hay D, et al. Characterizing the ADHD phenotype for genetic studies. Dev Sci 2005;8(2):115–21.

99. Wang B, Wang Y, Zhou R, et al. Possible association of the alpha-2A adrenergic receptor gene (ADRA2A) with symptoms of attention-deficit/hyperactivity disorder. Am J Med Genet B Neuropsychiatr Genet 2006;141(2):130–4.

100. Deupree JD, Smith SD, Kratochvil CJ, et al. Possible involvement of alpha-2A adrenergic receptors in attention deficit hyperactivity disorder: Radioligand

binding and polymorphism studies. Am J Med Genet B Neuropsychiatr Genet 2006;141(8):877–84.

101. Roman T, Polanczyk GV, Zeni C, et al. Further evidence of the involvement of alpha-2A-adrenergic receptor gene (ADRA2A) in inattentive dimensional scores of attention-deficit/hyperactivity disorder. Mol Psychiatry 2006;11(1):8–10.

102. Waldman ID, Nigg JT, Gizer IR, et al. The adrenergic receptor alpha-2A gene (ADRA2A) and neuropsychological executive functions as putative endopheno-types for childhood ADHD. Cogn Affect Behav Neurosci 2006;6(1):18–30.

103. Safford SM, Kendall PC, Flannery-Schroeder E, et al. A longitudinal look at parent-child diagnostic agreement in youth treated for anxiety disorders. J Clin Child Adolesc Psychol 2005;34(4):747–57.

104. Comings D, Gade-Andavolu R, Gonzalez N, et al. Additive effect of three nara-denergic genes (ADRA2A, ADRA2C, DBH) on attention-defecit hyperactivity disorder and learning disabilities an Tourette syndrome subjects. Clin Genet 1999;55(3):160–72.

105. Barr CL, Wigg K, Zai G, et al. Attention-deficit hyperactivity disorder and the adrenergic receptors alpha1C and alpha2C. Mol Psychiatry 2001;6(3):334–7.

106. De Luca V, Muglia P, Vincent JB, et al. Adrenergic alpha 2C receptor genomic organization: association study in adult ADHD. Am J Med Genet B Neuro-psychiatr Genet 2004;127B(1):65–7.

107. Biederman J, Spencer T. Non-stimulant treatments for ADHD. Eur Child Adolesc Psychiatry 2000;9(Suppl 1):I51–9.

108. Barr CL, Kroft J, Feng Y, et al. The norepinephrine transporter gene and atten-tion-deficit hyperactivity disorder. Am J Med Genet 2002;114(3):255–9.

109. McEvoy B, Hawi Z, Fitzgerald M, et al. No evidence of linkage or association between the norepinephrine transporter (NET) gene polymorphisms and ADHD in the Irish population. Am J Med Genet 2002;114(6):665–6.

110. Xu X, Knight J, Brookes K, et al. DNA pooling analysis of 21 norepinephrine transporter gene SNPs with attention deficit hyperactivity disorder: no evidence for association. Am J Med Genet B Neuropsychiatr Genet 2005;134(1):115–8.

111. Bobb AJ, Addington AM, Sidransky E, et al. Support for association between ADHD and two candidate genes: NET1 and DRD1. Am J Med Genet B Neuro-psychiatr Genet 2005;134(1):67–72.

112. Kim CH, Hahn MK, Joung Y, et al. A polymorphism in the norepinephrine trans-porter gene alters promoter activity and is associated with attention-deficit hyperactivity disorder. Proc Natl Acad Sci U S A 2006;103(50):19164–9.

113. Hawi Z, Dring M, Kirley A, et al. Serotonergic system and attention deficit hyper-activity disorder (ADHD): a potential susceptibility locus at the 5-HT(1B) receptor gene in 273 nuclear families from a multi-centre sample. Mol Psychiatry 2002;7(7):718–25.

114. Quist JF, Barr CL, Schachar R, et al. The serotonin 5-HT1B receptor gene and attention deficit hyperactivity disorder. Mol Psychiatry 2003;8(1):98–102.

115. Smoller JW, Biederman J, Arbeitman L, et al. Association between the 5HT1B Receptor Gene (HTR1B) and the Inattentive Subtype of ADHD. Biol Psychiatry 2006;59(5):460–7.

116. Heiser P, Dempfle A, Friedel S, et al. Family-based association study of seroto-nergic candidate genes and attention-deficit/hyperactivity disorder in a German sample. J Neural Transm 2007;114(4):513–21.

117. Li J, Wang Y, Zhou R, et al. Serotonin 5-HT1B receptor gene and attention deficit hyperactivity disorder in Chinese Han subjects. Am J Med Genet B Neuro-psychiatr Genet 2005;132B(1):59–63.

118. Quist JF, Barr CL, Schachar R, et al. Evidence for the serotonin HTR2A receptor gene as a susceptibility factor in attention deficit hyperactivity disorder (ADHD). Mol Psychiatry 2000;5(5):537–41.
119. Zoroglu SS, Erdal ME, Alasehirli B, et al. Significance of serotonin transporter gene 5-HTTLPR and variable number of tandem repeat polymorphism in attention deficit hyperactivity disorder. Neuropsychobiology 2002;45(4):176–81.
120. Li J, Wang Y, Zhou R, et al. No association of attention-deficit/hyperactivity disorder with genes of the serotonergic pathway in Han Chinese subjects. Neurosci Lett 2006;403(1–2):172–5.
121. Li J, Kang C, Wang Y, et al. Contribution of 5-HT2A receptor gene -1438A>G polymorphism to outcome of attention-deficit/hyperactivity disorder in adolescents. Am J Med Genet B Neuropsychiatr Genet 2006;141B(5):473–6.
122. Guimaraes AP, Zeni C, Polanczyk GV, et al. Serotonin genes and attention deficit/hyperactivity disorder in a Brazilian sample: Preferential transmission of the HTR2A 452His allele to affected boys. Am J Med Genet B Neuropsychiatr Genet 2007;144(1):69–73.
123. Levitan R, Masellis M, Basile V, et al. Polymorphism of the serotonin-2A receptor gene (HTR2A) associated with childhood attention deficit hyperactivity disorder (ADHD) in adult women with seasonal affective disorder. J Affect Disord 2002; 71(1–3):229–33.
124. Li J, Wang Y, Zhou R, et al. Association between polymorphisms in serotonin 2C receptor gene and attention-deficit/hyperactivity disorder in Han Chinese subjects. Neurosci Lett 2006;407(2):107–11.
125. Li J, Wang Y, Zhou R, et al. Association of attention-deficit/hyperactivity disorder with serotonin 4 receptor gene polymorphisms in Han Chinese subjects. Neurosci Lett 2006;401(1–2):6–9.
126. Li J, Zhang X, Wang Y, et al. The serotonin 5-HT1D receptor gene and attention-deficit hyperactivity disorder in Chinese Han subjects. Am J Med Genet B Neuropsychiatr Genet 2006;141(8):874–6.
127. Anguelova M, Benkelfat C, Turecki G. A systematic review of association studies investigating genes coding for serotonin receptors and the serotonin transporter: I. Affective disorders. Mol Psychiatry 2003;8(6):574–91.
128. Anguelova M, Benkelfat C, Turecki G. A systematic review of association studies investigating genes coding for serotonin receptors and the serotonin transporter: II. Suicidal behavior. Mol Psychiatry 2003;8(7):646–53.
129. Curran S, Purcell S, Craig I, et al. The serotonin transporter gene as a QTL for ADHD. Am J Med Genet B Neuropsychiatr Genet 2005;134(1):42–7.
130. Kim SJ, Badner J, Cheon KA, et al. Family-based association study of the serotonin transporter gene polymorphisms in Korean ADHD trios. Am J Med Genet B Neuropsychiatr Genet 2005;139(1):14–8.
131. Xu X, Mill J, Chen CK, et al. Family-based association study of serotonin transporter gene polymorphisms in attention deficit hyperactivity disorder: no evidence for association in UK and Taiwanese samples. Am J Med Genet B Neuropsychiatr Genet 2005;139(1):11–3.
132. Xu M, Hu XT, Copper DC, et al. Elimination of cocaine-induced hyperactivity and dopamine-mediated neurophysiological effects in dopamine D1 receptor mutant mice [see comments]. Cell 1994;79(6):945–55.
133. Banerjee E, Sinha S, Chatterjee A, et al. A family-based study of Indian subjects from Kolkata reveals allelic association of the serotonin transporter intron-2 (STin2) polymorphism and attention-deficit-hyperactivity disorder (ADHD). Am J Med Genet B Neuropsychiatr Genet 2006;141(4):361–6.

134. Wigg KG, Takhar A, Ickowicz A, et al. Gene for the serotonin transporter and ADHD: No association with two functional polymorphisms. Am J Med Genet B Neuropsychiatr Genet 2006;141B(6):566–70.
135. Li J, Wang Y, Zhou R, et al. Association between polymorphisms in serotonin transporter gene and attention deficit hyperactivity disorder in Chinese Han subjects. Am J Med Genet B Neuropsychiatr Genet 2007;144(1):14–9.
136. Manuck SB, Flory JD, Ferrell RE, et al. Aggression and anger-related traits associated with a polymorphism of the tryptophan hydroxylase gene. Biol Psychiatry 1999;45(5):603–14.
137. Tang G, Ren D, Xin R, et al. Lack of association between the tryptophan hydroxylase gene A218C polymorphism and attention-deficit hyperactivity disorder in Chinese Han population. Am J Med Genet 2001;105(6):485–8.
138. Li J, Wang YF, Zhou RL, et al. [Association between tryptophan hydroxylase gene polymorphisms and attention deficit hyperactivity disorder with or without learning disorder]. Zhonghua Yi Xue Za Zhi 2003;83(24):2114–8 [in Chinese].
139. Li J, Wang Y, Zhou R, et al. Association between tryptophan hydroxylase gene polymorphisms and attention deficit hyperactivity disorder in Chinese Han population. Am J Med Genet B Neuropsychiatr Genet 2006;141:126–9.
140. Sheehan K, Lowe N, Kirley A, et al. Tryptophan hydroxylase 2 (TPH2) gene variants associated with ADHD. Mol Psychiatry 2005;10(10):944–9.
141. Walitza S, Renner TJ, Dempfle A, et al. Transmission disequilibrium of polymorphic variants in the tryptophan hydroxylase-2 gene in attention-deficit/hyperactivity disorder. Mol Psychiatry 2005;10(12):1126–32.
142. Sheehan K, Hawi Z, Gill M, et al. No association between TPH2 gene polymorphisms and ADHD in a UK sample. Neurosci Lett 2007;412(2):105–7.
143. Wilson MC. Coloboma mouse mutant as an animal model of hyperkinesis and attention deficit hyperactivity disorder. Neurosci Biobehav Rev 2000;24(1): 51–7.
144. Barr CL, Feng Y, Wigg K, et al. Identification of DNA variants in the SNAP-25 gene and linkage study of these polymorphisms and attention-deficit hyperactivity disorder. Mol Psychiatry 2000;5(4):405–9.
145. Brophy K, Hawi Z, Kirley A, et al. Synaptosomal-associated protein 25 (SNAP-25) and attention deficit hyperactivity disorder (ADHD): evidence of linkage and association in the Irish population. Mol Psychiatry 2002;7(8):913–7.
146. Kustanovich V, Merriman V, McGough J, et al. Biased paternal transmission of SNAP-25 risk alleles in attention-deficit hyperactivity disorder. Mol Psychiatry 2003;8(3):309–15.
147. Mill J, Curran S, Kent L, et al. Association study of a SNAP-25 microsatellite and attention deficit hyperactivity disorder. Am J Med Genet 2002;114(3): 269–71.
148. Mill J, Richards S, Knight J, et al. Haplotype analysis of SNAP-25 suggests a role in the aetiology of ADHD. Mol Psychiatry 2004;9(8):801–10.
149. Feng Y, Crosbie J, Wigg K, et al. The SNAP25 gene as a susceptibility gene contributing to attention-deficit hyperactivity disorder. Mol Psychiatry 2005; 10(11):998–1005, 973.
150. Kim JW, Biederman J, Arbeitman L, et al. Investigation of variation in SNAP-25 and ADHD and relationship to co-morbid major depressive disorder. Am J Med Genet B Neuropsychiatr Genet 2007;144B(6):781–90.
151. Comings DE, Gade-Andavolu R, Gonzalez N, et al. Multivariate analysis of associations of 42 genes in ADHD, ODD and conduct disorder. Clin Genet 2000; 58(1):31–40.

152. Kent L, Middle F, Hawi Z, et al. Nicotinic acetylcholine receptor alpha4 subunit gene polymorphism and attention deficit hyperactivity disorder. Psychiatr Genet 2001;11(1):37–40.
153. Todd RD, Lobos EA, Sun LW, et al. Mutational analysis of the nicotinic acetylcholine receptor alpha 4 subunit gene in attention deficit/hyperactivity disorder: evidence for association of an intronic polymorphism with attention problems. Mol Psychiatry 2003;8(1):103–8.
154. Lee J, Laurin N, Crosbie J, et al. Association study of the nicotinic acetylcholine receptor alpha4 subunit gene, CHRNA4, in attention-deficit hyperactivity disorder. Genes Brain Behav 2008;7(1):53–60.
155. Turic D, Langley K, Mills S, et al. Follow-up of genetic linkage findings on chromosome 16p13: evidence of association of N-methyl-D aspartate glutamate receptor 2A gene polymorphism with ADHD. Mol Psychiatry 2004;9(2):169–73.
156. Adams J, Crosbie J, Wigg K, et al. Glutamate receptor, ionotropic, N-methyl D-aspartate 2A (GRIN2A) gene as a positional candidate for attention-deficit/hyperactivity disorder in the 16p13 region. Mol Psychiatry 2004;9(5):494–9.
157. Egan MF, Kojima M, Callicott JH, et al. The BDNF val66met polymorphism affects activity-dependent secretion of BDNF and human memory and hippocampal function. Cell 2003;112(2):257–69.
158. Kent L, Green E, Hawi Z, et al. Association of the paternally transmitted copy of common Valine allele of the Val66Met polymorphism of the brain-derived neurotrophic factor (BDNF) gene with susceptibility to ADHD. Mol Psychiatry 2005; 10(10):939–43.
159. Xu X, Mill J, Zhou K, et al. Family-based association study between brain-derived neurotrophic factor gene polymorphisms and attention deficit hyperactivity disorder in UK and Taiwanese samples. Am J Med Genet B Neuropsychiatr Genet 2007;144(1):83–6.
160. Neale BM, Lasky-Su J, Anney R, et al. Genome-wide association scan of attention deficit hyperactivity disorder. Am J Med Genet B Neuropsychiatr Genet 2008;147(8):1337–44.
161. Lasky-Su J, Anney RJ, Neale BM, et al. Genome-wide association scan of the time to onset of attention deficit hyperactivity disorder. Am J Med Genet B Neuropsychiatr Genet 2008;147(8):1355–8.
162. Lasky-Su J, Neale BM, Franke B, et al. Genome-wide association scan of quantitative traits for attention deficit hyperactivity disorder identifies novel associations and confirms candidate gene associations. Am J Med Genet B Neuropsychiatr Genet 2008;147(8):1345–54.
163. Lesch KP, Timmesfeld N, Renner TJ, et al. Molecular genetics of adult ADHD: converging evidence from genome-wide association and extended pedigree linkage studies. J Neural Transm 2008;115(11):1573–85.
164. Doyle AE, Faraone SV, Seidman LJ, et al. Are endophenotypes based on measures of executive functions useful for molecular genetic studies of ADHD? J Child Psychol Psychiatry 2005;46(7):774–803.
165. Doyle AE, Willcutt EG, Seidman LJ, et al. Attention-deficit/hyperactivity disorder endophenotypes. Biol Psychiatry 2005;57(11):1324–35.
166. Rommelse NN, Arias-Vasquez A, Altink ME, et al. Neuropsychological endophenotype approach to genome-wide linkage analysis identifies susceptibility loci for ADHD on 2q21.1 and 13q12.11. Am J Hum Genet 2008;83(1):99–105.

The Promise and Reality of Pharmacogenetics in Psychiatry

Peter P. Zandi, PhD*, Jennifer T. Judy, MS

KEYWORDS

- Pharmacogenetics • Pharmacogenomics • Antidepressants
- Antipsychotics • Mood stabilizers
- Genome-wide association study • Efficacy • Side effects

The primary means of treating mental illnesses is with an arsenal of psychotropic medications, including antidepressants, antipsychotics, and mood stabilizers. Despite progress over the past several decades in developing new classes of such medications that are presumably safer and more effective, the ability to treat mental illnesses remains clinically suboptimal. These medications are effective in only a subset of patients or produce partial responses, and they are often associated with debilitating side effects that discourage adherence.[1]

The results from the latest and largest treatment effectiveness trials of psychotropic medications sponsored by the National Institute of Mental Health reinforce the notion that there is still a long way to go in the war against mental illnesses. In the recently completed Sequenced Treatment Alternatives to Relieve Depression (STAR*D) study in which patients with nonpsychotic major depression were followed for up to 6 years through a sequence of alternative treatment regimens, only 37% achieved remission on first-line therapy with a selective serotonin reuptake inhibitor (SSRI), whereas another 16.3% withdrew completely from treatment because of drug intolerance.[2] Even worse, in the Clinical Antipsychotic Trials of Intervention Effectiveness (CATIE) in which patients with schizophrenia were treated with a menu of leading antipsychotics under conditions meant to reflect realistic clinical practice and followed for up to 18 months, over 74% eventually discontinued their study medication either because of lack of efficacy or tolerability.[3] Similarly, in the Systematic Treatment Enhancement Program for Bipolar Disorder (STEP-BD) trial in which patients with bipolar disorder were enrolled and provided treatments with mood stabilizers and

The work of Peter P. Zandi is supported by National Institute of Mental Health grant K01 MH072866-01. The work of Jennifer T. Judy is supported by National Institute of Mental Health grant T32-MH14592.

Department of Mental Health, Johns Hopkins Bloomberg School of Public Health, Hampton House, Room 857, 624 North Broadway, Baltimore, MD 21205, USA

* Corresponding author.

E-mail address: pzandi@jhsph.edu (P.P. Zandi).

antidepressants that followed expert consensus guidelines, up to 75% experienced symptom relapse sometime over the course of follow-up.[4] These figures are sobering and suggest considerable room for improvement in psychiatric treatments.

With the advent of the genomics revolution, there has been growing excitement that pharmacogenetics can pave the way to improved treatments. The term "pharmacogenetics" was first coined nearly a half century ago when it was recognized that inherited variation can influence responses to medications.[5] Since then, an evergrowing number of pharmacogenetic traits have been studied. Earlier studies focused on variation in candidate genes or gene systems believed to influence the absorption, distribution, or clearance of drugs (ie, pharmacokinetics) or mediate their mechanisms of actions by interactions with receptors or transporters and downstream second messengers (ie, pharmacodynamics). Completion of the Human Genome Project and the emergence of new tools to interrogate the entire genome on an unprecedented scale, however, have accelerated interest in studying the relevance of variation across the entire genome. These advances have spawned a new term, "pharmacogenomics." Pharmacogenomics and pharmacogenetics are used interchangeably, and in both cases refer to the study of how genetic variation influences response to drug treatments in terms of efficacy (ie, efficacy pharmacogenetics) or tolerability (ie, safety pharmacogenetics).

The hope is that through pharmacogenetics genetic profiles will be discovered that can be determined by simple genetic tests and that predict how patients respond to different psychotropic treatments before they are initiated. The benefits are that it would allow physicians to tailor medications to their patients in such a way that maximizes their efficacy and tolerability, ushering in an era of "personalized medicine." In addition, by elucidating the pathways by which drugs act to treat illness and provoke unwanted side effects, pharmacogenetics may inform the rational development of new treatments that are ever more safe and efficacious. The promise of pharmacogenetics in psychiatry is that it will lead to the smarter use of existing weapons and, in turn, the development of even smarter weapons to combat mental illness.

There is still a long way to go before the promise becomes a reality. This article reviews the progress that has been made in research toward understanding how genetic factors influence psychotropic drug response and the challenges that lie ahead in translating the research findings into clinical practice that yields tangible benefits for patients. Discussed are antidepressants, mood stabilizers, and antipsychotics, and for each are reviewed the pharmacogenetic studies that have been performed on them, including candidate gene studies of pharmacokinetic or pharmacodynamic factors and genome-wide studies. Next the few examples of pharmacogenetic biomarkers and corresponding tests that have begun to penetrate into clinical practice in psychiatry are examined and their impact on patient care assessed. The article concludes with a discussion of the challenges to advancing the goals of personalized care in psychiatry.

ANTIDEPRESSANTS

The monoamine oxidase inhibitors and tricyclics were the first antidepressants introduced, back in the 1950s. They heralded a major breakthrough in the treatment of depression, but their wider use was limited by partial efficacy and significant concerns about side effects, such as sedation.[6] In the late 1980s a new class of antidepressants became available known as the "selective serotonin reuptake inhibitors." Because of their improved efficacy and tolerability, the SSRIs quickly gained popularity and are now the most widely used antidepressants.[7] They are among the first-line choices for the treatment of depression,[8,9] but they are still only effective in a subset of patients[10] and are associated with certain common side effects, such as weight gain, insomnia, and sexual dysfunction, which are leading causes of nonadherence.[11] More recently, a number of other new classes of antidepressants have been introduced with mixed pharmacodynamic profiles. These include serotonin-norepinephrine reuptake inhibitors, the dopamine-norepinephrine reuptake inhibitors, serotonin modulators, norepinephrine-serotonin modulators, and selective norepinephrine reuptake inhibitors.

Overview of Pharmacogenetic Studies

At least 119 pharmacogenetic studies of candidate genes and the efficacy or tolerability of treatment with antidepressants have been reported in the literature.[12–130] Most of these have studied SSRIs, although several have examined serotonin-norepinephrine reuptake inhibitors or other older agents, such as the monoamine oxidase inhibitors or tricyclics. Approximately 65% of the studies have been on samples of whites, whereas the remaining studies have mostly studied Asian samples, including Chinese, Japanese, or Korean. The samples sizes have been generally small with a median of less than 150 subjects, and each of the studies have investigated no more than a handful of specific candidate gene polymorphisms at a time. The exceptions to this include several reports[71,87,90,97,108,115,123,124,127] from STAR*D in which pharmacogenetic studies with over 1900 subjects who provided a DNA sample have been performed to examine the association between a number of different candidate genes and treatment response to citalopram, including efficacy, treatment-emergent suicide ideation, and sexual dysfunction. In addition to these studies, three genome-wide association studies of antidepressant treatment response have recently been reported in the literature.[131–133] **Table 1** provides a description of candidate genes studies from STAR*D and genome-wide association studies of treatment responses to antidepressants.

Pharmacokinetic Studies

Multiple pharmacogenetic studies have been performed on the relationship between genes coding for CYP450 enzymes, which are involved in the metabolism of many different xenobiotics, and antidepressant treatment responses. CYP2D6 and CYP2C19, which together with CYP2C9 metabolize virtually all SSRIs,[134] have received the greatest attention.

CYP2D6 is constitutively expressed in the liver and is responsible for metabolizing approximately 25% of drugs known to be metabolized by CYP450 enzymes.[135] It is the key enzyme in the metabolic pathway of many antidepressants.[136] Because CYP2D6 is not inducible,[137] functional genetic variation and "environmental" inhibitors of the enzyme are the only factors that can modify its activity, making it a good candidate for pharmacogenetic testing.[138] Over 90 genetic variants have been identified in CYP2D6.[139] These variants have been functionally classified into four phenotypic groups based on their effects on enzyme activity: (1) poor metabolizers (PMs), (2) intermediate metabolizers (IMs), (3) extensive metabolizers (EMs), and (4) ultrarapid metabolizers (UMs). There are considerable differences in the frequencies of these classes across racial and ethnic groups.[138] CYP2C19 is also polymorphic with two main phenotypic groups: EMs and the rarer PMs.[138]

The contention is that CYP-related PMs are at an increased risk of side effects from antidepressants, whereas UMs and to a lesser extent IMs are less likely to show positive response to treatment.[138] A commercially available pharmacogenetic test has been clinically approved to test for the CYP2D6 and CYP2C19 genetic variants based

Table 1
Candidate gene studies from STAR*D and genome-wide association studies of treatment responses to antidepressants

Author (Year)	Drug	Genes	Outcome	Sample Size	Key Findings
*Candidate gene studies from STAR*D*					
McMahon (2006)	Citalopram	68 genes	Efficacy	1953 (split sample design)	Association with *5-HTR2A*
Hu (2007)	Citalopram	*5-HTT*	Efficacy Remission Tolerance Adverse effects	1775	Association with adverse effect burden
Kraft (2007)	Citalopram	*5-HTT*	Efficacy	1914	No association
Paddock (2007)	Citalopram	68 genes	Efficacy	1816 (full sample)	Association with *GRIK4*
Peters (2008)	Citalopram	*CYP2D6, CYP2C19, CYP3A4, CYP3A5, ABCB1*	Efficacy Tolerance	1953 (split sample design)	No associations
Lekman (2008)	Citalopram	*FKBP5*	Efficacy	1809	Association with response
Cabanero (2009)	Citalopram	*PDE11A, PDE1A, PDE9A*	Efficacy	1914	No association
Domschke (2009)	Citalopram	*BDNF*	Efficacy	1914	No association
Perlis (2009)	Citalopram	68 genes	Sexual dysfunction	1473	Associations with *GRIA3, GRIK2, GRIA1, GRIN3A*
Genome-wide association studies					
Laje (2009)	Citalopram	Illumina Human-1 Bead Chip	Treatment-emergent suicidal ideation	180	Association with *PAPLN*
Garriock (2009)	Citalopram	Affymetrix 500K and 5.0	Efficacy	1491	Suggestive associations with *UBE3C, BMP7, RORA*
Ising (2009)	Antidepressants	Illumina Human-1 and HumanHap300 Bead Chips	Efficacy	339	Association with a multifactorial SNP score

Abbreviation: SNP, single nucleotide polymorphism.

on this characterization.[140] At least 13 different studies have examined the relationship between variation in these genes and treatment response to antidepressants,[12,22,24,39,40,48,54,55,59,75,82,83,108] however, and the results have been decidedly mixed. The largest study from STAR*D included 1877 genotyped subjects and found no association between variation in *CYP2D6* or *CYP2C19* and either efficacy or tolerability.[108] Moreover, a recent review of existing studies found little overall evidence of an association between these two CYP450 genes and antidepressant response, calling into question the clinical use of testing for these variants.[141] The commercially available pharmacogenetic test and its potential use in clinic practice are discussed in further detail later.

Pharmacodynamic Studies

The therapeutic action of antidepressants is thought to be mediated at least partially through their effects on monoaminergic transmission and primarily the serotonergic pathway. Consequently, genes in the serotonergic pathway have been of great interest in pharmacogenetic studies of antidepressants. *5HTT*, which codes for the presynaptic membrane-bound serotonin transporter protein that is the target of SSRIs, is of these by far the most widely studied. It has a variable length repeat polymorphism in the promoter region (5HTTLPR), in which a 44-bp long stretch of DNA is either present in the "long" form of the gene or absent in the "short" form. Experimental data suggest the long form is associated with greater expression of the gene,[142] although recent findings have suggested this locus may actually be triallelic because of the presence of a single nucleotide polymorphism (SNP) nearby, which leads to further variability in the effect on gene expression.[143] Other common variants are found in the gene, including a variable number of tandem repeats in intron 2 (STin2), which has been shown to influence gene transcription[144] and has also been examined in multiple pharmacogenetic studies.

A systematic review of pharmacogenetic studies of antidepressants[145,146] was recently reported in which the published associations between treatment response and these two well-characterized *5HTT* variants were comprehensively examined. In this review, a meta-analysis of 15 studies[13–16,21,27,28,34,37,38,44,49,73,74,88] showed the long allele of the promoter polymorphism was associated with better response and remission rates, whereas another meta-analysis of nine studies[35,41,46,74,81,87,100,118,121] indicated the long allele was also associated with lower rates of side effects. The review of studies on the intronic variant was less clear, although a meta-analysis of seven studies[14,30,51,73,84,110,121] suggested an influence on efficacy, particularly among Asians. Enthusiasm for these findings is dampened by the fact that another study[90] from the STAR*D trial found no evidence of an association between any variants in *5HTT* and treatment outcomes, despite having one of the largest samples to test the relationship.

The systematic review[146] also examined variants in 16 other candidate genes thought to play a role in the pharmacodynamics of antidepressants and reported on by at least two different studies. Of these, variants in four of the genes were found on meta-analysis to be significantly associated with either efficacy or side effects. The four genes are (1) *5HT1A*, (2) *5HT2A*, (3) *TPH1*, and (4) *BDNF*. *5HT1A* and *5HT2A* code for serotonin receptors that are the targets of certain antidepressants and atypical antipsychotics. Interestingly, an association between *5HT2A* and antidepressant efficacy was one of the leading pharmacogenetic findings from STAR*D.[71] *TPH1* codes for tryptophan hydroxylase, which is the rate-limiting enzyme in the biosynthesis of serotonin. It is more commonly expressed in the periphery,[147] but there is some evidence from the mouse that it is also expressed in the brain during the late developmental stages.[148] *BDNF* is a neurotrophic factor that is involved in the development, survival, and functional maintenance of neurons.[149]

Genome-wide Studies

Three genome-wide association studies of antidepressant response have been published.[131–133] In the first study[131] 90 whites who developed treatment-emergent suicidal ideation with citalopram in STAR*D and an equal number of gender- and race-matched treated controls were genotyped at 109,365 SNPs on the Illumina Human-1 BeadChip (Illumina Inc, San Diego, CA, USA). One marker was significant after correction for multiple testing in the gene *PAPLN*. This gene encodes a proteoglycan-like sulfated glycoprotein, but little else is known about its function and potential relevance to treatment-emergent suicidal ideation.

The second study[132] examined efficacy responses to citalopram in 1491 STAR*D subjects who were genotyped at 430,198 SNPs with the Affymetrix (Santa Clara, CA, USA) 500K and 5.0 platforms. No SNPs met criteria for genome-wide significance, but there were three with suggestive evidence in or near the genes *UBE3C*, *BMP7*, and *RORA*. The biological relevance of these genes to treatment response is not immediately obvious.

The most recent study[133] was performed in the Munich Antidepressant Response Signature project in which patients who were treated with antidepressants according to the choice of their physicians were naturalistically followed for efficacy response. A total of 339 patients were genotyped on almost 410,000 nonoverlapping SNPs with the Illumina Sentrix Human-1 and HumanHap300 BeadChip arrays. A multilocus genetic variable that described the individual number of alleles of select SNPs associated with beneficial treatment outcome was constructed and then dichotomized. The dichotomized variable describing carriers with high and low number of response alleles was associated with positive outcome in the Munich Antidepressant Response Signature sample and in a replication sample derived from STAR*D. This finding suggests that treatment response may be multifactorial and under the control of a number of additive genetic loci instead of a limited number with large effects.

MOOD STABILIZERS

The leading mood stabilizers include lithium and the anticonvulsants, such as valproate, carbamazepine, and lamotrigine. Lithium has been a remarkably successful drug, but its introduction into psychiatry has had a complicated and somewhat controversial history.[150] Its use in practice dates back to the mid-nineteenth century, but it was not until the 1970s that it was finally approved in the United States for the treatment and prophylaxis of mania. Considerable evidence has accumulated since then about the positive benefits of lithium,[151] yet it lacks universal effectiveness and can provoke side effects, such as hand tremor, frequent urination, and weight gain. Despite the benefits and relatively cheap cost of lithium, its use has been steadily eclipsed over the past couple decades by the introduction of the anticonvulsants.[152] The comparative safety and efficacy of lithium versus the rival anticonvulsants, however, remains a matter of debate.[153]

Overview of Pharmacogenetic Studies

There is a relative dearth of pharmacogenetic studies of mood stabilizers. Some 36 candidate gene studies have been reported.[154–189] Almost all of these examined lithium. With few exceptions, the studies were based on samples of whites with exceedingly small numbers (median = 111), and in most cases they relied on retrospective characterization of response to lithium. One genome-wide association study of lithium responsiveness was recently reported.[190] **Table 2** provides a description of the genome-wide association study of treatment response to mood stabilizers.

Pharmacodynamic Studies

As far as the authors are aware, no pharmacogenetic studies have been reported on the pharmacokinetics of mood stabilizers. Published studies have instead concentrated on pharmacodynamic factors. Although the mechanisms of action of lithium and the other anticonvulsant mood stabilizers are not completely known, there are two leading hypotheses. The first involves the phosphoinositide pathway and has been referred to as the "inositol depletion hypothesis."[191] It posits that lithium, and perhaps valproate and carbamazepine,[192] inhibit the activity of two enzymes, inositol monophosphatase and inositol-polyphosphate 1-polyphosphatase, which causes a reduction in the amount of free inositol available for the regeneration of phosphatidylinositol 4,5-bisphosphate (PIP_2). PIP_2 is a substrate needed for the generation of important intracellular signaling molecules, inositol 1,4,5-triphosphate (IP_3) and diacylglycerol by activation of the enzyme G-protein-coupled phospholipase C. IP_3 mediates $Ca+2$ release from intracellular stores and mediates a range of signaling pathways. Both $Ca+2$ and diacylglycerol further stimulate protein kinase C, which is also a component of other signaling pathways. There have been at least seven studies[156,157,159,167,169,179,181] on the relationship between variation in genes coding for key enzymes in this pathway and treatment response to lithium, but the findings have been largely inconclusive.

The leading alternative hypothesis for lithium's mechanism of action is its effects on cell survival through the inhibition of GSK3b.[193] Lithium acts in the same manner as the Wnt pathway to inhibit GSK3b, leading to the translocation of β-catenin to the cell nucleus where it becomes part of complexes that regulate the transcription of genetic components involved in cell survival.[194,195] It has been shown that valproate may have similar effects.[196] Motivated by these considerations, several pharmacogenetic studies of GSK3b[175,176] have been reported, again with mixed findings.

There has also been interest in examining some of the usual suspects in psychiatric genetics, such as MAOA, COMT, 5HTT, TPH1, and BDNF.[161,163,168,170,173,174,177,179,182,184] As yet, there remains no conclusive evidence that variation in any of these genes influences treatment response to mood stabilizers.

Genome-wide Studies

One genome-wide association study of lithium response has been reported.[190] In this prospective study from STEP-BD, the associations between 1.4 million genotyped and imputed SNPs and the risk of mood disorder recurrence were examined among

Table 2
Genome-wide association studies of treatment responses to mood stabilizers

Author (Year)	Drug	Genes	Outcome	Sample Size	Key Findings
Perlis (2009)	Lithium (alone or in combination with other psychotropic medications)	Affymetrix 500K	Efficacy (recurrence)	458	Suggestive associations with GRIA2, SDC2, ODZ4

1177 patients with bipolar disorder, including 458 who were treated with lithium alone or in combination with other psychotropic medications. SNPs found to be associated at the threshold of $P<5 \times 10^{-4}$ were examined in a replication sample from the University College London in which 359 patients with bipolar disorder were retrospectively assessed for lithium response. These SNPs were also tested to determine if their association with recurrence was specific to treatment lithium in the STEP-BD cohort. None of the SNPs tested in the STEP-BD cohort met genome-wide significant criteria for association. A total of 140 SNPs were carried forward for replication, however, and of these nine were significant in the University College London sample at $P<.05$. Of these, five had the same direction of effect as in the STEP-BD cohort, and three displayed associations that were specific to lithium treatment. The latter three SNPs point to associations with GRIA2, which has been found to be downregulated by chronic lithium treatment in a human neuronal cell line[197,198]; SDC2, which codes for a cell-surface proteoglycan that may play a role in dendritic spine formation in the hippocampus[197]; and ODZ4, which has been implicated in brain patterning.[199] These findings implicate novel candidate genes for lithium response that merit further investigation, but more generally they suggest there are few if any genes with large effects on lithium response and, instead, as with other complex traits, multiple loci may be involved.

ANTIPSYCHOTICS

The first generation of antipsychotics (FGAs), including the phenothiazine derivates, such as chlorpromazine, dates back to the 1950s. Their introduction was responsible for large decreases in psychiatric inpatient populations.[200] Because of side effects, however, such as extrapyramidal symptoms including parkinsonism, akathisia, and tardive dyskinesia (TD), their appeal was limited. In the 1990s a second generation of antipsychotics (SGAs) with a more diverse mechanism of action that targeted various serotonin and dopamine receptors was developed. The first of these, clozapine, has been shown to be effective against treatment-resistant schizophrenia,[201] but it is also associated with life-threatening agranulocytosis. Several other SGAs, such as risperidone, olanzapine, and quetiapine, have since been introduced. The conventional notion is that compared with FGAs these so-called "atypical antipsychotics" have better safety profiles and greater efficacy, particularly against the negative symptoms of schizophrenia.[200] A recent meta-analysis suggested, however, that only a few are actually more effective at reducing symptoms and have less tendency for inducing extrapyramidal symptoms.[202] SGAs are also associated with notable adverse effects of their own, such as weight gain, diabetes, metabolic syndrome, and sedation.[203]

Overview of Pharmacogenetic Studies

At least 273 pharmacogenetic studies of candidate genes and antipsychotic treatment response have been published.[204–476] Most of these studies examined the use of multiple antipsychotics, although FGAs were typically considered separately from SGAs. Approximately 40% of the studies examined only one antipsychotic, with clozapine being the most widely studied, followed by olanzapine and risperidone. The outcomes of interest were split evenly between efficacy and side effects. Among the latter, TD and weight gain were most commonly studied, with a subset of studies focused on agranulocytosis associated with clozapine. Just over half the studies were on samples of whites, whereas the rest were mostly of Chinese, Japanese, or Korean samples. As with the pharmacogenetic studies of antidepressants and mood stabilizers, the sample sizes were generally small with a median of 115, not counting four reports[398,403,441,442] from the CATIE trial, which each included approximately 700 patients. Five genome-wide association studies of antipsychotic treatment response have been published.[477–481] **Table 3** provides a description of candidate genes studies from CATIE and genome-wide association studies of treatment responses to antipsychotics.

Table 3
Candidate gene studies from CATIE and genome-wide association studies of treatment responses to antipsychotics

Author (Year)	Drug	Genes	Outcome	Sample Size	Key Findings
Candidate gene studies from CATIE					
Grossman (2008)	CATIE[a]	CYP2D6, CYP1A2, CYP2C8, CYP2C9, CYP2C19, CYP1A4, CYP3A5, CYP3A4, ABCB1, FMO3, UGT1A4	Optimized dose Treatment stop because of side effects Tardive dyskinesia	750	No associations
Campbell (2008)	CATIE[a]	RGS4	Efficacy	678	Suggestive association
Need (2009)	CATIE[a]	118 genes	21 phenotypes	756	Multiple suggestive associations
Tsai (2009)	CATIE[a]	128 genes	Tardive dyskinesia	710	No associations
Genome-wide association studies					
McClay (2009)	CATIE[a]	Affymetrix 500K	Efficacy	738	Significant association in 4p15
Alkelai (2009)	CATIE[a]	Affymetrix 500K plus custom 164K fill-in chip	Antipsychotic-induced parkinsonism	397	Suggesitve associations in EPF1, NOVA1, FIGN
Aberg (2009)	CATIE[a]	Affymetrix 500K	Extrapyramidal side effects	738	Significant associations in 11q24 and ZNF202
Lavedan (2009)	Iloperidone	Affymetrix 500K	Efficacy	426	Suggestive association with NPAS3
Volpi (2009)	Iloperidone	Affymetrix 500K	QT interval prolongation	183	Suggestive association with CERKL and SLCO3A1

[a] In CATIE, patients were treated with up to five different antipsychotics: olanzapine, quetiapine, risperidone, ziprasidone, and perphenazine.

Pharmacokinetics

Just as they do with antidepressants, the CYP450 enzymes play a leading role in the pharmacokinetics of antipsychotics. Along with CYP2D6, CYP1A2, CYP3A4, and CYP3A5 are the key enzymes responsible for metabolizing most commonly used antipsychotics.[482] A number of studies[205,222,232,236,245,260,262,270,271,281,292,294,310,311,324,331,341,342,348,367,377,388,389,404,420,451,459,461,463] have examined the association between variants in the genes coding for these enzymes and antipsychotic response. Most of these have studied adverse effects, and in particular TD. A meta-analysis[483] of studies on TD provided evidence of an increased risk with loss of function alleles in *CYP2D6*. Further analysis suggested, however, that publication bias could not be entirely ruled out. In addition, a recent report[398] from the CATIE trial in which a number of variants across the key CYP450 genes, and several other Phase II and transporter genes, were examined found no strong associations with dosing, safety, or efficacy of the antipsychotic treatments used in the trial.

Pharmacodynamics

Dysregulation of the dopaminergic system was among the first pathological findings observed in schizophrenia, and dopamine inhibition is a common feature of most antipsychotics, particularly the FGAs. Evidence suggests that dopamine antagonism may be required for antipsychotic activity, with positron emission tomography studies showing that a certain level of blockade of dopaminergic receptors in the striatum is needed to sustain a therapeutic effect, whereas excess blockade can lead to extrapyramidal side effects.[484–486] There are five subtypes of dopamine receptors (D1–D5), and of these D2 and D3 are the most widely implicated in pharmacogenetic studies of antipsychotics.

Three polymorphisms in *DRD2*, which encodes the D2 receptor, have received the greatest attention. These include the Taq1A polymorphism, which is located approximately 10 kb from the 3' end of the gene and has no known functional effect; the -141-C Ins/Del polymorphism in the promoter region, which has been associated with lower expression of the D2 receptor in vitro[487] and higher D2 density in the striatum in vivo[488]; and Ser311Cys, a relatively common coding polymorphism that has been shown to reduce signal transduction by the receptor.[489] At least 14 studies[250,261,265,273,306,330,345,349,351,390,392,411,420,421] have examined the relationship between *DRD2* polymorphisms and efficacy of both FGAs and SGAs, whereas 20 studies[243,255,259,264,274,278,289,293,295,300,352,372,375,382,395,401,421,422,444,452] have investigated adverse effects, including TD, weight gain, and neuromalignant syndrome. In a recent meta-analysis[490] of four different genes and TD, a significant association was found with the Taq1A polymorphism in *DRD2*.

The *DRD3* gene, which has also been extensively studied, contains a Ser9Gly polymorphism that has been shown in vitro to influence dopamine binding affinity.[491] Several studies have examined the association between this polymorphism and efficacy[227,238,250,284,316,334,339,400,418,420,439,446,449] and adverse effects like TD.[211,215,223,228,237,242,244,252,257,278,286,375,401,416,443,452,473,492] A mega-analysis of combined data from several studies on 780 patients[276] suggested the Gly9 allele conferred a small, but significant, increase in risk of TD. This finding was corroborated by a later meta-analysis,[492] which suggested the association was stronger in non-Asian versus Asian populations.

The serotonergic system has also been implicated in treatment responses to antipsychotics. SGAs in particular display high affinities for serotonin receptors, which have been hypothesized to mediate, at least partially, their therapeutic action.[493,494]

Seven distinct families of serotonin receptors have been identified (5HT1–5HT7).[495] Of greatest interest is the 5HT2 receptor family, especially 5-HT2A and 5-HT2C. Several polymorphisms in both *5HT2A* (-1438-G/A and 102-T/C in the promoter and His425Tyr in the coding region) and *5HT2C* (a VNTR, -759-T/C, and -995-G/A in the promoter and Cys23Ser in the coding region) have been investigated in multiple studies of treatment response and adverse effects.[204,206,210,212,214,218,220,225,226,230,246,248,249,263,266,268, 269,275,280,283,285,288,290,297,308,320,327,329,336,365,367,370,375,384,385,387,401,402,409,413,418,429, 430,443,445,448,453,456,468,473] Several meta-analyses of these studies have been conducted including one showing an association between the 102-T/C and His425Tyr polymorphisms in *5HT2A* and treatment response to clozpaine,[496] a second showing an association between the 102-T/C polymorphism in *5HT2A* and TD,[497] and a third showing an association between the -759C/T polymorphism in *5HT2C* and weight gain.[498]

A number of other genes have been investigated in relation to antipsychotic responses. These studies have been motivated by various hypotheses about the mechanisms of action of antipsychotics, such as the role of the glutamatergic system or neuronal genesis and plasticity.[482] In addition, several pharmacogenetic studies from the CATIE trial have examined a range of candidate genes with inconclusive results.[441,442]

Genome-wide Studies

Five genome-wide association studies of antipsychotic treatment response have been reported in the literature.[477–481] Three of these came from the CATIE trial in which patients with schizophrenia were randomized to treatment with either a SGA (olanzapine, quetiapine, risperidone, or ziprasidone) or a FGA (perphenazine). The first study[477] tested for genome-wide predictors of efficacy among 738 patients genotyped using the Affymetrix 500K genotyping platform supplemented with a custom 164K chip to improve genome-wide coverage. Efficacy was measured by changes over time in positive and negative symptom scores. Because the patients were allowed to switch among treatments because of lack of efficacy or tolerability, associations were examined relative to the first drug to which the patient was randomized. Only one finding, in an intergenic region on chromosome 4p15, reached the prespecified threshold for genome-wide significance. Two other findings were close to this threshold in *ANKS1B* and *CNTNAP5*, which were found to mediate negative symptom response to olanzapine and risperidone, respectively.

The two other studies[478,479] from CATIE were partially overlapping. The more inclusive study[479] examined symptoms of parkinsonism, akathasia, and abnormal involuntary movements among the 738 patients included in the efficacy study described previously. Three findings met genome-wide significance in novel regions that have not been previously implicated in the pharmacogenetics of extrapyramidal symptoms. Two were located in an intergenic region on chromosome 11q24, and the other was in *ZNF202*, which is a transcriptional repressor controlling PLP1, a major component of myelin.

The remaining two genome-wide association studies[480,481] came from a Phase 3 randomized trial of iloperidone, an investigational new drug for the treatment of schizophrenia from Vanda Pharmaceuticals. The 28-day trial was double-blinded and placebo- and ziprasidone-controlled. In the first study,[480] genome-wide associations with efficacy were examined. A total of 426 patients genotyped on the Affymetrix 500K platform were included, including 218 on iloperidone, 103 on active comparator, and 103 on placebo. The outcome was change from baseline to last scheduled observation in positive and negative total symptom scores. Three complimentary analyses were performed, and six loci were identified with consistent findings across these analyses. The single best finding was in *NPAS3*, a gene that circumstantial evidence has previously implicated in schizophrenia. In the second study,[481] genome-wide associations with QT interval prolongation, a potentially life-threatening side effect of treatment with iloperidone and other antipsychotics, were examined. A total of 183 patients on iloperidone treatment with QT interval measurements at day 14 of the trial were included in this analysis. The top findings implicated two genes in particular, *CERKL* and *SLCO3A1*, with plausible roles in this adverse effect. CERKL is thought to be part of the ceramide pathway, which regulates currents conducted by various potassium channels including the hERG channel, which when inhibited can prolong the QT interval. SLCO3A1 plays a role in translocation of prostaglandins, which may have cardioprotective effects.

PHARMACOGENETICS IN CLINICAL PRACTICE

Only one pharmacogenetics test has been approved by the Food and Drug Administration (FDA) for clinical use in psychiatry.[140] This is the AmpliChip CYP450 Test marketed by Roche Molecular Systems. It uses Affymetrix microarray-based genotyping technology with more than 15,000 oligonucleotide probes to assay for 20 *CYP2D6* alleles, 7 *CYP2D6* duplications, and 3 *CYP2C19* alleles. The test includes software with an algorithm to predict CYP2D6 and CYP2C19 phenotypes (ie, PM, IM, EM, and UM) based on the identified alleles.

The intended use of the chip cleared by the FDA is very general and does not refer to any specific drug. Instead, it states that information about the two CYP450 genes assayed, "may be used as an aid to clinicians in determining therapeutic strategy and treatment dose for therapeutics that are metabolized" by-products of these genes.[499] Consequently, the FDA cleared the Roche AmpliChip without clinical studies demonstrating that it is actually beneficial for selection or dosing of any psychotropic medication, despite the fact that it has been marketed, often direct-to-consumer, for use with these medications, especially the SSRIs.[500] This is consistent with the FDA's approach to other diagnostic devices, such as MRIs, where it has left demonstration of clinical benefit to clinicians and payers.

The Centers for Disease Control and Prevention commissioned an independent panel to examine the analytic validity, clinical validity, and clinical use of CYP450 genotyping when prescribing SSRI antidepressants.[501] These three key characteristics of a pharmacogenetics test are defined, respectively, as the ability to (1) detect different alleles accurately, (2) predict clinically meaningful outcomes, and (3) provide information that improves the risk/benefit ratio of clinical treatment. In their review, the independent panel determined there was strong evidence for the analytic validity of CYP450 genotyping, but only marginal evidence for its clinical validity and almost no evidence for its clinical use.[141] The independent panel concluded[501] there was, "insufficient evidence to support a recommendation for or against use of CYP450 testing in adults beginning SSRI treatment," and further noted that, "in the absence of supporting evidence, and with consideration of other contextual issues, EGAPP discourages use of CYP450 testing for patients beginning SSRI treatment until further clinical trials are completed."

In addition to regulating pharmacogenetic tests, the FDA also oversees the incorporation of information about relevant pharmacogenetic biomarkers into the drug labels. Biomarkers are defined as characteristics that can be objectively measured and evaluated as indicators of normal biological processes, pathogenic processes, or pharmacologic responses to a therapeutic intervention.[502] Genetic variants associated with therapeutic responses to a pharmacological agent are pharmacogenetics biomarkers. The FDA collects information on pharmacogenetic biomarkers and their analytic validity, clinical validity, and clinical use from pharmaceutical companies during the drug application process,[503] and then incorporates this information into approved drug labels as deemed appropriate.

In a recent survey[504] of drug labels approved between 1945 and 2005, it was reported that a total of 121 contained pharmacogenetic information. Of these, 69 labels referred to human genomic biomarkers, and the remainder referred to microbial genomic biomarkers. Of the labels referring to human genomic biomarkers, 43 (62%) pertained to polymorphisms in CYP450 genes, with *CYP2D6* being the most common. Approximately 17% of the labels were for psychiatric drugs. In most cases the drug labels merely provided pharmacogenetic information. Only one label went further and recommended, but did not require, a specific action before making a therapeutic decision. This was for testing urea cycle enzyme deficiencies before prescribing valproic acid. Although pharmacogenetic information has begun to penetrate into clinical practice, it has not yet had a meaningful impact on therapeutic decision making in psychiatry.

CHALLENGES TO CLINICAL TRANSLATION

Despite notable progress in research over the past decade, the promise of pharmacogenetics in psychiatry has not yet been fully realized. The biggest obstacle to translating the promise into reality is that there is still no clear understanding of how genetic factors influence treatment response to psychotropic medications. The studies performed to date suggest a number of intriguing hypotheses that merit further investigation, but they do not point to any definitive associations that can be used with confidence to predict how a patient responds to a particular treatment. The difficulty with the pharmacogenetic associations thus far reported is the lack of consistent findings. For every positive association, there are typically several negative studies that cast doubt on the finding. As a result, it is difficult to draw firm conclusions about the clinical relevance of any genes that may be implicated.

There are several reasons for the difficulty. First, treatment responses to psychotropic medications are complex phenotypes. They may be as complex as the diseases for which they are used to treat. Psychotropic medications may act on a number of different molecular pathways to exert their therapeutic effect, and in turn they may be acted on by a number of different molecular pathways in the process of their absorption, distribution, and elimination. Consequently, multiple variants in distinct and converging genetic pathways may independently and interactively contribute to a particular drug response. In addition, multiple environmental factors may further contribute to variability in the response. Demographic factors, diet, substance abuse, smoking, concomitant treatments, and comorbidities may all affect the actions of psychotropic drugs.[505] For example, it has been shown that smoking induces CYP450 activity and promotes the metabolism of substrate drugs,[506,507] whereas SSRIs are known to inhibit CYP450 activity and may disrupt the metabolism of other concomitant medications.[508] Treatment responses may be the sum of a number of impinging genetic and environmental factors, making it difficult to identify any one factor in isolation and to construct more complete models of the determinants of drug response.

Second, it is particularly challenging to conduct appropriately designed pharmacogenetic studies that can illuminate the complex architecture of treatment responses. The studies performed to date have had rather small sample sizes and short periods of follow-up, largely because it is costly and logistically challenging to ascertain and prospectively evaluate patients in such studies. Even the largest studies that have been reported are significantly underpowered to detect genes with effect sizes likely involved in treatment responses. To address this issue, efforts have been made to combine data across studies in meta- or mega-analyses. Although this can be a useful strategy, existing studies frequently differ so considerably in design, patient populations, and outcome measures that it raises serious questions about the comparability of results across studies. Finally, to complicate matters, within each study patients often take multiple medications and have erratic patterns of adherence. As a result, the responses to any one drug during follow-up may be hopelessly obscured. Clearly, new approaches are needed to overcome these limitations to further advance the goals of pharmacogenetics.

SUMMARY

By personalizing treatments to psychotropic medications, pharmacogenetics holds great promise to dramatically improve care in psychiatry. The genomics revolution has provided an unprecedented set of tools to pursue the goal of pharmacogenetics. As reviewed here, a great deal of work has begun to use these tools to unravel the complex pharmacogenetic underpinnings of treatment responses. Although considerable progress has been made, much work remains to be done. It seems this is only the end of the beginning of a long venture.

REFERENCES

1. Liu-Seifert H, Adams DH, Kinon BJ. Discontinuation of treatment of schizophrenic patients is driven by poor symptom response: a pooled post-hoc analysis of four atypical antipsychotic drugs. BMC Microbiol 2005;3:21.
2. Rush AJ, Trivedi MH, Wisniewski SR, et al. Acute and longer-term outcomes in depressed outpatients requiring one or several treatment steps: a STAR*D report. Am J Pharmacogenomics 2006;163:1905–17.
3. Lieberman JA, Stroup TS, McEvoy JP, et al. Effectiveness of antipsychotic drugs in patients with chronic schizophrenia. N Engl J Med 2005;353:1209–23.
4. Thase ME. STEP-BD and bipolar depression: what have we learned? Curr Psychiatry Rep 2007;9:497–503.
5. Weinshilboum R, Wang L. Pharmacogenomics: bench to bedside. Nat Rev Drug Discov 2004;3:739–48.
6. Lieberman JA III. History of the use of antidepressants in primary care. Prim Care Companion J Clin Psychiatry 2003;5:6–10.
7. Preskorn SH, Stanga CY, Ross R. Selective serotonin reuptake inhibitor. In: Preskorn SH, Stanga CY, Feighner JP, et al, editors. Antidepressants, past, present and future. New York: Springer; 2004. p. 242.
8. Anderson IM, Ferrier IN, Baldwin RC, et al. Evidence-based guidelines for treating depressive disorders with antidepressants: a revision of the 2000 British Association for Psychopharmacology guidelines. J Psychopharmacol 2008;22: 343–96.
9. Crismon ML, Trivedi M, Pigott TA, et al. The texas medication algorithm project: report of the texas consensus conference panel on medication treatment of major depressive disorder. J Clin Psychiatry 1999;60:142–56.
10. Thase ME, Rush AJ. Treatment-resistant depression. In: Bloom FE, Kupfer DJ, editors. Psychopharmacology: the fourth generation of progress. New York: Raven Press Ltd; 1995. p. 1081–97.

11. Lin EH, Von KM, Katon W, et al. The role of the primary care physician in patients' adherence to antidepressant therapy. Med Care 1995;33:67–74.

12. Chen S, Chou WH, Blouin RA, et al. The cytochrome P450 2D6 (CYP2D6) enzyme polymorphism: screening costs and influence on clinical outcomes in psychiatry. Clin Pharmacol Ther 1996;60:522–34.

13. Smeraldi E, Zanardi R, Benedetti F, et al. Polymorphism within the promoter of the serotonin transporter gene and antidepressant efficacy of fluvoxamine. Mol Psychiatry 1998;3:508–11.

14. Kim DK, Lim SW, Lee S, et al. Serotonin transporter gene polymorphism and antidepressant response. Neuroreport 2000;11:215–9.

15. Pollock BG, Ferrell RE, Mulsant BH, et al. Allelic variation in the serotonin transporter promoter affects onset of paroxetine treatment response in late-life depression. Neuropsychopharmacology 2000;23:587–90.

16. Zanardi R, Benedetti F, Di BD, et al. Efficacy of paroxetine in depression is influenced by a functional polymorphism within the promoter of the serotonin transporter gene. J Clin Psychopharmacol 2000;20:105–7.

17. Zill P, Baghai TC, Zwanzger P, et al. Evidence for an association between a G-protein beta3-gene variant with depression and response to antidepressant treatment. Neuroreport 2000;11:1893–7.

18. Minov C, Baghai TC, Schule C, et al. Serotonin-2A-receptor and -transporter polymorphisms: lack of association in patients with major depression. Neurosci Lett 2001;303:119–22.

19. Serretti A, Zanardi R, Cusin C, et al. Tryptophan hydroxylase gene associated with paroxetine antidepressant activity. Eur Neuropsychopharmacol 2001;11:375–80.

20. Serretti A, Zanardi R, Rossini D, et al. Influence of tryptophan hydroxylase and serotonin transporter genes on fluvoxamine antidepressant activity. Mol Psychiatry 2001;6:586–92.

21. Zanardi R, Serretti A, Rossini D, et al. Factors affecting fluvoxamine antidepressant activity: influence of pindolol and 5-HTTLPR in delusional and nondelusional depression. Biol Psychiatry 2001;50:323–30.

22. Allgulander C, Nilsson B. A prospective study of 86 new patients with social anxiety disorder. Acta Psychiatr Scand 2001;103:447–52.

23. Baghai TC, Schule C, Zwanzger P, et al. Possible influence of the insertion/deletion polymorphism in the angiotensin I-converting enzyme gene on therapeutic outcome in affective disorders. Mol Psychiatry 2001;6:258–9.

24. Wang JH, Liu ZQ, Wang W, et al. Pharmacokinetics of sertraline in relation to genetic polymorphism of CYP2C19. Clin Pharmacol Ther 2001;70:42–7.

25. Wu WH, Huo SJ, Cheng CY, et al. Association study of the 5-HT(6) receptor polymorphism (C267T) and symptomatology and antidepressant response in major depressive disorders. Neuropsychobiology 2001;44:172–5.

26. Cusin C, Serretti A, Zanardi R, et al. Influence of monoamine oxidase a and serotonin receptor 2A polymorphisms in SSRI antidepressant activity. Int J Neuropsychopharmacol 2002;5:27–35.

27. Yoshida K, Ito K, Sato K, et al. Influence of the serotonin transporter gene-linked polymorphic region on the antidepressant response to fluvoxamine in Japanese depressed patients. Prog Neuropsychopharmacol Biol Psychiatry 2002;26:383–6.

28. Yu YW, Tsai SJ, Chen TJ, et al. Association study of the serotonin transporter promoter polymorphism and symptomatology and antidepressant response in major depressive disorders. Mol Psychiatry 2002;7:1115–9.

29. Hong CJ, Wang YC, Tsai SJ. Association study of angiotensin I-converting enzyme polymorphism and symptomatology and antidepressant response in major depressive disorders. J Neural Transm 2002;109:1209–14.

30. Ito K, Yoshida K, Sato K, et al. A variable number of tandem repeats in the serotonin transporter gene does not affect the antidepressant response to fluvoxamine. Psychiatry Res 2002;111:235–9.

31. Muller DJ, Schulze TG, Macciardi F, et al. Moclobemide response in depressed patients: association study with a functional polymorphism in the monoamine oxidase a promoter. Pharmacopsychiatry 2002;35:157–8.

32. Sato K, Yoshida K, Takahashi H, et al. Association between -1438G/A promoter polymorphism in the 5-HT(2A) receptor gene and fluvoxamine response in Japanese patients with major depressive disorder. Neuropsychobiology 2002; 46:136–40.

33. Yoshida K, Naito S, Takahashi H, et al. Monoamine oxidase: a gene polymorphism, tryptophan hydroxylase gene polymorphism and antidepressant response to fluvoxamine in Japanese patients with major depressive disorder. Prog Neuropsychopharmacol Biol Psychiatry 2002;26:1279–83.

34. Rausch JL, Johnson ME, Fei YJ, et al. Initial conditions of serotonin transporter kinetics and genotype: influence on SSRI treatment trial outcome. Biol Psychiatry 2002;51:723–32.

35. Takahashi H, Yoshida K, Ito K, et al. No association between the serotonergic polymorphisms and incidence of nausea induced by fluvoxamine treatment. Eur Neuropsychopharmacol 2002;12:477–81.

36. Serretti A, Lorenzi C, Cusin C, et al. SSRIs antidepressant activity is influenced by G beta 3 variants. Eur Neuropsychopharmacol 2003;13:117–22.

37. Arias B, Catalan R, Gasto C, et al. 5-HTTLPR polymorphism of the serotonin transporter gene predicts non-remission in major depression patients treated with citalopram in a 12-weeks follow up study. J Clin Psychopharmacol 2003;23:563–7.

38. Joyce PR, Mulder RT, Luty SE, et al. Age-dependent antidepressant pharmacogenomics: polymorphisms of the serotonin transporter and G protein beta3 subunit as predictors of response to fluoxetine and nortriptyline. Int J Neuropsychopharmacol 2003;6:339–46.

39. Murphy GM Jr, Kremer C, Rodrigues HE, et al. Pharmacogenetics of antidepressant medication intolerance. Am J Psychiatry 2003;160:1830–5.

40. Gerstenberg G, Aoshima T, Fukasawa T, et al. Relationship between clinical effects of fluvoxamine and the steady-state plasma concentrations of fluvoxamine and its major metabolite fluvoxamino acid in Japanese depressed patients. Psychopharmacology (Berl) 2003;167:443–8.

41. Perlis RH, Mischoulon D, Smoller JW, et al. Serotonin transporter polymorphisms and adverse effects with fluoxetine treatment. Biol Psychiatry 2003;54:879–83.

42. Tsai SJ, Cheng CY, Yu YW, et al. Association study of a brain-derived neurotrophic-factor genetic polymorphism and major depressive disorders, symptomatology, and antidepressant response. Am J Med Genet B NeuroPsychiatr Genet 2003;123B:19–22.

43. Yoshida K, Naito S, Takahashi H, et al. Monoamine oxidase a gene polymorphism, 5-HT 2A receptor gene polymorphism and incidence of nausea induced by fluvoxamine. Neuropsychobiology 2003;48:10–3.

44. Durham LK, Webb SM, Milos PM, et al. The serotonin transporter polymorphism, 5HTTLPR, is associated with a faster response time to sertraline in an elderly population with major depressive disorder. Psychopharmacology (Berl) 2004; 174:525–9.

45. Lee MS, Lee HY, Lee HJ, et al. Serotonin transporter promoter gene polymorphism and long-term outcome of antidepressant treatment. Psychiatr Genet 2004;14:111–5.
46. Murphy GM Jr, Hollander SB, Rodrigues HE, et al. Effects of the serotonin transporter gene promoter polymorphism on mirtazapine and paroxetine efficacy and adverse events in geriatric major depression. Arch Gen Psychiatry 2004;61:1163–9.
47. Peters EJ, Slager SL, McGrath PJ, et al. Investigation of serotonin-related genes in antidepressant response. Mol Psychiatry 2004;9:879–89.
48. Rau T, Wohlleben G, Wuttke H, et al. CYP2D6 genotype: impact on adverse effects and nonresponse during treatment with antidepressants: a pilot study. Clin Pharmacol Ther 2004;75:386–93.
49. Serretti A, Cusin C, Rossini D, et al. Further evidence of a combined effect of SERTPR and TPH on SSRIs response in mood disorders. Am J Med Genet B NeuroPsychiatr Genet 2004;129B:36–40.
50. Serretti A, Artioli P, Lorenzi C, et al. The C(-1019)G polymorphism of the 5-HT1A gene promoter and antidepressant response in mood disorders: preliminary findings. Int J Neuropsychopharmacol 2004;7:453–60.
51. Yoshida K, Takahashi H, Higuchi H, et al. Prediction of antidepressant response to milnacipran by norepinephrine transporter gene polymorphisms. Am J Psychiatry 2004;161:1575–80.
52. Baghai TC, Schule C, Zill P, et al. The angiotensin I converting enzyme insertion/deletion polymorphism influences therapeutic outcome in major depressed women, but not in men. Neurosci Lett 2004;363:38–42.
53. Binder EB, Salyakina D, Lichtner P, et al. Polymorphisms in FKBP5 are associated with increased recurrence of depressive episodes and rapid response to antidepressant treatment. Nat Genet 2004;36:1319–25.
54. Grasmader K, Verwohlt PL, Rietschel M, et al. Impact of polymorphisms of cytochrome-P450 isoenzymes 2C9, 2C19 and 2D6 on plasma concentrations and clinical effects of antidepressants in a naturalistic clinical setting. Eur J Clin Pharmacol 2004;60:329–36.
55. Kawanishi C, Lundgren S, Agren H, et al. Increased incidence of CYP2D6 gene duplication in patients with persistent mood disorders: ultrarapid metabolism of antidepressants as a cause of nonresponse: a pilot study. Eur J Clin Pharmacol 2004;59:803–7.
56. Lee HJ, Cha JH, Ham BJ, et al. Association between a G-protein beta 3 subunit gene polymorphism and the symptomatology and treatment responses of major depressive disorders. Pharmacogenomics J 2004;4:29–33.
57. Lemonde S, Du L, Bakish D, et al. Association of the C(-1019)G 5-HT1A functional promoter polymorphism with antidepressant response. Int J Neuropsychopharmacol 2004;7:501–6.
58. Licinio J, O'Kirwan F, Irizarry K, et al. Association of a corticotropin-releasing hormone receptor 1 haplotype and antidepressant treatment response in Mexican-Americans. Mol Psychiatry 2004;9:1075–82.
59. Roberts RL, Mulder RT, Joyce PR, et al. No evidence of increased adverse drug reactions in cytochrome P450 CYP2D6 poor metabolizers treated with fluoxetine or nortriptyline. Hum Psychopharmacol 2004;19:17–23.
60. Suzuki Y, Sawamura K, Someya T. The effects of a 5-hydroxytryptamine 1A receptor gene polymorphism on the clinical response to fluvoxamine in depressed patients. Pharmacogenomics J 2004;4:283–6.
61. Zill P, Baghai TC, Engel R, et al. The dysbindin gene in major depression: an association study. Am J Med Genet B NeuroPsychiatr Genet 2004;129B:55–8.

62. Arias B, Catalan R, Gasto C, et al. Evidence for a combined genetic effect of the 5-HT(1A) receptor and serotonin transporter genes in the clinical outcome of major depressive patients treated with citalopram. J Psychopharmacol 2005; 19:166–72.

63. Ham BJ, Lee MS, Lee HJ, et al. No association between the tryptophan hydroxylase gene polymorphism and major depressive disorders and antidepressant response in a Korean population. Psychiatr Genet 2005;15:299–301.

64. Szegedi A, Rujescu D, Tadic A, et al. The catechol-O-methyltransferase Val108/158Met polymorphism affects short-term treatment response to mirtazapine, but not to paroxetine in major depression. Pharmacogenomics J 2005;5:49–53.

65. Choi MJ, Kang RH, Ham BJ, et al. Serotonin receptor 2A gene polymorphism (-1438A/G) and short-term treatment response to citalopram. Neuropsychobiology 2005;52:155–62.

66. Garriock HA, Allen JJ, Delgado P, et al. Lack of association of TPH2 exon XI polymorphisms with major depression and treatment resistance. Mol Psychiatry 2005;10:976–7.

67. Kato M, Ikenaga Y, Wakeno M, et al. Controlled clinical comparison of paroxetine and fluvoxamine considering the serotonin transporter promoter polymorphism. Int Clin Psychopharmacol 2005;20:151–6.

68. Kraft JB, Slager SL, McGrath PJ, et al. Sequence analysis of the serotonin transporter and associations with antidepressant response. Biol Psychiatry 2005;58: 374–81.

69. Lee SH, Lee KJ, Lee HJ, et al. Association between the 5-HT6 receptor C267T polymorphism and response to antidepressant treatment in major depressive disorder. Psychiatry Clin Neurosci 2005;59:140–5.

70. Yu YW, Tsai SJ, Hong CJ, et al. Association study of a monoamine oxidase a gene promoter polymorphism with major depressive disorder and antidepressant response. Neuropsychopharmacology 2005;30:1719–23.

71. McMahon FJ, Buervenich S, Charney D, et al. Variation in the gene encoding the serotonin 2A receptor is associated with outcome of antidepressant treatment. Am J Hum Genet 2006;78:804–14.

72. Arias B, Serretti A, Lorenzi C, et al. Analysis of COMT gene (Val 158 Met polymorphism) in the clinical response to SSRIs in depressive patients of European origin. J Atten Disord 2006;90:251–6.

73. Hong CJ, Chen TJ, Yu YW, et al. Response to fluoxetine and serotonin 1A receptor (C-1019G) polymorphism in Taiwan Chinese major depressive disorder. Pharmacogenomics J 2006;6:27–33.

74. Kato M, Fukuda T, Wakeno M, et al. Effects of the serotonin type 2A, 3A and 3B receptor and the serotonin transporter genes on paroxetine and fluvoxamine efficacy and adverse drug reactions in depressed Japanese patients. Neuropsychobiology 2006;53:186–95.

75. Shams ME, Arneth B, Hiemke C, et al. CYP2D6 polymorphism and clinical effect of the antidepressant venlafaxine. J Clin Pharm Ther 2006;31:493–502.

76. Smeraldi E, Serretti A, Artioli P, et al. Serotonin transporter gene-linked polymorphic region: possible pharmacogenetic implications of rare variants. Psychiatr Genet 2006;16:153–8.

77. Yu YW, Tsai SJ, Liou YJ, et al. Association study of two serotonin 1A receptor gene polymorphisms and fluoxetine treatment response in Chinese major depressive disorders. Eur Neuropsychopharmacol 2006;16:498–503.

78. Bishop JR, Moline J, Ellingrod VL, et al. Serotonin 2A -1438 G/A and G-protein Beta3 subunit C825T polymorphisms in patients with depression and

SSRI-associated sexual side-effects. Neuropsychopharmacology 2006;31: 2281–8.

79. Choi MJ, Kang RH, Lim SW, et al. Brain-derived neurotrophic factor gene polymorphism (Val66Met) and citalopram response in major depressive disorder. Brain Res 2006;1118:176–82.

80. Ng CH, Easteal S, Tan S, et al. Serotonin transporter polymorphisms and clinical response to sertraline across ethnicities. Prog Neuropsychopharmacol Biol Psychiatry 2006;30:953–7.

81. Popp J, Leucht S, Heres S, et al. Serotonin transporter polymorphisms and side effects in antidepressant therapy: a pilot study. Pharmacogenomics 2006;7: 159–66.

82. Sugai T, Suzuki Y, Sawamura K, et al. The effect of 5-hydroxytryptamine 3A and 3B receptor genes on nausea induced by paroxetine. Pharmacogenomics J 2006;6:351–6.

83. Suzuki Y, Sawamura K, Someya T. Polymorphisms in the 5-hydroxytryptamine 2A receptor and cytochrome P4502D6 genes synergistically predict fluvoxamine-induced side effects in japanese depressed patients. Neuropsychopharmacology 2006;31:825–31.

84. Kim H, Lim SW, Kim S, et al. Monoamine transporter gene polymorphisms and antidepressant response in koreans with late-life depression. JAMA 2006;296: 1609–18.

85. Perlis RH, Purcell S, Fava M, et al. Association between treatment-emergent suicidal ideation with citalopram and polymorphisms near cyclic adenosine monophosphate response element binding protein in the STAR*D study. Arch Gen Psychiatry 2007;64:689–97.

86. Ham BJ, Lee BC, Paik JW, et al. Association between the tryptophan hydroxylase-1 gene A218C polymorphism and citalopram antidepressant response in a Korean population. Prog Neuropsychopharmacol Biol Psychiatry 2007;31: 104–7.

87. Hu XZ, Rush AJ, Charney D, et al. Association between a functional serotonin transporter promoter polymorphism and citalopram treatment in adult outpatients with major depression. Arch Gen Psychiatry 2007;64:783–92.

88. Kirchheiner J, Nickchen K, Sasse J, et al. A 40-basepair VNTR polymorphism in the dopamine transporter (DAT1) gene and the rapid response to antidepressant treatment. Pharmacogenomics J 2007;7:48–55.

89. Levin GM, Bowles TM, Ehret MJ, et al. Assessment of human serotonin 1A receptor polymorphisms and SSRI responsiveness. Mol Diagn Ther 2007;11: 155–60.

90. Kraft JB, Peters EJ, Slager SL, et al. Analysis of association between the serotonin transporter and antidepressant response in a large clinical sample. Biol Psychiatry 2007;61:734–42.

91. Kang RH, Wong ML, Choi MJ, et al. Association study of the serotonin transporter promoter polymorphism and mirtazapine antidepressant response in major depressive disorder. Prog Neuropsychopharmacol Biol Psychiatry 2007; 31:1317–21.

92. Kang RH, Hahn SW, Choi MJ, et al. Relationship between G-protein beta-3 subunit C825T polymorphism and mirtazapine responses in Korean patients with major depression. Neuropsychobiology 2007;56:1–5.

93. Kato M, Wakeno M, Okugawa G, et al. No association of TPH1 218A/C polymorphism with treatment response and intolerance to SSRIs in Japanese patients with major depression. Neuropsychobiology 2007;56:167–71.

94. Kronenberg S, Apter A, Brent D, et al. Serotonin transporter polymorphism (5-HTTLPR) and citalopram effectiveness and side effects in children with depression and/or anxiety disorders. J Child Adolesc Psychopharmacol 2007; 17:741–50.

95. Laje G, Paddock S, Manji H, et al. Genetic markers of suicidal ideation emerging during citalopram treatment of major depression. Am J Psychiatry 2007;164: 1530–8.

96. Liu Z, Zhu F, Wang G, et al. Association study of corticotropin-releasing hormone receptor1 gene polymorphisms and antidepressant response in major depressive disorders. Neurosci Lett 2007;414:155–8.

97. Paddock S, Laje G, Charney D, et al. Association of GRIK4 with outcome of antidepressant treatment in the STAR*D cohort. Am J Psychiatry 2007;164:1181–8.

98. Pae CU, Serretti A, Mandelli L, et al. Dysbindin associated with selective serotonin reuptake inhibitor antidepressant efficacy. Pharmacogenet Genomics 2007;17:69–75.

99. Papiol S, Arias B, Gasto C, et al. Genetic variability at HPA axis in major depression and clinical response to antidepressant treatment. J Affect Disord 2007; 104:83–90.

100. Smits K, Smits L, Peeters F, et al. Serotonin transporter polymorphisms and the occurrence of adverse events during treatment with selective serotonin reuptake inhibitors. Int Clin Psychopharmacol 2007;22:137–43.

101. Tadic A, Muller MJ, Rujescu D, et al. The MAOA T941G polymorphism and short-term treatment response to mirtazapine and paroxetine in major depression. Am J Med Genet B Neuropsychiatr Genet 2007;144:325–31.

102. Tsai SJ, Hong CJ, Chen TJ, et al. Lack of supporting evidence for a genetic association of the FKBP5 polymorphism and response to antidepressant treatment. Am J Med Genet B Neuropsychiatr Genet 2007;144:1097–8.

103. Wilkie MJ, Smith D, Reid IC, et al. A splice site polymorphism in the G-protein beta subunit influences antidepressant efficacy in depression. Pharmacogenet Genomics 2007;17:207–15.

104. Yoshida K, Higuchi H, Kamata M, et al. The G196A polymorphism of the brain-derived neurotrophic factor gene and the antidepressant effect of milnacipran and fluvoxamine. J Psychopharmacol 2007;21:650–6.

105. Benedetti F, Barbini B, Bernasconi A, et al. Lithium overcomes the influence of 5-HTTLPR gene polymorphism on antidepressant response to sleep deprivation. J Clin Psychopharmacol 2008;28:249–51.

106. Lotrich FE, Pollock BG, Kirshner M, et al. Serotonin transporter genotype interacts with paroxetine plasma levels to influence depression treatment response in geriatric patients. J Psychiatry Neurosci 2008;33:123–30.

107. Uhr M, Tontsch A, Namendorf C, et al. Polymorphisms in the drug transporter gene ABCB1 predict antidepressant treatment response in depression. Neuron 2008;57:203–9.

108. Peters EJ, Slager SL, Kraft JB, et al. Pharmacokinetic genes do not influence response or tolerance to citalopram in the STAR*D sample. PLoS One 2008;3: e1872.

109. Baune BT, Hohoff C, Roehrs T, et al. Serotonin receptor 1A-1019C/G variant: impact on antidepressant pharmacoresponse in melancholic depression? Neurosci Lett 2008;436:111–5.

110. Bozina N, Peles AM, Sagud M, et al. Association study of paroxetine therapeutic response with SERT gene polymorphisms in patients with major depressive disorder. World J Biol Psychiatry 2008;9:190–7.

111. Gex-Fabry M, Eap CB, Oneda B, et al. CYP2D6 and ABCB1 genetic variability: influence on paroxetine plasma level and therapeutic response. Ther Drug Monit 2008;30:474–82.
112. Gratacos M, Soria V, Urretavizcaya M, et al. A brain-derived neurotrophic factor (BDNF) haplotype is associated with antidepressant treatment outcome in mood disorders. Pharmacogenomics J 2008;8:101–12.
113. Kato M, Fukuda T, Serretti A, et al. ABCB1 (MDR1) gene polymorphisms are associated with the clinical response to paroxetine in patients with major depressive disorder. Prog Neuropsychopharmacol Biol Psychiatry 2008;32: 398–404.
114. Kato M, Wakeno M, Okugawa G, et al. Antidepressant response and intolerance to SSRI is not influenced by G-protein beta3 subunit gene C825T polymorphism in Japanese major depressive patients. Prog Neuropsychopharmacol Biol Psychiatry 2008;32:1041–4.
115. Lekman M, Laje G, Charney D, et al. The FKBP5-gene in depression and treatment response: an association study in the Sequenced Treatment Alternatives to Relieve Depression (STAR*D). Cohort Biol Psychiatry 2008;63: 1103–10.
116. Mihaljevic PA, Bozina N, Sagud M, et al. MDR1 gene polymorphism: therapeutic response to paroxetine among patients with major depression. Prog Neuropsychopharmacol Biol Psychiatry 2008;32:1439–44.
117. Smits KM, Smits LJ, Peeters FP, et al. The influence of 5-HTTLPR and STin2 polymorphisms in the serotonin transporter gene on treatment effect of selective serotonin reuptake inhibitors in depressive patients. Psychiatr Genet 2008;18: 184–90.
118. Tanaka M, Kobayashi D, Murakami Y, et al. Genetic polymorphisms in the 5-hydroxytryptamine type 3B receptor gene and paroxetine-induced nausea. Int J Neuropsychopharmacol 2008;11:261–7.
119. Yoshida K, Higuchi H, Takahashi H, et al. Influence of the tyrosine hydroxylase val81met polymorphism and catechol-O-methyltransferase val158met polymorphism on the antidepressant effect of milnacipran. Hum Psychopharmacol 2008;23:121–8.
120. Bishop JR, Ellingrod VL, Akroush M, et al. The association of serotonin transporter genotypes and selective serotonin reuptake inhibitor (SSRI)-associated sexual side effects: possible relationship to oral contraceptives. Hum Psychopharmacol 2009;24:207–15.
121. Wilkie MJ, Smith G, Day RK, et al. Polymorphisms in the SLC6A4 and HTR2A genes influence treatment outcome following antidepressant therapy. Pharmacogenomics J 2009;9:61–70.
122. Arias B, Serretti A, Mandelli L, et al. Dysbindin gene (DTNBP1) in major depression: association with clinical response to selective serotonin reuptake inhibitors. Pharmacogenet Genomics 2009;19:121–8.
123. Cabanero M, Laje G, Detera-Wadleigh S, et al. Association study of phosphodiesterase genes in the sequenced treatment alternatives to relieve depression sample. Pharmacogenet Genomics 2009;19:235–8.
124. Domschke K, Lawford B, Laje G, et al. Brain-derived neurotrophic factor (BDNF) gene: no major impact on antidepressant treatment response. Int J Neuropsychopharmacol 2009;1–9. [Epub ahead of print].
125. Kang R, Chang H, Wong M, et al. Brain-derived neurotrophic factor gene polymorphisms and mirtazapine responses in Koreans with major depression. J Psychopharmacol 2009. [Epub ahead of print].

126. Kato M, Fukuda T, Wakeno M, et al. Effect of 5-HT1A gene polymorphisms on antidepressant response in major depressive disorder. Am J Med Genet B Neuropsychiatr Genet 2009;150:115–23.

127. Mrazek DA, Rush AJ, Biernacka JM, et al. SLC6A4 variation and citalopram response. Am J Med Genet B Neuropsychiatr Genet 2009;150:341–51.

128. Perlis RH, Fijal B, Adams DH, et al. Variation in catechol-O-methyltransferase is associated with duloxetine response in a clinical trial for major depressive disorder. Biol Psychiatry 2009;65:785–91.

129. Perlis RH, Laje G, Smoller JW, et al. Genetic and clinical predictors of sexual dysfunction in citalopram-treated depressed patients. Neuropsychopharmacology 2009;34:1819–28.

130. Secher A, Bukh J, Bock C, et al. Antidepressive-drug-induced bodyweight gain is associated with polymorphisms in genes coding for COMT and TPH1. Int Clin Psychopharmacol 2009;24:199–203.

131. Laje G, Allen AS, Akula N, et al. Genome-wide association study of suicidal ideation emerging during citalopram treatment of depressed outpatients. Pharmacogenet Genomics 2009;19:666–74.

132. Garriock HA, Kraft JB, Shyn SI, et al. A genome-wide association study of citalopram response in major depressive disorder. Biol Psychiatry 2010;67:133–8.

133. Ising M, Lucae S, Binder EB, et al. A genome-wide association study points to multiple loci that predict antidepressant drug treatment outcome in depression. Arch Gen Psychiatry 2009;66:966–75.

134. Brosen K. Some aspects of genetic polymorphism in the biotransformation of antidepressants. Therapiewoche 2004;59:5–12.

135. Ingelman-Sundberg M. Genetic polymorphisms of cytochrome P450 2D6 (CYP2D6): clinical consequences, evolutionary aspects and functional diversity. Pharmacogenomics J 2005;5:6–13.

136. Bertilsson L, Dahl ML, Dalen P, et al. Molecular genetics of CYP2D6: clinical relevance with focus on psychotropic drugs. Br J Clin Pharmacol 2002;53:111–22.

137. Madan A, Graham RA, Carroll KM, et al. Effects of prototypical microsomal enzyme inducers on cytochrome P450 expression in cultured human hepatocytes. Drug Metab Dispos 2003;31:421–31.

138. de LJ, Armstrong SC, Cozza KL. Clinical guidelines for psychiatrists for the use of pharmacogenetic testing for CYP450 2D6 and CYP450 2C19. Psychosomatics 2006;47:75–85.

139. Nebert DW, Dieter MZ. The evolution of drug metabolism. Pharmacology 2000; 61:124–35.

140. de LJ. AmpliChip CYP450 test: personalized medicine has arrived in psychiatry. Expert Rev Mol Diagn 2006;6:277–86.

141. Thakur M, Grossman I, McCrory DC, et al. Review of evidence for genetic testing for CYP450 polymorphisms in management of patients with nonpsychotic depression with selective serotonin reuptake inhibitors. Genet Med 2007;9:826–35.

142. Heils A, Teufel A, Petri S, et al. Allelic variation of human serotonin transporter gene expression. J Neurochem 1996;66:2621–4.

143. Hu XZ, Lipsky RH, Zhu G, et al. Serotonin transporter promoter gain-of-function genotypes are linked to obsessive-compulsive disorder. Am J Hum Genet 2006; 78:815–26.

144. Hranilovic D, Stefulj J, Schwab S, et al. Serotonin transporter promoter and intron 2 polymorphisms: relationship between allelic variants and gene expression. Biol Psychiatry 2004;55:1090–4.

145. Serretti A, Kato M, De RD, et al. Meta-analysis of serotonin transporter gene promoter polymorphism (5-HTTLPR) association with selective serotonin re-uptake inhibitor efficacy in depressed patients. Mol Psychiatry 2007;12: 247–57.

146. Kato M, Serretti A. Review and meta-analysis of antidepressant pharmacogenetic findings in major depressive disorder. Mol Psychiatry 2008. [Epub ahead of print].

147. Walther DJ, Peter JU, Bashammakh S, et al. Synthesis of serotonin by a second tryptophan hydroxylase isoform. Science 2003;299:76.

148. Nakamura K, Sugawara Y, Sawabe K, et al. Late developmental stage-specific role of tryptophan hydroxylase 1 in brain serotonin levels. J Neurosci 2006;26: 530–4.

149. Binder DK, Scharfman HE. Brain-derived neurotrophic factor. Growth Factors 2004;22:123–31.

150. Shorter E. The history of lithium therapy. Bipolar Disord 2009;11(Suppl 2):4–9.

151. Grof P, Muller-Oerlinghausen B. A critical appraisal of lithium's efficacy and effectiveness: the last 60 years. Bipolar Disord 2009;11(Suppl 2):10–9.

152. Young AH, Hammond JM. Lithium in mood disorders: increasing evidence base, declining use? Br J Psychiatry 2007;191:474–6.

153. Coryell W. Maintenance treatment in bipolar disorder: a reassessment of lithium as the first choice. Bipolar Disord 2009;11(Suppl 2):77–83.

154. Cavazzoni P, Alda M, Turecki G, et al. Lithium-responsive affective disorders: no association with the tyrosine hydroxylase gene. Psychiatry Res 1996;64:91–6.

155. Turecki G, Alda M, Grof P, et al. No association between chromosome-18 markers and lithium-responsive affective disorders. Psychiatry Res 1996;63: 17–23.

156. Steen VM, Gulbrandsen AK, Eiken HG, et al. Lack of genetic variation in the coding region of the myo-inositol monophosphatase gene in lithium-treated patients with manic depressive illness. Pharmacogenetics 1996;6:113–6.

157. Turecki G, Grof P, Cavazzoni P, et al. Evidence for a role of phospholipase C-gamma1 in the pathogenesis of bipolar disorder. Mol Psychiatry 1998;3: 534–8.

158. Alda M, Grof P, Grof E. MN blood groups and bipolar disorder: evidence of genotypic association and Hardy-Weinberg disequilibrium. Biol Psychiatry 1998;44:361–3.

159. Steen VM, Lovlie R, Osher Y, et al. The polymorphic inositol polyphosphate 1-phosphatase gene as a candidate for pharmacogenetic prediction of lithium-responsive manic-depressive illness. Pharmacogenetics 1998;8:259–68.

160. Serretti A, Lilli R, Lorenzi C, et al. Dopamine receptor D3 gene and response to lithium prophylaxis in mood disorders. Int J Neuropsychopharmacol 1998;1: 125–9.

161. Turecki G, Grof P, Cavazzoni P, et al. association and linkage studies with lithium responsive bipolar disorder. Psychiatr Genet 1999;9:13–6.

162. Serretti A, Lilli R, Lorenzi C, et al. Dopamine receptor D2 and D4 genes, GABA(A) alpha-1 subunit genes and response to lithium prophylaxis in mood disorders. Psychiatry Res 1999;87:7–19.

163. Serretti A, Lilli R, Lorenzi C, et al. Tryptophan hydroxylase gene and response to lithium prophylaxis in mood disorders. J Psychiatr Res 1999;33:371–7.

164. Duffy A, Turecki G, Grof P, et al. Association and linkage studies of candidate genes involved in GABAergic neurotransmission in lithium-responsive bipolar disorder. J Psychiatry Neurosci 2000;25:353–8.

165. Alda M, Turecki G, Grof P, et al. Association and linkage studies of CRH and PENK genes in bipolar disorder: a collaborative IGSLI study. Am J Med Genet 2000;96:178–81.
166. Serretti A, Lorenzi C, Lilli R, et al. Serotonin receptor 2A, 2C, 1A genes and response to lithium prophylaxis in mood disorders. J Psychiatr Res 2000;34:89–98.
167. Ftouhi-Paquin N, Alda M, Grof P, et al. Identification of three polymorphisms in the translated region of PLC-gamma1 and their investigation in lithium responsive bipolar disorder. Am J Med Genet 2001;105:301–5.
168. Serretti A, Lilli R, Mandelli L, et al. Serotonin transporter gene associated with lithium prophylaxis in mood disorders. Pharmacogenomics J 2001;1:71–7.
169. Lovlie R, Berle JO, Stordal E, et al. The phospholipase C-gamma1 gene (PLCG1) and lithium-responsive bipolar disorder: re-examination of an intronic dinucleotide repeat polymorphism. Psychiatr Genet 2001;11:41–3.
170. Serretti A, Lorenzi C, Lilli R, et al. Pharmacogenetics of lithium prophylaxis in mood disorders: analysis of COMT, MAO-A, and Gbeta3 variants. Am J Med Genet 2002;114:370–9.
171. Washizuka S, Ikeda A, Kato N, et al. Possible relationship between mitochondrial DNA polymorphisms and lithium response in bipolar disorder. Int J Neuropsychopharmacol 2003;6:421–4.
172. Dmitrzak-Weglarz M, Rybakowski JK, Suwalska A, et al. Association studies of 5-HT2A and 5-HT2C serotonin receptor gene polymorphisms with prophylactic lithium response in bipolar patients. Pharmacol Rep 2005;57:761–5.
173. Rybakowski JK, Suwalska A, Skibinska M, et al. Prophylactic lithium response and polymorphism of the brain-derived neurotrophic factor gene. Pharmacopsychiatry 2005;38:166–70.
174. Rybakowski JK, Suwalska A, Czerski PM, et al. Prophylactic effect of lithium in bipolar affective illness may be related to serotonin transporter genotype. Pharmacol Rep 2005;57:124–7.
175. Benedetti F, Serretti A, Pontiggia A, et al. Long-term response to lithium salts in bipolar illness is influenced by the glycogen synthase kinase 3-beta -50 T/C SNP. Neurosci Lett 2005;376:51–5.
176. Szczepankiewicz A, Rybakowski JK, Suwalska A, et al. Association study of the glycogen synthase kinase-3beta gene polymorphism with prophylactic lithium response in bipolar patients. World J Biol Psychiatry 2006;7:158–61.
177. Masui T, Hashimoto R, Kusumi I, et al. Lithium response and Val66Met polymorphism of the brain-derived neurotrophic factor gene in Japanese patients with bipolar disorder. Psychiatr Genet 2006;16:49–50.
178. Masui T, Hashimoto R, Kusumi I, et al. A possible association between the -116C/G single nucleotide polymorphism of the XBP1 gene and lithium prophylaxis in bipolar disorder. Int J Neuropsychopharmacol 2006;9:83–8.
179. Michelon L, Meira-Lima I, Cordeiro Q, et al. Association study of the INPP1, 5HTT, BDNF, AP-2beta and GSK-3beta GENE variants and restrospectively scored response to lithium prophylaxis in bipolar disorder. Neurosci Lett 2006; 403:288–93.
180. Mamdani F, Sequeira A, Alda M, et al. No association between the PREP gene and lithium responsive bipolar disorder. BMC Psychiatry 2007;7:9.
181. Bremer T, Diamond C, McKinney R, et al. The pharmacogenetics of lithium response depends upon clinical co-morbidity. Mol Diagn Ther 2007;11:161–70.
182. Rybakowski JK, Suwalska A, Skibinska M, et al. Response to lithium prophylaxis: interaction between serotonin transporter and BDNF genes. Am J Med Genet B Neuropsychiatr Genet 2007;144B:820–3.

183. Mamdani F, Alda M, Grof P, et al. Lithium response and genetic variation in the CREB family of genes. Am J Med Genet B Neuropsychiatr Genet 2008;147B:500–4.
184. Dmitrzak-Weglarz M, Rybakowski JK, Suwalska A, et al. Association studies of the BDNF and the NTRK2 gene polymorphisms with prophylactic lithium response in bipolar patients. Pharmacogenomics 2008;9:1595–603.
185. Masui T, Hashimoto R, Kusumi I, et al. A possible association between missense polymorphism of the breakpoint cluster region gene and lithium prophylaxis in bipolar disorder. Prog Neuropsychopharmacol Biol Psychiatry 2008;32:204–8.
186. Kim B, Kim CY, Lee MJ, et al. Preliminary evidence on the association between XBP1-116C/G polymorphism and response to prophylactic treatment with valproate in bipolar disorders. Psychiatry Res 2009;168:209–12.
187. Szczepankiewicz A, Skibinska M, Suwalska A, et al. No association of three GRIN2B polymorphisms with lithium response in bipolar patients. Pharmacol Rep 2009;61:448–52.
188. Szczepankiewicz A, Skibinska M, Suwalska A, et al. The association study of three FYN polymorphisms with prophylactic lithium response in bipolar patients. Hum Psychopharmacol 2009;24:287–91.
189. Rybakowski JK, Dmitrzak-Weglarz M, Suwalska A, et al. Dopamine D1 receptor gene polymorphism is associated with prophylactic lithium response in bipolar disorder. Pharmacopsychiatry 2009;42:20–2.
190. Perlis RH, Smoller JW, Ferreira MA, et al. A genome-wide association study of response to lithium for prevention of recurrence in bipolar disorder. Am J Psychiatry 2009;166:718–25.
191. Berridge MJ, Downes CP, Hanley MR. Neural and developmental actions of lithium: a unifying hypothesis. Cell 1989;59:411–9.
192. Harwood AJ. Lithium and bipolar mood disorder: the inositol-depletion hypothesis revisited. Mol Psychiatry 2005;10:117–26.
193. Klein PS, Melton DA. A molecular mechanism for the effect of lithium on development. Proc Natl Acad Sci U S A 1996;93:8455–9.
194. Williams RS, Harwood AJ. Lithium therapy and signal transduction. Trends Pharmacol Sci 2000;21:61–4.
195. Jope RS, Bijur GN. Mood stabilizers, glycogen synthase kinase-3beta and cell survival. Mol Psychiatry 2002;7(Suppl 1):S35–45.
196. Chen G, Huang LD, Jiang YM, et al. The mood-stabilizing agent valproate inhibits the activity of glycogen synthase kinase-3. J Neurochem 1999;72:1327–30.
197. Bajjalieh SM, Peterson K, Linial M, et al. Brain contains two forms of synaptic vesicle protein 2. Proc Natl Acad Sci U S A 1993;90:2150–4.
198. Seelan RS, Khalyfa A, Lakshmanan J, et al. Deciphering the lithium transcriptome: microarray profiling of lithium-modulated gene expression in human neuronal cells. Neuroscience 2008;151:1184–97.
199. Ben-Zur T, Feige E, Motro B, et al. The mammalian Odz gene family: homologs of a Drosophila pair-rule gene with expression implying distinct yet overlapping developmental roles. Dev Biol 2000;217:107–20.
200. Shen WW. A history of antipsychotic drug development. Compr Psychiatry 1999; 40:407–14.
201. Kane J, Honigfeld G, Singer J, et al. Clozapine for the treatment-resistant schizophrenic: a double-blind comparison with chlorpromazine. Arch Gen Psychiatry 1988;45:789–96.
202. Leucht S, Corves C, Arbter D, et al. Second-generation versus first-generation antipsychotic drugs for schizophrenia: a meta-analysis. Lancet 2009;373:31–41.

203. Sharif Z. Side effects as influencers of treatment outcome. J Clin Psychiatry 2008;69(Suppl 3):38–43.
204. Arranz M, Collier D, Sodhi M, et al. Association between clozapine response and allelic variation in 5-HT2A receptor gene. Lancet 1995;346:281–2.
205. Arranz MJ, Dawson E, Shaikh S, et al. Cytochrome P4502D6 genotype does not determine response to clozapine. Br J Clin Psychol 1995;39:417–20.
206. Masellis M, Paterson AD, Badri F, et al. Genetic variation of 5-HT2A receptor and response to clozapine. Lancet 1995;346:1108.
207. Nothen MM, Rietschel M, Erdmann J, et al. Genetic variation of the 5-HT2A receptor and response to clozapine. Lancet 1995;346:908–9.
208. Sodhi MS, Arranz MJ, Curtis D, et al. Association between clozapine response and allelic variation in the 5-HT2C receptor gene. Neuroreport 1995;7:169–72.
209. Malhotra AK, Goldman D, Ozaki N, et al. Lack of association between polymorphisms in the 5-HT2A receptor gene and the antipsychotic response to clozapine. Am J Psychiatry 1996;153:1092–4.
210. Arranz MJ, Collier DA, Munro J, et al. Analysis of a structural polymorphism in the 5-HT2A receptor and clinical response to clozapine. Neurosci Lett 1996; 217:177–8.
211. Gaitonde EJ, Morris A, Sivagnanasundaram S, et al. Assessment of association of D3 dopamine receptor Mscl polymorphism with schizophrenia: analysis of symptom ratings, family history, age at onset, and movement disorders. Am J Med Genet 1996;67:455–8.
212. Jonsson E, Nothen MM, Bunzel R, et al. 5HT 2a receptor T102C polymorphism and schizophrenia. Lancet 1996;347:1831.
213. Rietschel M, Naber D, Oberlander H, et al. Efficacy and side-effects of clozapine: testing for association with allelic variation in the dopamine D4 receptor gene. Neuropsychopharmacology 1996;15:491–6.
214. Rietschel M, Naber D, Fimmers R, et al. Efficacy and side-effects of clozapine not associated with variation in the 5-HT2C receptor. Neuroreport 1997;8: 1999–2003.
215. Steen VM, Lovlie R, MacEwan T, et al. Dopamine D3-receptor gene variant and susceptibility to tardive dyskinesia in schizophrenic patients. Mol Psychiatry 1997;2:139–45.
216. Turbay D, Lieberman J, Alper CA, et al. Tumor necrosis factor constellation polymorphism and clozapine-induced agranulocytosis in two different ethnic groups. Blood 1997;89:4167–74.
217. Amar A, Segman RH, Shtrussberg S, et al. An association between clozapine-induced agranulocytosis in schizophrenics and HLA-DQB1*0201. Int J Neuropsychopharmacol 1998;1:41–4.
218. Arranz MJ, Munro J, Owen MJ, et al. Evidence for association between polymorphisms in the promoter and coding regions of the 5-HT2A receptor gene and response to clozapine. Mol Psychiatry 1998;3:61–6.
219. Hwu HG, Hong CJ, Lee YL, et al. Dopamine D4 receptor gene polymorphisms and neuroleptic response in schizophrenia. Biol Psychiatry 1998;44: 483–7.
220. Masellis M, Basile V, Meltzer HY, et al. Serotonin subtype 2 receptor genes and clinical response to clozapine in schizophrenia patients. Neuropsychopharmacology 1998;19:123–32.
221. Valevski A, Klein T, Gazit E, et al. HLA-B38 and clozapine-induced agranulocytosis in Israeli Jewish schizophrenic patients. Eur J Immunol 1998;25:11–3.

222. Aitchison KJ, Munro J, Wright P, et al. Failure to respond to treatment with typical antipsychotics is not associated with CYP2D6 ultrarapid hydroxylation. Br J Clin Pharmacol 1999;48:388–94.

223. Basile VS, Masellis M, Badri F, et al. Association of the Mscl polymorphism of the dopamine D3 receptor gene with tardive dyskinesia in schizophrenia. Neuropsychopharmacology 1999;21:17–27.

224. Cohen BM, Ennulat DJ, Centorrino F, et al. Polymorphisms of the dopamine D4 receptor and response to antipsychotic drugs. Psychopharmacology (Berl) 1999;141:6–10.

225. Joober R, Benkelfat C, Brisebois K, et al. T102C polymorphism in the 5HT2A gene and schizophrenia: relation to phenotype and drug response variability. J Psychiatry Neurosci 1999;24:141–6.

226. Lin CH, Tsai SJ, Yu YW, et al. No evidence for association of serotonin-2A receptor variant (102T/C) with schizophrenia or clozapine response in a Chinese population. Neuroreport 1999;10:57–60.

227. Scharfetter J, Chaudhry HR, Hornik K, et al. Dopamine D3 receptor gene polymorphism and response to clozapine in schizophrenic Pakastani patients. Eur Neuropsychopharmacol 1999;10:17–20.

228. Segman R, Neeman T, Heresco-Levy U, et al. Genotypic association between the dopamine D3 receptor and tardive dyskinesia in chronic schizophrenia. Mol Psychiatry 1999;4:247–53.

229. Yu YW, Tsai SJ, Lin CH, et al. Serotonin-6 receptor variant (C267T) and clinical response to clozapine. Neuroreport 1999;10:1231–3.

230. Arranz MJ, Munro J, Birkett J, et al. Pharmacogenetic prediction of clozapine response. Lancet 2000;355:1615–6.

231. Arranz MJ, Bolonna AA, Munro J, et al. The serotonin transporter and clozapine response. Mol Psychiatry 2000;5:124–5.

232. Basile VS, Ozdemir V, Masellis M, et al. A functional polymorphism of the cytochrome P450 1A2 (CYP1A2) gene: association with tardive dyskinesia in schizophrenia. Mol Psychiatry 2000;5:410–7.

233. Birkett JT, Arranz MJ, Munro J, et al. Association analysis of the 5-HT5A gene in depression, psychosis and antipsychotic response. Neuroreport 2000;11:2017–20.

234. Bolonna AA, Arranz MJ, Munro J, et al. No influence of adrenergic receptor polymorphisms on schizophrenia and antipsychotic response. Neurosci Lett 2000; 280:65–8.

235. Chong SA, Tan EC, Tan CH, et al. Tardive dyskinesia is not associated with the serotonin gene polymorphism (5-HTTLPR) in Chinese. Am J Med Genet 2000; 96:712–5.

236. Dettling M, Sachse C, Muller-Oerlinghausen B, et al. Clozapine-induced agranulocytosis and hereditary polymorphisms of clozapine metabolizing enzymes: no association with myeloperoxidase and cytochrome P4502D6. Pharmacopsychiatry 2000;33:218–20.

237. Eichhammer P, Albus M, Borrmann-Hassenbach M, et al. Association of dopamine D3-receptor gene variants with neuroleptic induced akathisia in schizophrenic patients: a generalization of Steen's study on DRD3 and tardive dyskinesia. Am J Med Genet 2000;96:187–91.

238. Joober R, Toulouse A, Benkelfat C, et al. DRD3 and DAT1 genes in schizophrenia: an association study. J Psychiatr Res 2000;34:285–91.

239. Joober R, Benkelfat C, Lal S, et al. Association between the methylenetetrahydrofolate reductase 677C–>T missense mutation and schizophrenia. Mol Psychiatry 2000;5:323–6.

240. Kaiser R, Konneker M, Henneken M, et al. Dopamine D4 receptor 48-bp repeat polymorphism: no association with response to antipsychotic treatment, but association with catatonic schizophrenia. Mol Psychiatry 2000;5:418–24.
241. Krebs MO, Guillin O, Bourdell MC, et al. Brain derived neurotrophic factor (BDNF) gene variants association with age at onset and therapeutic response in schizophrenia. Mol Psychiatry 2000;5:558–62.
242. Lovlie R, Daly AK, Blennerhassett R, et al. Homozygosity for the Gly-9 variant of the dopamine D3 receptor and risk for tardive dyskinesia in schizophrenic patients. Int J Neuropsychopharmacol 2000;3:61–5.
243. Mihara K, Suzuki A, Kondo T, et al. No relationship between Taq1 a polymorphism of dopamine D(2) receptor gene and extrapyramidal adverse effects of selective dopamine D(2) antagonists, bromperidol, and nemonapride in schizophrenia: a preliminary study. Am J Med Genet 2000;96:422–4.
244. Rietschel M, Krauss H, Muller DJ, et al. Dopamine D3 receptor variant and tardive dyskinesia. Eur Arch Psychiatry Clin Neurosci 2000;250:31–5.
245. Scordo MG, Spina E, Romeo P, et al. CYP2D6 genotype and antipsychotic-induced extrapyramidal side effects in schizophrenic patients. Eur J Clin Pharmacol 2000;56:679–83.
246. Segman RH, Heresco-Levy U, Finkel B, et al. Association between the serotonin 2C receptor gene and tardive dyskinesia in chronic schizophrenia: additive contribution of 5-HT2Cser and DRD3gly alleles to susceptibility. Psychopharmacology (Berl) 2000;152:408–13.
247. Tsai SJ, Hong CJ, Yu YW, et al. Association study of a functional serotonin transporter gene polymorphism with schizophrenia, psychopathology and clozapine response. Schizophr Res 2000;44:177–81.
248. Basile VS, Ozdemir V, Masellis M, et al. Lack of association between serotonin-2A receptor gene (HTR2A) polymorphisms and tardive dyskinesia in schizophrenia. Mol Psychiatry 2001;6:230–4.
249. Basile VS, Masellis M, McIntyre RS, et al. Genetic dissection of atypical antipsychotic-induced weight gain: novel preliminary data on the pharmacogenetic puzzle. J Clin Psychiatry 2001;62(Suppl 23):45–66.
250. Dahmen N, Muller MJ, Germeyer S, et al. Genetic polymorphisms of the dopamine D2 and D3 receptor and neuroleptic drug effects in schizophrenic patients. Schizophr Res 2001;49:223–5.
251. Dettling M, Cascorbi I, Roots I, et al. Genetic determinants of clozapine-induced agranulocytosis: recent results of HLA subtyping in a non-Jewish caucasian sample. Arch Gen Psychiatry 2001;58:93–4.
252. Garcia-Barcelo MM, Lam LC, Ungvari GS, et al. Dopamine D3 receptor gene and tardive dyskinesia in Chinese schizophrenic patients. J Neural Transm 2001;108:671–7.
253. Hong CJ, Lin CH, Yu YW, et al. Genetic variants of the serotonin system and weight change during clozapine treatment. Pharmacogenetics 2001;11:265–8.
254. Hong CJ, Yu YW, Lin CH, et al. Association analysis for NMDA receptor subunit 2B (GRIN2B) genetic variants and psychopathology and clozapine response in schizophrenia. Psychiatr Genet 2001;11:219–22.
255. Hori H, Ohmori O, Shinkai T, et al. Association between three functional polymorphisms of dopamine D2 receptor gene and tardive dyskinesia in schizophrenia. Am J Med Genet 2001;105:774–8.
256. Kaiser R, Tremblay PB, Schmider J, et al. Serotonin transporter polymorphisms: no association with response to antipsychotic treatment, but associations with

the schizoparanoid and residual subtypes of schizophrenia. Mol Psychiatry 2001;6:179–85.

257. Liao DL, Yeh YC, Chen HM, et al. Association between the Ser9Gly polymorphism of the dopamine D3 receptor gene and tardive dyskinesia in Chinese schizophrenic patients. Neuropsychobiology 2001;44:95–8.

258. Masellis M, Basile VS, Meltzer HY, et al. Lack of association between the T->C 267 serotonin 5-HT6 receptor gene (HTR6) polymorphism and prediction of response to clozapine in schizophrenia. Schizophr Res 2001;47:49–58.

259. Mihara K, Kondo T, Suzuki A, et al. No relationship between–141C Ins/Del polymorphism in the promoter region of dopamine D2 receptor and extrapyramidal adverse effects of selective dopamine D2 antagonists in schizophrenic patients: a preliminary study. Psychiatry Res 2001;101:33–8.

260. Roh HK, Kim CE, Chung WG, et al. Risperidone metabolism in relation to CYP2D6*10 allele in Korean schizophrenic patients. Eur J Clin Pharmacol 2001;57:671–5.

261. Schafer M, Rujescu D, Giegling I, et al. Association of short-term response to haloperidol treatment with a polymorphism in the dopamine D(2) receptor gene. Am J Psychiatry 2001;158:802–4.

262. Schulze TG, Schumacher J, Muller DJ, et al. Lack of association between a functional polymorphism of the cytochrome P450 1A2 (CYP1A2) gene and tardive dyskinesia in schizophrenia. Am J Med Genet 2001;105:498–501.

263. Segman RH, Heresco-Levy U, Finkel B, et al. Association between the serotonin 2A receptor gene and tardive dyskinesia in chronic schizophrenia. Mol Psychiatry 2001;6:225–9.

264. Suzuki A, Kondo T, Otani K, et al. Association of the TaqI A polymorphism of the dopamine D(2) receptor gene with predisposition to neuroleptic malignant syndrome. Am J Psychiatry 2001;158:1714–6.

265. Suzuki A, Kondo T, Mihara K, et al. The -141C Ins/Del polymorphism in the dopamine D2 receptor gene promoter region is associated with anxiolytic and antidepressive effects during treatment with dopamine antagonists in schizophrenic patients. Pharmacogenetics 2001;11:545–50.

266. Tan EC, Chong SA, Mahendran R, et al. Susceptibility to neuroleptic-induced tardive dyskinesia and the T102C polymorphism in the serotonin type 2A receptor. Biol Psychiatry 2001;50:144–7.

267. Tsai SJ, Wang YC, Yu Younger WY, et al. Association analysis of polymorphism in the promoter region of the alpha2a-adrenoceptor gene with schizophrenia and clozapine response. Schizophr Res 2001;49:53–8.

268. Yu YW, Tsai SJ, Yang KH, et al. Evidence for an association between polymorphism in the serotonin-2A receptor variant (102T/C) and increment of N100 amplitude in schizophrenics treated with clozapine. Neuropsychobiology 2001;43:79–82.

269. Basile VS, Masellis M, De LV, et al. 759C/T genetic variation of 5HT(2C) receptor and clozapine-induced weight gain. Lancet 2002;360:1790–1.

270. Brockmoller J, Kirchheiner J, Schmider J, et al. The impact of the CYP2D6 polymorphism on haloperidol pharmacokinetics and on the outcome of haloperidol treatment. Clin Pharmacol Ther 2002;72:438–52.

271. Ellingrod VL, Miller D, Schultz SK, et al. CYP2D6 polymorphisms and atypical antipsychotic weight gain. Psychiatr Genet 2002;12:55–8.

272. Gutierrez B, Arranz MJ, Huezo-Diaz P, et al. Novel mutations in 5-HT3A and 5-HT3B receptor genes not associated with clozapine response. Schizophr Res 2002;58:93–7.

273. Himei A, Koh J, Sakai J, et al. The influence on the schizophrenic symptoms by the DRD2Ser/Cys311 and -141C Ins/Del polymorphisms. Psychiatry Clin Neurosci 2002;56:97–102.
274. Kaiser R, Tremblay PB, Klufmoller F, et al. Relationship between adverse effects of antipsychotic treatment and dopamine D(2) receptor polymorphisms in patients with schizophrenia. Mol Psychiatry 2002;7:695–705.
275. Lane HY, Chang YC, Chiu CC, et al. Association of risperidone treatment response with a polymorphism in the 5-HT(2A) receptor gene. Am J Psychiatry 2002;159:1593–5.
276. Lerer B, Segman RH, Fangerau H, et al. Pharmacogenetics of tardive dyskinesia: combined analysis of 780 patients supports association with dopamine D3 receptor gene Ser9Gly polymorphism. Neuropsychopharmacology 2002; 27:105–19.
277. Mancama D, Arranz MJ, Munro J, et al. Investigation of promoter variants of the histamine 1 and 2 receptors in schizophrenia and clozapine response. Neurosci Lett 2002;333:207–11.
278. Mihara K, Kondo T, Higuchi H, et al. Tardive dystonia and genetic polymorphisms of cytochrome P4502D6 and dopamine D2 and D3 receptors: a preliminary finding. Am J Med Genet 2002;114:693–5.
279. Ohmori O, Shinkai T, Hori H, et al. Genetic association analysis of 5-HT(6) receptor gene polymorphism (267C/T) with tardive dyskinesia. Psychiatry Res 2002;110:97–102.
280. Reynolds GP, Zhang ZJ, Zhang XB. Association of antipsychotic drug-induced weight gain with a 5-HT2C receptor gene polymorphism. Lancet 2002;359: 2086–7.
281. Schillevoort I, de BA, van der Weide J, et al. Antipsychotic-induced extrapyramidal syndromes and cytochrome P450 2D6 genotype: a case-control study. Pharmacogenetics 2002;12:235–40.
282. Segman RH, Heresco-Levy U, Yakir A, et al. Interactive effect of cytochrome P450 17alpha-hydroxylase and dopamine D3 receptor gene polymorphisms on abnormal involuntary movements in chronic schizophrenia. Biol Psychiatry 2002;51:261–3.
283. Segman RH, Lerer B. Age and the relationship of dopamine D3, serotonin 2C and serotonin 2A receptor genes to abnormal involuntary movements in chronic schizophrenia. Mol Psychiatry 2002;7:137–9.
284. Staddon S, Arranz MJ, Mancama D, et al. Clinical applications of pharmacogenetics in psychiatry. Psychopharmacology (Berl) 2002;162:18–23.
285. Tsai SJ, Hong CJ, Yu YW, et al. 759C/T genetic variation of 5HT(2C) receptor and clozapine-induced weight gain. Lancet 2002;360:1790.
286. Woo SI, Kim JW, Rha E, et al. Association of the Ser9Gly polymorphism in the dopamine D3 receptor gene with tardive dyskinesia in Korean schizophrenics. Psychiatry Clin Neurosci 2002;56:469–74.
287. Zhang Z, Zhang X, Hou G, et al. The increased activity of plasma manganese superoxide dismutase in tardive dyskinesia is unrelated to the Ala-9Val polymorphism. J Psychiatr Res 2002;36:317–24.
288. Zhang ZJ, Zhang XB, Sha WW, et al. Association of a polymorphism in the promoter region of the serotonin 5-HT2C receptor gene with tardive dyskinesia in patients with schizophrenia. Mol Psychiatry 2002;7:670–1.
289. Chong SA, Tan EC, Tan CH, et al. Polymorphisms of dopamine receptors and tardive dyskinesia among Chinese patients with schizophrenia. Am J Med Genet B Neuropsychiatr Genet. 2003;116B:51–4.

290. Herken H, Erdal ME, Boke O, et al. Tardive dyskinesia is not associated with the polymorphisms of 5-HT2A receptor gene, serotonin transporter gene and cate-chol-o-methyltransferase gene. Eur Psychiatry 2003;18:77–81.
291. Hong CJ, Yu YW, Lin CH, et al. An association study of a brain-derived neuro-trophic factor Val66Met polymorphism and clozapine response of schizophrenic patients. Neurosci Lett 2003;349:206–8.
292. Inada T, Senoo H, Iijima Y, et al. Cytochrome P450 II D6 gene polymorphisms and the neuroleptic-induced extrapyramidal symptoms in Japanese schizo-phrenic patients. Psychiatr Genet 2003;13:163–8.
293. Kishida I, Kawanishi C, Furuno T, et al. Lack of association in Japanese patients between neuroleptic malignant syndrome and the TaqI A polymorphism of the dopamine D2 receptor gene. Psychiatr Genet 2003;13:55–7.
294. Lohmann PL, Bagli M, Krauss H, et al. CYP2D6 polymorphism and tardive dyski-nesia in schizophrenic patients. Pharmacopsychiatry 2003;36:73–8.
295. Mihara K, Kondo T, Suzuki A, et al. Relationship between functional dopamine D2 and D3 receptors gene polymorphisms and neuroleptic malignant syndrome. Am J Med Genet B Neuropsychiatr Genet 2003;117B:57–60.
296. Ostrousky O, Meged S, Loewenthal R, et al. NQO2 gene is associated with clo-zapine-induced agranulocytosis. Tissue Antigens 2003;62:483–91.
297. Reynolds GP, Zhang Z, Zhang X. Polymorphism of the promoter region of the serotonin 5-HT(2C) receptor gene and clozapine-induced weight gain. Am J Psychiatry 2003;160:677–9.
298. Tsai SJ, Hong CJ, Yu YW, et al. No association of tumor necrosis factor alpha gene polymorphisms with schizophrenia or response to clozapine. Schizophr Res 2003;65:27–32.
299. Zalsman G, Frisch A, Lev-Ran S, et al. DRD4 exon III polymorphism and response to risperidone in Israeli adolescents with schizophrenia: a pilot phar-macogenetic study. Eur Neuropsychopharmacol 2003;13:183–5.
300. Zhang ZJ, Yao ZJ, Zhang XB, et al. No association of antipsychotic agent-induced weight gain with a DA receptor gene polymorphism and therapeutic response. Acta Pharmacol Sin 2003;24:235–40.
301. Anttila S, Illi A, Kampman O, et al. Interaction between NOTCH4 and catechol-O-methyltransferase genotypes in schizophrenia patients with poor response to typical neuroleptics. Pharmacogenetics 2004;14:303–7.
302. Bertolino A, Caforio G, Blasi G, et al. Interaction of COMT (Val(108/158)Met) genotype and olanzapine treatment on prefrontal cortical function in patients with schizophrenia. Am J Psychiatry 2004;161:1798–805.
303. Huezo-Diaz P, Arranz MJ, Munro J, et al. An association study of the neurotensin receptor gene with schizophrenia and clozapine response. Schizophr Res 2004;66:193–5.
304. Kampman O, Anttila S, Illi A, et al. Neuregulin genotype and medication response in Finnish patients with schizophrenia. Neuroreport 2004;15:2517–20.
305. Kishida I, Kawanishi C, Furuno T, et al. Association in Japanese patients between neuroleptic malignant syndrome and functional polymorphisms of the dopamine D(2) receptor gene. Mol Psychiatry 2004;9:293–8.
306. Lane HY, Lee CC, Chang YC, et al. Effects of dopamine D2 receptor Ser311Cys polymorphism and clinical factors on risperidone efficacy for positive and nega-tive symptoms and social function. Int J Neuropsychopharmacol 2004;7:461–70.
307. Lane HY, Lin CC, Huang CH, et al. Risperidone response and 5-HT6 receptor gene variance: genetic association analysis with adjustment for nongenetic confounders. Schizophr Res 2004;67:63–70.

308. Lattuada E, Cavallaro R, Serretti A, et al. Tardive dyskinesia and DRD2, DRD3, DRD4, 5-HT2A variants in schizophrenia: an association study with repeated assessment. Int J Neuropsychopharmacol 2004;7:489–93.

309. Liou YJ, Liao DL, Chen JY, et al. Association analysis of the dopamine D3 receptor gene ser9gly and brain-derived neurotrophic factor gene val66met polymorphisms with antipsychotic-induced persistent tardive dyskinesia and clinical expression in Chinese schizophrenic patients. Neuromolecular Med 2004;5:243–51.

310. Liou YJ, Wang YC, Bai YM, et al. Cytochrome P-450 2D6*10 C188T polymorphism is associated with antipsychotic-induced persistent tardive dyskinesia in Chinese schizophrenic patients. Neuropsychobiology 2004;49:167–73.

311. Matsumoto C, Ohmori O, Shinkai T, et al. Genetic association analysis of functional polymorphisms in the cytochrome P450 1A2 (CYP1A2) gene with tardive dyskinesia in Japanese patients with schizophrenia. Psychiatr Genet 2004;14: 209–13.

312. Matsumoto C, Shinkai T, Hori H, et al. Polymorphisms of dopamine degradation enzyme (COMT and MAO) genes and tardive dyskinesia in patients with schizophrenia. Psychiatry Res 2004;127:1–7.

313. Mosyagin I, Dettling M, Roots I, et al. Impact of myeloperoxidase and NADPH-oxidase polymorphisms in drug-induced agranulocytosis. J Clin Psychopharmacol 2004;24:613–7.

314. Pae CU, Yu HS, Kim JJ, et al. Quinone oxidoreductase (NQO1) gene polymorphism (609C/T) may be associated with tardive dyskinesia, but not with the development of schizophrenia. Int J Neuropsychopharmacol 2004;7:495–500.

315. Shinkai T, Ohmori O, Matsumoto C, et al. Genetic association analysis of neuronal nitric oxide synthase gene polymorphism with tardive dyskinesia. Neuromolecular Med 2004;5:163–70.

316. Szekeres G, Keri S, Juhasz A, et al. Role of dopamine D3 receptor (DRD3) and dopamine transporter (DAT) polymorphism in cognitive dysfunctions and therapeutic response to atypical antipsychotics in patients with schizophrenia. Am J Med Genet B Neuropsychiatr Genet 2004;124B:1–5.

317. Tsai SJ, Yu YW, Lin CH, et al. Association study of adrenergic beta3 receptor (Trp64Arg) and G-protein beta3 subunit gene (C825T) polymorphisms and weight change during clozapine treatment. Neuropsychobiology 2004;50: 37–40.

318. Wang YC, Liou YJ, Liao DL, et al. Association analysis of a neural nitric oxide synthase gene polymorphism and antipsychotics-induced tardive dyskinesia in Chinese schizophrenic patients. J Neural Transm 2004;111:623–9.

319. Weickert TW, Goldberg TE, Mishara A, et al. Catechol-O-methyltransferase val108/158met genotype predicts working memory response to antipsychotic medications. Biol Psychiatry 2004;56:677–82.

320. Templeman LA, Reynolds GP, Arranz B, et al. Polymorphisms of the 5-HT2C receptor and leptin genes are associated with antipsychotic drug-induced weight gain in caucasian subjects with a first-episode psychosis. Pharmacogenet Genomics 2005;15:195–200.

321. Theisen FM, Gebhardt S, Haberhausen M, et al. Clozapine-induced weight gain: a study in monozygotic twins and same-sex sib pairs. Psychiatr Genet 2005;15: 285–9.

322. Anttila S, Illi A, Kampman O, et al. Lack of association between two polymorphisms of brain-derived neurotrophic factor and response to typical neuroleptics. J Neural Transm 2005;112:885–90.

323. Bishop JR, Ellingrod VL, Moline J, et al. Association between the polymorphic GRM3 gene and negative symptom improvement during olanzapine treatment. Schizophr Res 2005;77:253–60.

324. de LJ, Susce MT, Pan RM, et al. The CYP2D6 poor metabolizer phenotype may be associated with risperidone adverse drug reactions and discontinuation. J Clin Psychiatry 2005;66:15–27.

325. de LJ, Susce MT, Pan RM, et al. Polymorphic variations in GSTM1, GSTT1, PgP, CYP2D6, CYP3A5, and dopamine D2 and D3 receptors and their association with tardive dyskinesia in severe mental illness. J Clin Psychopharmacol 2005;25:448–56.

326. De LV, Vincent JB, Muller DJ, et al. Identification of a naturally occurring 21 bp deletion in alpha 2c noradrenergic receptor gene and cognitive correlates to antipsychotic treatment. Pharm Res 2005;51:381–4.

327. Deshpande SN, Varma PG, Semwal P, et al. Serotonin receptor gene polymorphisms and their association with tardive dyskinesia among schizophrenia patients from North India. Psychiatr Genet 2005;15:157–8.

328. Ellingrod VL, Perry PJ, Ringold JC, et al. Weight gain associated with the -759C/T polymorphism of the 5HT2C receptor and olanzapine. Am J Med Genet B Neuropsychiatr Genet 2005;134B:76–8.

329. Hamdani N, Bonniere M, Ades J, et al. Negative symptoms of schizophrenia could explain discrepant data on the association between the 5-HT2A receptor gene and response to antipsychotics. Neurosci Lett 2005;377:69–74.

330. Hwang R, Shinkai T, De LV, et al. Association study of 12 polymorphisms spanning the dopamine D(2) receptor gene and clozapine treatment response in two treatment refractory/intolerant populations. Psychopharmacology (Berl) 2005;181:179–87.

331. Kakihara S, Yoshimura R, Shinkai K, et al. Prediction of response to risperidone treatment with respect to plasma concencentrations of risperidone, catecholamine metabolites, and polymorphism of cytochrome P450 2D6. Int Clin Psychopharmacol 2005;20:71–8.

332. Kim JY, Jung IK, Han C, et al. Antipsychotics and dopamine transporter gene polymorphisms in delirium patients. Psychiatry Clin Neurosci 2005;59:183–8.

333. Lai IC, Wang YC, Lin CC, et al. Negative association between catechol-O-methyltransferase (COMT) gene Val158Met polymorphism and persistent tardive dyskinesia in schizophrenia. J Neural Transm 2005;112:1107–13.

334. Lane HY, Hsu SK, Liu YC, et al. Dopamine D3 receptor Ser9Gly polymorphism and risperidone response. J Clin Psychopharmacol 2005;25:6–11.

335. Liou YJ, Wang YC, Lin CC, et al. Association analysis of NAD(P)Hratioquinone oxidoreductase (NQO1) Pro187Ser genetic polymorphism and tardive dyskinesia in patients with schizophrenia in Taiwan. Int J Neuropsychopharmacol 2005;8:483–6.

336. Miller DD, Ellingrod VL, Holman TL, et al. Clozapine-induced weight gain associated with the 5HT2C receptor -759C/T polymorphism. Am J Med Genet B Neuropsychiatr Genet 2005;133B:97–100.

337. Muller DJ, Klempan TA, De LV, et al. The SNAP-25 gene may be associated with clinical response and weight gain in antipsychotic treatment of schizophrenia. Neurosci Lett 2005;379:81–9.

338. Muller DJ, De LV, Sicard T, et al. Suggestive association between the C825T polymorphism of the G-protein beta3 subunit gene (GNB3) and clinical improvement with antipsychotics in schizophrenia. Eur Neuropsychopharmacol 2005;15:525–31.

339. Reynolds GP, Yao Z, Zhang X, et al. Pharmacogenetics of treatment in first-episode schizophrenia: D3 and 5-HT2C receptor polymorphisms separately associate with positive and negative symptom response. Eur Neurol 2005;15:143–51.

340. Shinkai T, De LV, Hwang R, et al. Association study between a functional glutathione S-transferase (GSTP1) gene polymorphism (Ile105Val) and tardive dyskinesia. Neurosci Lett 2005;388:116–20.

341. Tiwari AK, Deshpande SN, Rao AR, et al. Genetic susceptibility to tardive dyskinesia in chronic schizophrenia subjects: I. Association of CYP1A2 gene polymorphism. Pharmacogenomics J 2005;5:60–9.

342. Tiwari AK, Deshpande SN, Rao AR, et al. Genetic susceptibility to tardive dyskinesia in chronic schizophrenia subjects: III. Lack of association of CYP3A4 and CYP2D6 gene polymorphisms. Schizophr Res 2005;75:21–6.

343. Wang YC, Bai YM, Chen JY, et al. Polymorphism of the adrenergic receptor alpha 2a -1291C>G genetic variation and clozapine-induced weight gain. J Neural Transm 2005;112:1463–8.

344. Wang YC, Bai YM, Chen JY, et al. C825T polymorphism in the human G protein beta3 subunit gene is associated with long-term clozapine treatment-induced body weight change in the Chinese population. Pharmacogenet Genomics 2005;15:743–8.

345. Wu S, Xing Q, Gao R, et al. Response to chlorpromazine treatment may be associated with polymorphisms of the DRD2 gene in Chinese schizophrenic patients. Neurosci Lett 2005;376:1–4.

346. Zhao AL, Zhao JP, Zhang YH, et al. Dopamine D4 receptor gene exon III polymorphism and interindividual variation in response to clozapine. Int J Neurosci 2005;115:1539–47.

347. Bishop JR, Ellingrod VL, Moline J, et al. Pilot study of the G-protein beta3 subunit gene (C825T) polymorphism and clinical response to olanzapine or olanzapine-related weight gain in persons with schizophrenia. Med Sci Monit 2006;12:BR47–50.

348. Fu Y, Fan CH, Deng HH, et al. Association of CYP2D6 and CYP1A2 gene polymorphism with tardive dyskinesia in Chinese schizophrenic patients. Acta Pharmacol Sin 2006;27:328–32.

349. Hwang R, Shinkai T, Deluca V, et al. Dopamine D2 receptor gene variants and quantitative measures of positive and negative symptom response following clozapine treatment. Eur Neuropsychopharmacol 2006;16:248–59.

350. Kampman O, Illi A, Hanninen K, et al. RGS4 genotype is not associated with antipsychotic medication response in schizophrenia. J Neural Transm 2006; 113:1563–8.

351. Lencz T, Robinson DG, Xu K, et al. DRD2 promoter region variation as a predictor of sustained response to antipsychotic medication in first-episode schizophrenia patients. Am J Psychiatry 2006;163:529–31.

352. Liou YJ, Lai IC, Liao DL, et al. The human dopamine receptor D2 (DRD2) gene is associated with tardive dyskinesia in patients with schizophrenia. Schizophr Res 2006;86:323–5.

353. Liou YJ, Lai IC, Lin MW, et al. Haplotype analysis of endothelial nitric oxide synthase (NOS3) genetic variants and tardive dyskinesia in patients with schizophrenia. Pharmacogenet Genomics 2006;16:151–7.

354. Mata I, Crespo-Facorro B, Perez-Iglesias R, et al. Association between the interleukin-1 receptor antagonist gene and negative symptom improvement during antipsychotic treatment. Am J Med Genet B Neuropsychiatr Genet 2006; 141B:939–43.

355. Park YM, Chung YC, Lee SH, et al. Weight gain associated with the alpha2a-adrenergic receptor -1,291 C/G polymorphism and olanzapine treatment. Am J Med Genet B Neuropsychiatr Genet 2006;141B:394–7.

356. Reynolds GP, Arranz B, Templeman LA, et al. Effect of 5-HT1A receptor gene polymorphism on negative and depressive symptom response to antipsychotic treatment of drug-naive psychotic patients. Am J Psychiatry 2006;163:1826–9.

357. Richardson MA, Chao HM, Read LL, et al. Investigation of the phenylalanine hydroxylase gene and tardive dyskinesia. Am J Med Genet B Neuropsychiatr Genet 2006;141B:195–7.

358. Shinkai T, Muller DJ, De LV, et al. Genetic association analysis of the glutathione peroxidase (GPX1) gene polymorphism (Pro197Leu) with tardive dyskinesia. Psychiatry Res 2006;141:123–8.

359. Srivastava V, Varma PG, Prasad S, et al. Genetic susceptibility to tardive dyskinesia among schizophrenia subjects: IV. Role of dopaminergic pathway gene polymorphisms. Pharmacogenet Genomics 2006;16:111–7.

360. Takao T, Tachikawa H, Kawanishi Y, et al. Association of treatment-resistant schizophrenia with the G2677A/T and C3435T polymorphisms in the ATP-binding cassette subfamily B member 1 gene. Psychiatr Genet 2006;16:47–8.

361. Yasui-Furukori N, Saito M, Nakagami T, et al. Association between multidrug resistance 1 (MDR1) gene polymorphisms and therapeutic response to bromperidol in schizophrenic patients: a preliminary study. Prog Neuropsychopharmacol Biol Psychiatry 2006;30:286–91.

362. Zai G, Muller DJ, Volavka J, et al. Family and case-control association study of the tumor necrosis factor-alpha (TNF-alpha) gene with schizophrenia and response to antipsychotic medication. Psychopharmacology (Berl) 2006;188:171–82.

363. Strous RD, Greenbaum L, Kanyas K, et al. Association of the dopamine receptor interacting protein gene, NEF3, with early response to antipsychotic medication. Int J Neuropsychopharmacol 2007;10:321–33.

364. Woodward ND, Jayathilake K, Meltzer HY. COMT val108/158met genotype, cognitive function, and cognitive improvement with clozapine in schizophrenia. Schizophr Res 2007;90:86–96.

365. Anttila S, Kampman O, Illi A, et al. Association between 5-HT2A, TPH1 and GNB3 genotypes and response to typical neuroleptics: a serotonergic approach. BMC Psychiatry 2007;7:22.

366. Bertolino A, Caforio G, Blasi G, et al. COMT Val158Met polymorphism predicts negative symptoms response to treatment with olanzapine in schizophrenia. Schizophr Res 2007;95:253–5.

367. Boke O, Gunes S, Kara N, et al. Association of serotonin 2A receptor and lack of association of CYP1A2 gene polymorphism with tardive dyskinesia in a Turkish population. DNA Cell Biol 2007;26:527–31.

368. Bozina N, Medved V, Kuzman MR, et al. Association study of olanzapine-induced weight gain and therapeutic response with SERT gene polymorphisms in female schizophrenic patients. J Psychopharmacol 2007;21:728–34.

369. Chagnon YC, Bureau A, Gendron D, et al. Possible association of the pro-melanin-concentrating hormone gene with a greater body mass index as a side effect of the antipsychotic olanzapine. Am J Med Genet B Neuropsychiatr Genet 2007;144B:1063–9.

370. De LV, Muller DJ, Hwang R, et al. HTR2C haplotypes and antipsychotics-induced weight gain: X-linked multimarker analysis. Hum Psychopharmacol. 2007;22:463–7.

371. Dettling M, Cascorbi I, Opgen-Rhein C, et al. Clozapine-induced agranulocytosis in schizophrenic caucasians: confirming clues for associations with human leukocyte class I and II antigens. Pharmacogenomics J 2007;7: 325–32.
372. Dolzan V, Plesnicar BK, Serretti A, et al. Polymorphisms in dopamine receptor DRD1 and DRD2 genes and psychopathological and extrapyramidal symptoms in patients on long-term antipsychotic treatment. Am J Med Genet B Neuropsychiatr Genet 2007;144B:809–15.
373. Ellingrod VL, Bishop JR, Moline J, et al. Leptin and leptin receptor gene polymorphisms and increases in body mass index (BMI) from olanzapine treatment in persons with schizophrenia. Psychopharmacol Bull 2007;40:57–62.
374. Greenbaum L, Strous RD, Kanyas K, et al. Association of the RGS2 gene with extrapyramidal symptoms induced by treatment with antipsychotic medication. Pharmacogenet Genomics 2007;17:519–28.
375. Gunes A, Scordo MG, Jaanson P, et al. Serotonin and dopamine receptor gene polymorphisms and the risk of extrapyramidal side effects in perphenazine-treated schizophrenic patients. Psychopharmacology (Berl) 2007;190: 479–84.
376. Hwang R, Shinkai T, De LV, et al. Association study of four dopamine D1 receptor gene polymorphisms and clozapine treatment response. J Psychopharmacol 2007;21:718–27.
377. Kato D, Kawanishi C, Kishida I, et al. Effects of CYP2D6 polymorphisms on neuroleptic malignant syndrome. Eur J Clin Pharmacol 2007;63:991–6.
378. Lee HJ, Kang SG, Paik JW, et al. No evidence for an association between G protein beta3 subunit gene C825T polymorphism and tardive dyskinesia in schizophrenia. Hum Psychopharmacol 2007;22:501–4.
379. Lee HJ, Kang SG, Choi JE, et al. No association between dopamine D4 receptor gene -521 C/T polymorphism and tardive dyskinesia in schizophrenia. Neuropsychobiology 2007;55:47–51.
380. Liou YJ, Wang YC, Chen JY, et al. Association analysis of polymorphisms in the N-methyl-D-aspartate (NMDA) receptor subunit 2B (GRIN2B) gene and tardive dyskinesia in schizophrenia. Psychiatry Res 2007;153:271–5.
381. Mancama D, Mata I, Kerwin RW, et al. Choline acetyltransferase variants and their influence in schizophrenia and olanzapine response. Am J Med Genet B Neuropsychiatr Genet 2007;144B:849–53.
382. Mo GH, Lai IC, Wang YC, et al. Support for an association of the C939T polymorphism in the human DRD2 gene with tardive dyskinesia in schizophrenia. Schizophr Res 2007;97:302–4.
383. Molero P, Ortuno F, Zalacain M, et al. Clinical involvement of catechol-O-methyltransferase polymorphisms in schizophrenia spectrum disorders: influence on the severity of psychotic symptoms and on the response to neuroleptic treatment. Pharmacogenomics J 2007;7:418–26.
384. Mulder H, Franke B, van der-Beek van der AA, et al. The association between HTR2C gene polymorphisms and the metabolic syndrome in patients with schizophrenia. J Clin Psychopharmacol 2007;27:338–43.
385. Mulder H, Franke B, van der-Beek van der AA, et al. The association between HTR2C polymorphisms and obesity in psychiatric patients using antipsychotics: a cross-sectional study. Pharmacogenomics J 2007;7:318–24.
386. Pae CU, Kim TS, Patkar AA, et al. Manganese superoxide dismutase (MnSOD: Ala-9Val) gene polymorphism may not be associated with schizophrenia and tardive dyskinesia. Psychiatry Res 2007;153:77–81.

387. Ryu S, Cho EY, Park T, et al. 759 C/T polymorphism of 5-HT2C receptor gene and early phase weight gain associated with antipsychotic drug treatment. Prog Neuropsychopharmacol Biol Psychiatry 2007;31:673–7.
388. Tay JK, Tan CH, Chong SA, et al. Functional polymorphisms of the cytochrome P450 1A2 (CYP1A2) gene and prolonged QTc interval in schizophrenia. Prog Neuropsychopharmacol Biol Psychiatry 2007;31:1297–302.
389. Tiwari AK, Deshpande SN, Lerer B, et al. Genetic susceptibility to tardive dyskinesia in chronic schizophrenia subjects: V. Association of CYP1A2 1545 C>T polymorphism. Pharmacogenomics J 2007;7:305–11.
390. Vijayan NN, Bhaskaran S, Koshy LV, et al. Association of dopamine receptor polymorphisms with schizophrenia and antipsychotic response in a South Indian population. Behav Brain Funct 2007;3:34.
391. Wang L, Yu L, He G, et al. Response of risperidone treatment may be associated with polymorphisms of HTT gene in Chinese schizophrenia patients. Neurosci Lett 2007;414:1–4.
392. Xing Q, Qian X, Li H, et al. The relationship between the therapeutic response to risperidone and the dopamine D2 receptor polymorphism in Chinese schizophrenia patients. Int J Neuropsychopharmacol 2007;10:631–7.
393. Xu MQ, Xing QH, Zheng YL, et al. Association of AKT1 gene polymorphisms with risk of schizophrenia and with response to antipsychotics in the Chinese population. J Clin Psychiatry 2007;68:1358–67.
394. Yue W, Kang G, Zhang Y, et al. Association of DAOA polymorphisms with schizophrenia and clinical symptoms or therapeutic effects. Neurosci Lett 2007;416:96–100.
395. Zai CC, Hwang RW, De LV, et al. Association study of tardive dyskinesia and twelve DRD2 polymorphisms in schizophrenia patients. Int J Neuropsychopharmacol 2007;10:639–51.
396. Zhang A, Xing Q, Wang L, et al. Dopamine transporter polymorphisms and risperidone response in Chinese schizophrenia patients: an association study. Pharmacogenomics 2007;8:1337–45.
397. Zhang XY, Tan YL, Zhou DF, et al. Association of clozapine-induced weight gain with a polymorphism in the leptin promoter region in patients with chronic schizophrenia in a Chinese population. J Clin Psychopharmacol 2007;27:246–51.
398. Grossman I, Sullivan PF, Walley N, et al. Genetic determinants of variable metabolism have little impact on the clinical use of leading antipsychotics in the CATIE study. Genet Med 2008;10:720–9.
399. Bozina N, Kuzman MR, Medved V, et al. Associations between MDR1 gene polymorphisms and schizophrenia and therapeutic response to olanzapine in female schizophrenic patients. J Psychiatr Res 2008;42:89–97.
400. Adams DH, Close S, Farmen M, et al. Dopamine receptor D3 genotype association with greater acute positive symptom remission with olanzapine therapy in predominately caucasian patients with chronic schizophrenia or schizoaffective disorder. Hum Psychopharmacol 2008;23:267–74.
401. Al Hadithy AF, Wilffert B, Stewart RE, et al. Pharmacogenetics of parkinsonism, rigidity, rest tremor, and bradykinesia in African-Caribbean inpatients: differences in association with dopamine and serotonin receptors. Am J Med Genet B Neuropsychiatr Genet 2008;147B:890–7.
402. Benmessaoud D, Hamdani N, Boni C, et al. Excess of transmission of the G allele of the -1438A/G polymorphism of the 5-HT2A receptor gene in patients with schizophrenia responsive to antipsychotics. BMC Psychiatry 2008;8:40.

403. Campbell DB, Ebert PJ, Skelly T, et al. Ethnic stratification of the association of RGS4 variants with antipsychotic treatment response in schizophrenia. Biol Psychiatry 2008;63:32–41.

404. Crescenti A, Mas S, Gasso P, et al. Cyp2d6*3, *4, *5 and *6 polymorphisms and antipsychotic-induced extrapyramidal side-effects in patients receiving antipsychotic therapy. Clin Exp Pharmacol Physiol 2008;35:807–11.

405. de LJ, Correa JC, Ruano G, et al. Exploring genetic variations that may be associated with the direct effects of some antipsychotics on lipid levels. Schizophr Res 2008;98:40–6.

406. Dolzan V, Serretti A, Mandelli L, et al. Acute antipyschotic efficacy and side effects in schizophrenia: association with serotonin transporter promoter genotypes. Prog Neuropsychopharmacol Biol Psychiatry 2008;32:1562–6.

407. Ellingrod VL, Miller DD, Taylor SF, et al. Metabolic syndrome and insulin resistance in schizophrenia patients receiving antipsychotics genotyped for the methylenetetrahydrofolate reductase (MTHFR) 677C/T and 1298A/C variants. Schizophr Res 2008;98:47–54.

408. Gu B, Wang L, Zhang AP, et al. Association between a polymorphism of the HTR3A gene and therapeutic response to risperidone treatment in drug-naive Chinese schizophrenia patients. Pharmacogenet Genomics 2008;18:721–7.

409. Gunes A, Dahl ML, Spina E, et al. Further evidence for the association between 5-HT2C receptor gene polymorphisms and extrapyramidal side effects in male schizophrenic patients. Eur J Clin Pharmacol 2008;64:477–82.

410. Hamdani N, Tabeze JP, Ramoz N, et al. The CNR1 gene as a pharmacogenetic factor for antipsychotics rather than a susceptibility gene for schizophrenia. Eur Neuropsychopharmacol 2008;18:34–40.

411. Ikeda M, Yamanouchi Y, Kinoshita Y, et al. Variants of dopamine and serotonin candidate genes as predictors of response to risperidone treatment in first-episode schizophrenia. Pharmacogenomics 2008;9:1437–43.

412. Ji X, Takahashi N, Branko A, et al. An association between serotonin receptor 3B gene (HTR3B) and treatment-resistant schizophrenia (TRS) in a Japanese population. Nagoya J Med Sci 2008;70:11–7.

413. Ji X, Takahashi N, Saito S, et al. Relationship between three serotonin receptor subtypes (HTR3A, HTR2A and HTR4) and treatment-resistant schizophrenia in the Japanese population. Neurosci Lett 2008;435:95–8.

414. Kang SG, Choi JE, An H, et al. Manganese superoxide dismutase gene Ala-9Val polymorphism might be related to the severity of abnormal involuntary movements in Korean schizophrenic patients. Prog Neuropsychopharmacol Biol Psychiatry 2008;32:1844–7.

415. Kang SG, Choi JE, An H, et al. No association between the brain-derived neurotrophic factor gene Val66Met polymorphism and tardive dyskinesia in schizophrenic patients. Prog Neuropsychopharmacol Biol Psychiatry 2008; 32:1545–8.

416. Kang SG, Lee HJ, Choi JE, et al. Association study between antipsychotics-induced restless legs syndrome and polymorphisms of dopamine D1, D2, D3, and D4 receptor genes in schizophrenia. Neuropsychobiology 2008;57: 49–54.

417. Kang SG, Lee HJ, Park YM, et al. Possible association between the -2548A/G polymorphism of the leptin gene and olanzapine-induced weight gain. Prog Neuropsychopharmacol Biol Psychiatry 2008;32:160–3.

418. Kim B, Choi EY, Kim CY, et al. Could HTR2A T102C and DRD3 Ser9Gly predict clinical improvement in patients with acutely exacerbated schizophrenia?

Results from treatment responses to risperidone in a naturalistic setting. Hum Psychopharmacol 2008;23:61–7.

419. Kohlrausch FB, Salatino-Oliveira A, Gama CS, et al. G-protein gene 825C>T polymorphism is associated with response to clozapine in Brazilian schizophrenics. Pharmacogenomics 2008;9:1429–36.

420. Kohlrausch FB, Gama CS, Lobato MI, et al. Naturalistic pharmacogenetic study of treatment resistance to typical neuroleptics in European-Brazilian schizophrenics. Pharmacogenet Genomics 2008;18:599–609.

421. Kwon JS, Kim E, Kang DH, et al. Taq1A polymorphism in the dopamine D2 receptor gene as a predictor of clinical response to aripiprazole. Eur Neuropsychopharmacol 2008;18:897–907.

422. Lafuente A, Bernardo M, Mas S, et al. Polymorphism of dopamine D2 receptor (TaqIA, TaqIB, and-141C Ins/Del) and dopamine degradation enzyme (COMT G158A, A-278G) genes and extrapyramidal symptoms in patients with schizophrenia and bipolar disorders. Psychiatry Res 2008;161:131–41.

423. Lane HY, Liu YC, Huang CL, et al. RGS4 polymorphisms predict clinical manifestations and responses to risperidone treatment in patients with schizophrenia. J Clin Psychopharmacol 2008;28:64–8.

424. Lavedan C, Volpi S, Polymeropoulos MH, et al. Effect of a ciliary neurotrophic factor polymorphism on schizophrenia symptom improvement in an iloperidone clinical trial. Pharmacogenomics 2008;9:289–301.

425. Liou YJ, Wang YC, Chen JY, et al. The coding-synonymous polymorphism rs1045280 (Ser280Ser) in beta-arrestin 2 (ARRB2) gene is associated with tardive dyskinesia in Chinese patients with schizophrenia. Eur J Neurol 2008;15:1406–8.

426. Meary A, Brousse G, Jamain S, et al. Pharmacogenetic study of atypical antipsychotic drug response: involvement of the norepinephrine transporter gene. Am J Med Genet B Neuropsychiatr Genet 2008;147B:491–4.

427. Mou XD, Zhang ZJ, Zhang XR, et al. [-2548G/A functional polymorphism in the promoter region of leptin gene and antipsychotic agent-induced weight gain in schizophrenic patients: a study of nuclear family-based association]. Zhong Nan Da Xue Xue Bao Yi Xue Ban 2008;33:316–20 [in Chinese].

428. Pae CU, Drago A, Kim JJ, et al. TAAR6 variation effect on clinic presentation and outcome in a sample of schizophrenic in-patients: an open label study. Eur Psychiatry 2008;23:390–5.

429. Park YM, Cho JH, Kang SG, et al. Lack of association between the -759C/T polymorphism of the 5-HT2C receptor gene and olanzapine-induced weight gain among Korean schizophrenic patients. J Clin Pharm Ther 2008;33:55–60.

430. Shao P, Zhao JP, Chen JD, et al. [Association of HTR2C-759C/T and -697G/C polymorphisms with antipsychotic agent-induced weight gain]. Zhong Nan Da Xue Xue Bao Yi Xue Ban 2008;33:312–5 [in Chinese].

431. Shinkai T, De LV, Utsunomiya K, et al. Functional polymorphism of the human multidrug resistance gene (MDR1) and polydipsia-hyponatremia in schizophrenia. Neuromolecular Med 2008;10:362–7.

432. Smith RC, Segman RH, Golcer-Dubner T, et al. Allelic variation in ApoC3, ApoA5 and LPL genes and first and second generation antipsychotic effects on serum lipids in patients with schizophrenia. Pharmacogenomics J 2008;8:228–36.

433. Souza RP, Romano-Silva MA, Lieberman JA, et al. Association study of GSK3 gene polymorphisms with schizophrenia and clozapine response. Psychopharmacology (Berl) 2008;200:177–86.

434. Spellmann I, Muller N, Musil R, et al. Associations of SNAP-25 polymorphisms with cognitive dysfunctions in caucasian patients with schizophrenia during

a brief trail of treatment with atypical antipsychotics. Eur Arch Psychiatry Clin Neurosci 2008;258:335–44.

435. Srivastava V, Deshpande SN, Nimgaonkar VL, et al. Genetic correlates of olanzapine-induced weight gain in schizophrenia subjects from north India: role of metabolic pathway genes. Pharmacogenomics 2008;9:1055–68.

436. Wang L, Fang C, Zhang A, et al. The –1019 C/G polymorphism of the 5-HT(1)A receptor gene is associated with negative symptom response to risperidone treatment in schizophrenia patients. J Psychopharmacol 2008;22:904–9.

437. Webb BT, Sullivan PF, Skelly T, et al. Model-based gene selection shows engrailed 1 is associated with antipsychotic response. Pharmacogenet Genomics 2008;18:751–9.

438. Xu MQ, St CD, Feng GY, et al. BDNF gene is a genetic risk factor for schizophrenia and is related to the chlorpromazine-induced extrapyramidal syndrome in the Chinese population. Pharmacogenet Genomics 2008;18:449–57.

439. Xuan J, Zhao X, He G, et al. Effects of the dopamine D3 receptor (DRD3) gene polymorphisms on risperidone response: a pharmacogenetic study. Neuropsychopharmacology 2008;33:305–11.

440. Zai CC, Romano-Silva MA, Hwang R, et al. Genetic study of eight AKT1 gene polymorphisms and their interaction with DRD2 gene polymorphisms in tardive dyskinesia. Schizophr Res 2008;106:248–52.

441. Need AC, Keefe RS, Ge D, et al. Pharmacogenetics of antipsychotic response in the CATIE trial: a candidate gene analysis. Eur J Hum Genet 2009;17:946–57.

442. Tsai HT, Caroff SN, Miller DD, et al. A candidate gene study of tardive dyskinesia in the CATIE schizophrenia trial. Am J Med Genet B Neuropsychiatr Genet 2010; 153B:336–40.

443. Al Hadithy AF, Ivanova SA, Pechlivanoglou P, et al. Tardive dyskinesia and DRD3, HTR2A and HTR2C gene polymorphisms in Russian psychiatric inpatients from Siberia. Prog Neuropsychopharmacol Biol Psychiatry 2009;33:475–81.

444. Al Hadithy AF, Wilffert B, Bruggeman R, et al. Lack of association between antipsychotic-induced Parkinsonism or its subsymptoms and rs4606 SNP of RGS2 gene in African-Caribbeans and the possible role of the medication: the Curacao extrapyramidal syndromes study X. Hum Psychopharmacol 2009;24:123–8.

445. Angelucci F, Bernardini S, Gravina P, et al. Delusion symptoms and response to antipsychotic treatment are associated with the 5-HT2A receptor polymorphism (102T/C) in Alzheimer's disease: a 3-year follow-up longitudinal study. J Alzheimers Dis 2009;17:203–11.

446. Barlas IO, Cetin M, Erdal ME, et al. Lack of association between DRD3 gene polymorphism and response to clozapine in Turkish schizoprenia patients. Am J Med Genet B Neuropsychiatr Genet 2009;150B:56–60.

447. Calarge CA, Ellingrod VL, Zimmerman B, et al. Leptin gene -2548G/A variants predict risperidone-associated weight gain in children and adolescents. Psychiatr Genet 2009;19:320–7.

448. Chen SF, Shen YC, Chen CH. HTR2A A-1438G/T102C polymorphisms predict negative symptoms performance upon aripiprazole treatment in schizophrenic patients. Psychopharmacology (Berl) 2009;205:285–92.

449. Chen SF, Shen YC, Chen CH. Effects of the DRD3 Ser9Gly polymorphism on aripiprazole efficacy in schizophrenic patients as modified by clinical factors. Prog Neuropsychopharmacol Biol Psychiatry 2009;33:470–4.

450. Consoli G, Lastella M, Ciapparelli A, et al. ABCB1 polymorphisms are associated with clozapine plasma levels in psychotic patients. Pharmacogenomics 2009;10:1267–76.

451. Du J, Zhang A, Wang L, et al. Relationship between response to risperidone, plasma concentrations of risperidone and CYP3A4 polymorphisms in schizophrenia patients. J Psychopharmacol 2009. [Epub ahead of print].

452. Gasso P, Mas S, Bernardo M, et al. A common variant in DRD3 gene is associated with risperidone-induced extrapyramidal symptoms. Pharmacogenomics J 2009; 9:404–10.

453. Godlewska BR, Olajossy-Hilkesberger L, Ciwoniuk M, et al. Olanzapine-induced weight gain is associated with the -759C/T and -697G/C polymorphisms of the HTR2C gene. Pharmacogenomics J 2009;9:234–41.

454. Greenbaum L, Smith RC, Rigbi A, et al. Further evidence for association of the RGS2 gene with antipsychotic-induced parkinsonism: protective role of a functional polymorphism in the 3'-untranslated region. Pharmacogenomics J 2009;9:103–10.

455. Gregoor JG, van der Weide J, Mulder H, et al. Polymorphisms of the LEP- and LEPR gene and obesity in patients using antipsychotic medication. J Clin Psychopharmacol 2009;29:21–5.

456. Gunes A, Melkersson KI, Scordo MG, et al. Association between HTR2C and HTR2A polymorphisms and metabolic abnormalities in patients treated with olanzapine or clozapine. J Clin Psychopharmacol 2009;29:65–8.

457. Gupta M, Bhatnagar P, Grover S, et al. Association studies of catechol-O-methyltransferase (COMT) gene with schizophrenia and response to antipsychotic treatment. Pharmacogenomics 2009;10:385–97.

458. Herken H, Erdal M, Aydin N, et al. The association of olanzapine-induced weight gain with peroxisome proliferator-activated receptor-gamma2 Pro12Ala polymorphism in patients with schizophrenia. DNA Cell Biol 2009;28:515–9.

459. Jaquenoud SE, Knezevic B, Morena GP, et al. ABCB1 and cytochrome P450 polymorphisms: clinical pharmacogenetics of clozapine. J Clin Psychopharmacol 2009;29:319–26.

460. Kang SG, Lee HJ, Choi JE, et al. Association study between glutathione S-transferase GST-M1, GST-T1, and GST-P1 polymorphisms and tardive dyskinesia. Hum Psychopharmacol 2009;24:55–60.

461. Kobylecki CJ, Jakobsen KD, Hansen T, et al. CYP2D6 genotype predicts antipsychotic side effects in schizophrenia inpatients: a retrospective matched case-control study. Neuropsychobiology 2009;59:222–6.

462. Kwon JS, Joo YH, Nam HJ, et al. Association of the glutamate transporter gene SLC1A1 with atypical antipsychotics-induced obsessive-compulsive symptoms. Arch Gen Psychiatry 2009;66:1233–41.

463. Laika B, Leucht S, Heres S, et al. Pharmacogenetics and olanzapine treatment: CYP1A2*1F and serotonergic polymorphisms influence therapeutic outcome. Pharmacogenomics J 2009. [Epub ahead of print].

464. Le HS, Theisen FM, Haberhausen M, et al. Association between the insulin-induced gene 2 (INSIG2) and weight gain in a German sample of antipsychotic-treated schizophrenic patients: perturbation of SREBP-controlled lipogenesis in drug-related metabolic adverse effects? Mol Psychiatry 2009; 14:308–17.

465. Lee HY, Kim DJ, Lee HJ, et al. No association of serotonin transporter polymorphism (5-HTTVNTR and 5-HTTLPR) with characteristics and treatment response to atypical antipsychotic agents in schizophrenic patients. Prog Neuropsychopharmacol Biol Psychiatry 2009;33:276–80.

466. Liou YJ, Chen ML, Wang YC, et al. Analysis of genetic variations in the RGS9 gene and antipsychotic-induced tardive dyskinesia in schizophrenia. Am J Med Genet B Neuropsychiatr Genet 2009;150B:239–42.

467. Mossner R, Schuhmacher A, Kuhn KU, et al. Functional serotonin 1A receptor variant influences treatment response to atypical antipsychotics in schizophrenia. Pharmacogenet Genomics 2009;19:91–4.

468. Mulder H, Cohen D, Scheffer H, et al. HTR2C gene polymorphisms and the metabolic syndrome in patients with schizophrenia: a replication study. J Clin Psychopharmacol 2009;29:16–20.

469. Park SW, Lee JG, Kong BG, et al. Genetic association of BDNF val66met and GSK-3beta-50T/C polymorphisms with tardive dyskinesia. Psychiatry Clin Neurosci 2009;63:433–9.

470. Sickert L, Muller DJ, Tiwari AK, et al. Association of the alpha2A adrenergic receptor -1291C/G polymorphism and antipsychotic-induced weight gain in European-Americans. Pharmacogenomics 2009;10:1169–76.

471. Volpi S, Potkin SG, Malhotra AK, et al. Applicability of a genetic signature for enhanced iloperidone efficacy in the treatment of schizophrenia. J Clin Psychiatry 2009;70:801–9.

472. Wei Z, Wang L, Xuan J, et al. Association analysis of serotonin receptor 7 gene (HTR7) and risperidone response in Chinese schizophrenia patients. Prog Neuropsychopharmacol Biol Psychiatry 2009;33:547–51.

473. Wilffert B, Al Hadithy AF, Sing VJ, et al. The role of dopamine D3, 5-HT2A and 5-HT2C receptor variants as pharmacogenetic determinants in tardive dyskinesia in African-Caribbean patients under chronic antipsychotic treatment: curacao extrapyramidal syndromes study IX. J Psychopharmacol 2009;23:652–9.

474. Zai CC, Tiwari AK, Basile V, et al. Association study of tardive dyskinesia and five DRD4 polymorphisms in schizophrenia patients. Pharmacogenomics J 2009;9:168–74.

475. Zai CC, Tiwari AK, Basile V, et al. Oxidative stress in tardive dyskinesia: genetic association study and meta-analysis of NADPH quinine oxidoreductase 1 (NQO1) and Superoxide dismutase 2 (SOD2, MnSOD) genes. Prog Neuropsychopharmacol Biol Psychiatry 2009. [Epub ahead of print].

476. Zuo L, Luo X, Krystal JH, et al. The efficacies of clozapine and haloperidol in refractory schizophrenia are related to DTNBP1 variation. Pharmacogenet Genomics 2009;19:437–46.

477. McClay JL, Adkins DE, Aberg K, et al. Genome-wide pharmacogenomic analysis of response to treatment with antipsychotics. Mol Psychiatry 2009. [Epub ahead of print].

478. Alkelai A, Greenbaum L, Rigbi A, et al. Genome-wide association study of antipsychotic-induced parkinsonism severity among schizophrenia patients. Psychopharmacology (Berl) 2009;206:491–9.

479. Aberg K, Adkins DE, Bukszar J, et al. Genome-wide association study of movement-related adverse antipsychotic effects. Biol Psychiatry 2009. [Epub ahead of print].

480. Lavedan C, Licamele L, Volpi S, et al. Association of the NPAS3 gene and five other loci with response to the antipsychotic iloperidone identified in a whole genome association study. Mol Psychiatry 2009;14:804–19.

481. Volpi S, Heaton C, Mack K, et al. Whole genome association study identifies polymorphisms associated with QT prolongation during iloperidone treatment of schizophrenia. Mol Psychiatry 2009;14:1024–31.

482. Arranz MJ, de LJ. Pharmacogenetics and pharmacogenomics of schizophrenia: a review of last decade of research. Mol Psychiatry 2007;12:707–47.

483. Patsopoulos NA, Ntzani EE, Zintzaras E, et al. CYP2D6 polymorphisms and the risk of tardive dyskinesia in schizophrenia: a meta-analysis. Pharmacogenet Genomics 2005;15:151–8.
484. Miyamoto S, Duncan GE, Marx CE, et al. Treatments for schizophrenia: a critical review of pharmacology and mechanisms of action of antipsychotic drugs. Mol Psychiatry 2005;10:79–104.
485. Lieberman JA. Dopamine partial agonists: a new class of antipsychotic. CNS Drugs 2004;18:251–67.
486. Mamo D, Kapur S, Shammi CM, et al. A PET study of dopamine D2 and serotonin 5-HT2 receptor occupancy in patients with schizophrenia treated with therapeutic doses of ziprasidone. Am J Psychiatry 2004;161:818–25.
487. Arinami T, Gao M, Hamaguchi H, et al. A functional polymorphism in the promoter region of the dopamine D2 receptor gene is associated with schizophrenia. Hum Mol Genet 1997;6:577–82.
488. Jonsson EG, Nothen MM, Grunhage F, et al. Polymorphisms in the dopamine D2 receptor gene and their relationships to striatal dopamine receptor density of healthy volunteers. Mol Psychiatry 1999;4:290–6.
489. Goldman D, Urbanek M, Guenther D, et al. A functionally deficient DRD2 variant [Ser311Cys] is not linked to alcoholism and substance abuse. Alcohol 1998;16:47–52.
490. Bakker PR, van Harten PN, van OJ. Antipsychotic-induced tardive dyskinesia and polymorphic variations in COMT, DRD2, CYP1A2 and MnSOD genes: a meta-analysis of pharmacogenetic interactions. Mol Psychiatry 2008;13:544–56.
491. Lundstrom K, Turpin MP. Proposed schizophrenia-related gene polymorphism: expression of the Ser9Gly mutant human dopamine D3 receptor with the Semliki forest virus system. Biochem Biophys Res Commun 1996;225:1068–72.
492. Bakker PR, van Harten PN, van OJ. Antipsychotic-induced tardive dyskinesia and the Ser9Gly polymorphism in the DRD3 gene: a meta analysis. Schizophr Res 2006;83:185–92.
493. Meltzer HY. Role of serotonin in the action of atypical antipsychotic drugs. Clin Neurosci 1995;3:64–75.
494. Meltzer HY, Li Z, Kaneda Y, et al. Serotonin receptors: their key role in drugs to treat schizophrenia. Prog Neuropsychopharmacol Biol Psychiatry 2003;27:1159–72.
495. Kroeze WK, Kristiansen K, Roth BL. Molecular biology of serotonin receptors structure and function at the molecular level. Curr Top Med Chem 2002;2:507–28.
496. Arranz MJ, Munro J, Sham P, et al. Meta-analysis of studies on genetic variation in 5-HT2A receptors and clozapine response. Schizophr Res 1998;32:93–9.
497. Lerer B, Segman RH, Tan EC, et al. Combined analysis of 635 patients confirms an age-related association of the serotonin 2A receptor gene with tardive dyskinesia and specificity for the non-orofacial subtype. Int J Neuropsychopharmacol 2005;8:411–25.
498. De LV, Mueller DJ, de BA, et al. Association of the HTR2C gene and antipsychotic induced weight gain: a meta-analysis. Int J Neuropsychopharmacol 2007;10:697–704.
499. Roche Molecular systems I. AmpliChip CYP450 test for in vitro diagnostic use. Roche Diagnostics 2006. [Epub ahead of print].
500. Katsanis SH, Javitt G, Hudson K. Public health: a case study of personalized medicine. Science 2008;320:53–4.

501. Evaluation of Genomic Applications in Practice and Prevention (EGAPP) Working Group. Recommendations from the EGAPP Working Group: testing for cytochrome P450 polymorphisms in adults with nonpsychotic depression treated with selective serotonin reuptake inhibitors. Genet Med 2007;9:819–25.

502. Wagner JA. Overview of biomarkers and surrogate endpoints in drug development. Dis Markers 2002;18:41–6.

503. FDA. Guidance for industry: pharmacogenomic data submission. FDA 2005.

504. Frueh FW, Amur S, Mummaneni P, et al. Pharmacogenomic biomarker information in drug labels approved by the United States Food and Drug Administration: prevalence of related drug use. Pharmacotherapy 2008;28:992–8.

505. Arranz MJ, Kapur S. Pharmacogenetics in psychiatry: are we ready for widespread clinical use? Schizophr Bull 2008;34:1130–44.

506. van der WJ, Steijns LS, van Weelden MJ. The effect of smoking and cytochrome P450 CYP1A2 genetic polymorphism on clozapine clearance and dose requirement. Pharmacogenetics 2003;13:169–72.

507. Desai HD, Seabolt J, Jann MW. Smoking in patients receiving psychotropic medications: a pharmacokinetic perspective. CNS Drugs 2001;15:469–94.

508. Spina E, de LJ. Metabolic drug interactions with newer antipsychotics: a comparative review. Basic Clin Pharmacol Toxicol 2007;100:4–22.

Predictive and Diagnostic Genetic Testing in Psychiatry

Philip B. Mitchell, MBBS, MD, FRANZCP, FRCPsych[a,b,c,]*,
Bettina Meiser, PhD[d], Alex Wilde, BSc, MA[e],
Janice Fullerton, BSc, PhD[f], Jennifer Donald, BA, PhD[g],
Kay Wilhelm, MBBS, MD, FRANZCP[h], Peter R. Schofield, PhD, DSc[c,i,j]

KEYWORDS

• Predictive • Diagnostic • Genetic testing
• Psychiatric • Mental

The announcement of commercially available genetic tests for the diagnosis of several mental illnesses in early 2008[1] has led to intense controversy amongst the psychiatric research community.

The main protagonist in this development was John Kelsoe of the University of California, San Diego. In conjunction with business partners, Kelsoe established a biotechnology company, Psynomics, in the words of its Web site

This work was supported by the Australian National Health and Medical Research Council (NHMRC) Program Grant (510135), Project Grant (510216), Public Health PhD scholarship (455414), and Career Development Award (350989).

a School of Psychiatry, Prince of Wales Hospital, University of New South Wales, Randwick, Sydney, NSW 2031, Australia
b Bipolar Disorders Clinic, Black Dog Institute, Hospital Road, Prince of Wales Hospital, Randwick, Sydney, NSW 2031, Australia
c Brain Sciences UNSW, University of New South Wales, Sydney, NSW 2052, Australia
d Psychosocial Research Group, Department of Medical Oncology, Prince of Wales Clinical School, Prince of Wales Hospital, University of New South Wales, Randwick, Sydney, NSW 2031, Australia
e School of Psychiatry, University of New South Wales, Black Dog Institute Building, Hospital Road, Prince of Wales Hospital, Randwick, Sydney, NSW 2031, Australia
f Prince of Wales Medical Research Centre, Prince of Wales Medical Research Institute, Barker Street, Randwick, Sydney, NSW 2031, Australia
g Department of Biological Sciences, Macquarie University, Sydney, NSW 2109, Australia
h School of Psychiatry, Consultation Liaison Psychiatry, St Vincent's Hospital Victoria Street, University of New South Wales, Sydney, NSW 2010, Australia
i Prince of Wales Medical Research Institute, Barker Street, Randwick, Sydney, NSW 2031, Australia
j School of Medical Sciences, University of New South Wales, Sydney, NSW 2052, Australia
* Corresponding author. School of Psychiatry, Prince of Wales Hospital, University of New South Wales, Randwick, Sydney, NSW 2031, Australia.
E-mail address: phil.mitchell@unsw.edu.au (P.B. Mitchell).

(https://psynomics.com/index.php), "the first and only company in the world to offer DNA-based diagnostic and therapeutic tests to help millions of people suffering from mental illness." Psynomics offered 2 initial products, Psynome (a diagnostic test) and Psynome2 (a pharmacogenomic test). Psynome was based on several single-nucleotide polymorphisms (SNPs) in the GRK3 (G-protein receptor kinase 3) gene on chromosome 22, which Kelsoe's group had reported to be associated with a doubling or tripling of risk for bipolar disorder.[2–4] This finding has not been replicated by other groups[5] nor has it been reported in genome-wide association studies. Psynomics offered the test for those with symptoms of depression, mania, or irritability "to help confirm your diagnosis and choose the best treatment." Furthermore, the Web site stated: "If you have this gene, you are more likely to have bipolar disorder," and: "This test will lead to a more accurate diagnosis." The Web site advised that patients would be mailed a "spit kit," which they would then return to the company, with the result in turn being communicated to a medical practitioner nominated by the patient, rather than to the patient directly.

In the same news report in Science,[1] 2 other biotechnology companies were listed as planning to market psychiatric diagnostic tests: Suregene (http://www.suregene.net/home.aspx) and Neuromark (http://www.neuromark.com/). Suregene (a Louisville, Kentucky-based company) proposed to market tests for risk to schizophrenia, while Neuromark (from Boulder, Colorado) planned to market pharmacogenomic tests for risk of suicidality with antidepressants. As detailed in Couzin's article, the advent of these tests was viewed as premature and inappropriate by many in the psychiatric genetics research community and the broader genetics arena, though some were strongly supportive of such developments.

In August 2008, a commentary in the American Journal of Psychiatry[6] voiced strong concern about these developments. While echoing the appropriateness of the "visionary goal" for psychiatry and genetics of identifying risk before the onset of illness and clarifying diagnosis in difficult cases, this editorial argued adamantly that "we still lack the requisite information to create genetic tests for psychiatric risk, diagnosis and treatment that are robust enough to use responsibly and in a valid manner in psychiatric practice." The investigators argued that "it is timely to begin a process for deciding when genetic information is robust enough to justify testing specifically and when test results correctly lead to an altered course of action ... We must move forward with developing responsible genomic testing in psychiatry."

Such major concerns from the field seem already to have had a tempering effect on these new biotechnology ventures. At the time of preparing this article, review of the aforementioned Web sites revealed that Psynomics was "not currently accepting orders." Furthermore, the Suregene and Neuromark websites did not indicate availability of the tests, which Couzin's report had stated would be available in 2009. Whereas many different reasons may have delayed the launch of these tests, for example, scientific, commercial, or financial, their announcement has placed great urgency on the need for the psychiatric genetics community to address these issues.

CURRENT STATUS OF GENETIC RESEARCH IN MENTAL ILLNESS

This article does not discuss in detail the current status of genetic findings in psychiatry, which are reviewed in other articles in this issue of Psychiatric Clinics of North America and elsewhere.[7] It should be noted specifically, though, that genome-wide association studies (GWAS) reported in the last few years have detected associations of common SNPs and rare copy number variants (CNVs) with several psychiatric disorders.[8] For schizophrenia, which has been the best studied psychiatric condition hitherto with large GWAS datasets, the data would suggest that: (1) a high proportion of the heritable risk is due to the interaction of combinations of common variants, none of which alone contributes a large effect to risk[9–11]; and (2) there are also rare CNVs that increase risk to that disorder.[12,13] This situation has been mirrored in the more limited GWAS and CNV studies that have been undertaken in bipolar disorder, autism,[14] and other disorders. Although recent findings in bipolar disorder have identified only a handful of specific genes that account for around 1% of the genetic variance[15] and hence show little to no predictive value for genetic testing, pathway analysis is beginning to reveal small effects at multiple genes within individual molecular pathways which, when combined, may have greater predictive value.[16]

Rather, this article provides an overview of the broader issues—across the whole of the health spectrum—related to the definitions and necessary prerequisites of genetic testing; the validity of genetic testing for complex disorders; the upsurge in the availability of commercial providers for such direct-to-consumer (DTC) tests, and the associated legal and ethical issues; and the pertinence of these developments for the future potential of predictive and diagnostic testing in psychiatry. The authors then explore the responses of patients, families, practitioners, and the general population to the possibility of such testing entering the psychiatric clinical arena. Related to this, the complex and important relationships between genetic testing for mental illness, stigma, and discrimination are examined.

CRITICAL DEFINITIONS

There has been much imprecision in the distinction between the concepts of assays and tests, and the definitions of a genetic test. Burke and Zimmern[17] define an *assay* as "a method for determining the presence or quantity of a component" or "a method to analyze or quantify a substance in a sample." The assay is to be distinguished from a *genetic test,* which is defined as a laboratory assay that is used to identify a particular genotype (or set of genotypes) for a particular disease in a particular population for a particular purpose. Definition of the population is critical, as the *positive predictive value* (PPV) of a test of known sensitivity and specificity is related to the prevalence of the disease in that particular population.

Clear definitions of the different types of validity are also important. Test evaluation involves: (1) the analytical validity of the test; (2) the clinical validity of the test; and (3) the clinical utility of the test.[17] *Analytical validity* is determined by the reliability and accuracy of the assay; in the context of genetic testing this is the capacity of the assay to measure the genotype(s) of interest. *Clinical validity* is determined by: (1) the strength of evidence for the link between genotype and disease; and (2) test performance characteristics such as sensitivity, specificity, positive and negative predictive values, and likelihood ratios.

Clinical utility is also an important concept that requires careful definition. Clinical utility is the measure of the health care value provided by the test or technology, that is, does the test provide information that assists in the care of patients? Burke and Zimmern[17] expand on this critical issue of clinical utility, which is of central concern in the current debate over DTC genetic tests. Burke and Zimmern propose 8 dimensions of clinical utility, the first 4 of which can be subsumed under *"test purpose,"* and the second 4 under *"feasibility of test delivery."* These terms are defined and detailed in **Box 1**.

Melzer and colleagues[18] also emphasize the importance of *clarifying the target patient group*, noting that some tests may only be valid for high-risk families. This

---

Box 1
Definitions of validity and utility

Analytical validity

The capacity of the assay to measure the genotype of interest, that is, its reliability and accuracy

Clinical validity

Clinical validity is determined by:

1. The strength of the evidence for the link between genotype and disease
2. Test performance characteristics such as sensitivity, specificity, positive and negative predictive values, and likelihood ratios

Clinical utility

The measure of the health care value provided by the test, that is, does the test provide information that assists in the care of patients?

Dimensions of clinical utility

1. Test purpose

    a. Legitimacy: Conformity of the test to social preferences
    b. Efficacy: Ability of the test to bring about the intended purpose when viewed under the most favorable circumstances
    c. Effectiveness: Degree to which attainable objectives are attained under routine conditions
    d. Appropriateness: Balance between the expected benefit and the expected negative consequences

2. Feasibility of test delivery

    a. Acceptability: Conformity of test to desires and expectations of patients and families
    b. Economic evaluation—efficiency: Ability of the test to lower costs without diminishing benefits
    c. Economic evaluation—optimality: Balance of improvements in health against the cost of such improvements
    d. Equity: Conformity of the test to the principle of just and fair distribution of health care and its benefits across the population

Data from Burke W, Zimmern R. Moving beyond ACCE: an expanded framework for genetic test evaluation. 2007; PHG Foundation.

---

defining of the population for the test is critical in determining the PPV of the proposed procedure.

GENOME-WIDE ASSOCIATION STUDIES ACROSS THE HEALTH SPECTRUM

Experience with GWAS in a range of complex physical disorders[19] has demonstrated that most significant findings are for common alleles with a genotypic relative risk (odds ratio) of between 1.1 and 1.4, that is, an increase in risk of 10% to 40%. The early experience with psychiatric disorders would suggest a similar level of increased risk for those genes identified in GWAS studies of schizophrenia and bipolar disorder.[9,10,15,20,21]

In an article published in the *New England Journal of Medicine*, Hardy and Singleton[22] recently reviewed progress in GWAS across the range of human disease, and discussed the current uncertainty regarding the relative contributions of common low-risk variants and rare high-risk variants for particular disorders. The ramifications of this rapidly developing technology, including the relevance of GWAS findings to the potential feasibility of genetic testing, were discussed in a series of accompanying commentaries.[23–25] Goldstein[23] argued that the GWAS studies have demonstrated that common gene variants only account for a small proportion of genetic variation. Using the example of studies of genetic contribution to the trait of height, he noted that the 20 polymorphisms reported by Weedon and colleagues[26] from large GWAS samples accounted only for less than 3% of the population variation in height. Goldstein's contention is that rare variants are likely to account for a significant proportion of the genetic variance for many diseases or traits. However, one should note that there is no a priori reason why individual rare variants should have any greater genetic effect than common variants for complex disorders. Rare variants with a large effect size would give rise to simple (Mendelian) patterns of inheritance.

Hirschhorn[24] was more optimistic, arguing that whereas the main benefit of GWAS studies is in identifying common biological pathways to disease, there is still a high probability of useful genetic predictive information being derived from the study of common variants; this being particularly so as it would seem likely that multiple independent causal variants may be found at each locus, accounting for additional increments in heritability.[24] Hirschhorn also noted that for conditions with effective preventive measures, even small increments in predictive power could help in effectively targeting preventive efforts. Kraft and Hunter[25] reflected on the recent advent of DTC SNP tests (see later discussion) in light of the GWAS findings, commenting that most newly identified risk-marker alleles only confer relatively small relative risks in the range of 1.1 to 1.5, and that even when combined, such alleles generally have low discriminatory and predictive power. Further, these investigators stated that it is becoming apparent that multiple common variant risk alleles are responsible for the majority of the inherited risk of each common disease, citing the examples of 16 loci already identified for diabetes and 30 for Crohn's disease.[25] Kraft and Hunter provided a hypothetical estimation of the approximate number of loci that would be needed to reach a level of risk equivalent to the sibling risk of complex diseases such as diabetes. For example, a sibling relative risk of 2.0 would require 347 to 867 risk alleles with a relative risk per allele of 1.1 or 87 to 231 alleles with a relative risk of 1.2. It should be noted that these estimates were premised on allele frequencies of 10% to 90%, and do not account for potentially higher relative risk rare variants. Kraft and Hunter[25] concluded from these figures that the current relatively small number of identified variants do not contribute more than a small fraction of the inherited predisposition. More optimistically, they believed that as more common variants conferring risk of disease are identified in coming years, the stability of individual risk benefits will increase, and the usefulness (or otherwise) of genetic screening will need to be reconsidered for each disease. Although they contend that testing for inherited susceptibility based on common risk alleles is currently premature for most disorders, the situation could well be very different in the not too distant future.

There have been several statistical models proposed for predicting individual genetic risk to disease using GWAS data.[27,28] The methodology outlined by Wray and colleagues[28] has been applied to recent studies demonstrating the presence of multiple causative common gene variants in schizophrenia.[12] The Wray model proposes that the 5% of individuals with the highest predicted risk are 3 to 7 times more likely to suffer the particular disease than the population average, depending on heritability and disease prevalence, and taking into account that whether an individual with known genetic risk develops the disease will depend on known and unknown environmental factors. For psychiatric disorders, relevant environmental factors would include stressful life events, childhood trauma (physical and sexual), and substance abuse.

DIRECT-TO-CONSUMER GENETIC TESTING

The current debate about the appropriateness of marketing genetic tests for psychiatric disorders is one facet of a broader controversy over the advent of DTC genetic testing across the field of health.[18,29–31] The term "DTC" can be used to refer to 2 distinct scenarios. The first comprises the advertising of such tests directly to the public, with the actual ordering of the investigation and receipt of results involving a health care provider; this situation is not unlike direct advertising of pharmaceuticals to the public in the United States. The second scenario is where, in addition to advertising to the public, the request for testing is initiated by the patient and results are, in turn, provided directly to the patient, independently of the person's usual medical practitioner. Sometimes, in this latter scenario, the genetic testing company may provide a practitioner employed by the company to order the tests to overcome any legal concerns, but there is no ongoing relationship between such practitioners and the patient concerned. The situation with Psynomics would seem to be more consistent with the first of these 2 scenarios.[1]

Worldwide, there has been a rapid increase in the availability of DTC genetic tests, for both Mendelian disorders and complex traits such as psychiatric illnesses although, with respect to the latter, unlike the situation several years ago there are currently no companies offering DTC availability of predictive genetic testing for depression risk. In 2008, Schmidt[32] estimated that there were some 1400 DTC genetic tests on the market. Some of these have been detailed by Melzer and colleagues.[18]

What are the potential benefits and risks of DTC testing? In a policy statement issued by the American Society for Human Genetics on DTC genetic testing,[29,33] the investigators summarized the benefits as: increased consumer access to testing, greater consumer autonomy and empowerment, and enhanced privacy. The following risks were mentioned: consumer choice uninformed by context or counseling; testing by laboratories of potentially dubious quality; and misleading claims of benefit. Hogarth and colleagues[30] focused on the lack of appropriate counseling and advice on the suitability of such DTC tests and the consequent potential implications, such as a lack of expert interpretation of test results, and a lack of guidance on actions to take as a consequence of such testing. Furthermore, these investigators argue that such adverse implications apply particularly to complex diseases (the mechanism of inheritance pertinent to most psychiatric illnesses) in which the relationship between specific gene variants and disease is less clear.[30]

In the United States, there has been limited governmental regulatory oversight of DTC testing. The Federal mechanism for oversight of proficiency testing of laboratories is the Centers for Medicare and Medicaid Services (CMS), which implements and enforces the Clinical Laboratory Improvement Amendments of 1988 (CLIA). However, CMS regulations implementing CLIA do not cover proficiency testing of genetic laboratories, despite concerns being raised about this.[30] Even if genetic testing were to come under the ambit of CLIA, CMS only certifies laboratories in terms of analytical validity, not clinical validity—a major limitation in relation to recently proposed diagnostic tests for mental illnesses. In addition, there are major differences between US states that have the legal capacity to enforce more stringent regulations. DTC testing is banned in approximately half of the states in the United States.[29]

In Europe, there are no common requirements for laboratory quality assurance, though several countries do have national legal accreditation frameworks. Laboratory regulation is largely undertaken by a voluntary system of accreditation. In 2006, Switzerland and France introduced a universal ban on DTC genetic testing due to concerns about fraud or error in the absence of proper regulation.[34] In the United Kingdom there are no prohibitions on DTC medical tests, with the exception of human immunodeficiency virus. In China there are no regulations concerning DTC testing, with a range of tests currently available from commercial providers for several medical conditions, and even some for prediction of childhood "developmental talent" (Yu Xin; personal communication, 2009).

These so-called in vitro diagnostic (IVD) genetic tests are generally considered as medical devices under most national regulatory regimes.[30] For example, they come under the auspices of the Food and Drug Administration (FDA) in the United States and the Therapeutic Goods Administration (TGA) in Australia. However, FDA regulation only holds for kits sold to clinical laboratories, and not for most genetic tests that have been developed "in house" by such clinical laboratories, and which are only accessible from the "home" laboratory; these are termed "laboratory-developed tests" (LDTs), known colloquially as "home brews."[32]

In general, the FDA does not review the majority of these LDTs, with the exception of IVD multivariate index assays (IVDMIAs)—LDTs that use algorithms for diagnosis, prevention, or treatment; this means that in the United States, most DTC genetic tests have no regulatory overview to assess their clinical validity. In the European Union and Australia, LDTs come under the purview of device regulation. However, in Europe such genetic tests are considered low risk and therefore not subject to review, whereas in Australia they are considered moderate to high risk and therefore require premarketing assessment.[30]

Concern over the need to regulate LDTs/DTC genetic tests has led to much activity in terms of proposed new legislation in various national jurisdictions. In the United States, 2 bills introduced into Congress (the Laboratory Test Improvement Act and the Genomics and Personalized Medicine Act) would, respectively, allow for FDA regulation of LDTs as medical devices (as in Europe and Australia) and improvement in the safety and efficacy of genetic tests.[30] In the United Kingdom, the *More* Genes Direct report of the Human Genetics Commission[34] has recommended stricter controls on direct genetic testing, including ensuring that certain tests are only offered by qualified health professionals; reclassifying IVD genetic tests such that premarketing review is required; and proscribing DTC marketing. In Europe, the Council of Europe Protocol on Genetic Testing for Health care Purposes[35,36] recommended that: (1) genetic tests need to meet accepted criteria of scientific and clinical validity; (2) demonstrated clinical utility should be an essential criterion; (3) appropriate genetic counseling should be available for predictive tests; and (4) persons providing genetic services must have appropriate qualifications.

In Australia, the TGA is planning to amend the Therapeutic Goods Act 1989 and other regulations to ensure that the supply and advertising of genetic tests directly to consumers is prohibited, except where specifically approved by the TGA. In addition, the TGA proposes that the Human Genetics Commission Australia (HGCA) develops a voluntary code of practice and other advice on DTC genetic testing. Such a code could include minimum technical standards for companies supplying products and minimum ethical standards for laboratories supplying the testing service. In Australia, it is an offense to advertise a genetic IVD DTC on the Internet unless the device is listed under the Therapeutic Goods Act, the Therapeutic Goods Regulations, and the Therapeutic Goods Advertising Code.

However, the TGA is unable to regulate advertisements when the Internet service provider is based overseas. In such cases, Australian jurisdiction is limited to liaising with consumer affairs bodies in the relevant country regarding DTC advertising material that is either posted on the Internet or mailed to Australian addresses.

What is the scientific evidence for the value of commercially available genomic profiles? In a rigorous review, Janssens and colleagues[37] identified 7 companies that offered predictive genetic testing using multiple markers for several physical illnesses via the Internet. The researchers undertook an extensive literature search of meta-analyses of gene-disease associations in which subjects with a disease were compared with those of a healthy population control group. Janssens and colleagues found that the 7 companies tested at least 69 different polymorphisms in 56 genes, 24 of which were not reported in the meta-analyses. For the remaining 32 genes, only 38% of the polymorphism-disease associations were significant, and for most the odds ratios were of modest effect.[37] Furthermore, for several conditions, such as cardiovascular or bone disease, a substantial number of the genes in the specific disease profiles did not show significant association with that particular condition. The investigators concluded that there was insufficient scientific evidence to conclude that such genomic profiling in these commercial packages were useful in measuring genetic risk for these common disorders or in developing personalized diet or lifestyle recommendations for disease prevention.[37]

What has been the response of professional bodies to the widespread availability of DTC genetic tests? The American Society of Human Genetics[29,33] has recommended: (1) *transparency*—companies offering DTC genetic testing should disclose: the sensitivity, specificity, and predictive value of the test, and the populations for which this information is known; the strength of scientific evidence on which the claims of benefit are based; and all risks associated with testing including psychological risks and risks to family members; (2) *provider education*—professional organizations should disseminate information to members on what tests are offered DTC and the potential benefits and limitations of these; and (3) *test and laboratory quality*—CMS (Centers for Medicare and Medicaid Services) should create a genetic testing specialty under CLIA ensuring the analytical validity of tests and the quality of related laboratories; and the United States federal government should ensure the clinical validity of DTC tests that make health-related claims. More recently, Zonno and Terry of the US Genetic Alliance[38] have called for a national registry of genetic tests, with test performance characteristics being made publicly available.

While discussing legal oversight of genetic testing, it is also necessary to refer to legislation concerned with the associated issues of privacy and discrimination on genetic grounds.[39] In 2008, the US Congress passed the Genetic Information Nondiscrimination Act, a landmark Act that protects consumers from discrimination by health insurers and employers on the basis of genetic information.[40] This Act specifically prohibits insurers from using a person's genetic information in determining eligibility or premiums, and requesting or requiring that a person undergo a genetic test; and employers from using a person's genetic information in making employment decisions such as hiring or firing, and requesting, requiring, or purchasing genetic information about persons or their family members.

Other related ethical and philosophical issues of recent interest have concerned the predictive genetic testing of asymptomatic minors,[41,42] prenatal predictive testing,[43] and the potential for a simplistic "neurogenetic determinism."[44–46]

CURRENT GENETIC TESTING FOR NEUROPSYCHIATRIC DISORDERS

In clinical practice, the most widely used neuropsychiatric predictive and diagnostic testing is for the Mendelian condition Huntington disease, the fully penetrant autosomal dominant gene that was discovered in the 1990s[47] and for which the mechanisms of genetic anticipation and triplet repeat expansion have been uncovered. However, even for this devastating condition, in practice uptake in at-risk individuals has been low, with rates of around 10% to 20% being commonly reported.[48] Some of the complexities in considerations concerning the decision to have testing, and disclosure of testing results in Huntington disease families, have been recently reported in qualitative studies.[49,50]

Another field for which genetic testing has become widely used is that of intellectual disability, particularly since the recent discovery of the etiological importance of abnormal CNVs.[51–53] However, there has been concern about the potential for the new genetics to perpetuate discrimination for those with these conditions by using prenatal testing to prevent the birth of children with disabilities.[54]

Another neuropsychiatric condition for which there have been major advances in understanding the genetic underpinnings has been Alzheimer disease. Although the major findings have been reported for the early-onset familial form, which occurs via autosomal dominant inheritance of mutations in the *APP*, *PSEN1*, and *PSEN2* genes, this is a relatively uncommon presentation of this condition. The highly prevalent and more common late-onset presentation is more genetically complex, with one of the most robustly replicated (in Caucasian populations) associations for a risk factor allele being for greater risk in those with the apolipoprotein E (APOE) ϵ-4 allele on chromosome 19.[55] At present, however, the association with the APOE genotype is not considered to be of sufficient clinical utility. There does, nonetheless, seem to be considerable interest in predictive testing among first-degree relatives,[56,57] and a recent randomized controlled trial found no adverse short-term psychological risks associated with such testing in first-degree relatives of people affected with the disease.[58] Although several companies are offering DTC testing for APOE for those at risk of Alzheimer disease,[58] it is currently not known how many individuals are accessing such tests.

ATTITUDES TOWARD THE POTENTIAL OF PREDICTIVE AND DIAGNOSTIC GENETIC TESTING FOR SCHIZOPHRENIA, BIPOLAR DISORDER, AND DEPRESSION

This section reviews the relatively small number of studies that have examined the attitudes of patients, relatives, and clinicians toward the future potential of genetic testing for bipolar disorder, schizophrenia, and depression. Most have used the methodology of providing hypothetical future genetic testing scenarios, and examining responses to these. All of these studies have been—as now viewed in retrospect—somewhat simplistic in considering single genes in isolation, rather than the more likely possibility of multiple interacting genes of small effect. Only 2 studies have examined responses of individuals who have actually been genotyped for a putative risk allele.[58,59] The aim of this research has been to systematically ascertain the important issues and societal implications of genetic risk determination for these conditions prior to these technological advances becoming widely available.

In one of the earliest studies examining this issue, by Trippitelli and colleagues,[60] patients with bipolar disorder and their unaffected spouses were questioned on their knowledge and attitudes about treatment response rates for bipolar disorder, probability of inheritance, genetic testing, disclosure of genetic information, abortion, marriage, and childbearing. The researchers found that the overwhelming majority of the patients and spouses said that they would take advantage of genetic tests for bipolar disorder if such tests were available.[60] Most patients and spouses agreed that the benefits of knowing whether one carries a gene for bipolar disorder would outweigh the risks. A majority of respondents also felt that they would not abort a fetus that carried a gene for bipolar disorder. Furthermore, most patients and spouses agreed that the knowledge that one of them carried a gene variation associated with bipolar disorder would not have deterred them from marriage or childbearing.

Studies of patients with bipolar disorder and their relatives by the authors' own group have replicated and enlarged on the findings of Trippitelli and colleagues.[60] In a qualitative hypothesis-generating study, Meiser and colleagues[61] explored, in a sample of families with a high density of bipolar disorder: (1) attitudes to predictive genetic and prenatal testing, using different risk frames; (2) attributions for bipolar disorder, in particular the degree to which a genetic model is endorsed; and (3) the impact of these attributions on the perceived stigma of bipolar disorder. In-depth interviews were conducted with 21 members of families with a high density of bipolar disorder. Most participants reported being interested in genetic testing if it were to give a definitive answer, while expressed interest in testing was lower if it gave a probable answer only. Almost all participants stressed that a genetic susceptibility and environmental factors interacted. Most felt that a genetic explanation was likely to decrease the stigma associated with bipolar disorder, as it shifted the locus of control and responsibility away from the individual toward the role of heredity. Findings indicated that expressed interest in genetic testing depended on the certainty imparted by the test, and suggested that families with bipolar disorder were likely to benefit psychologically from information about the genetic basis of bipolar disorder.

The findings of this qualitative report were then examined in a quantitative study of a large number of families with multiple cases of bipolar disorder.[62,63] Meiser and colleagues[62] explored attitudes toward childbearing; causal attributions for bipolar disorder, in particular the degree to which a genetic model is endorsed and its impact on the perceived stigma of bipolar disorder; and predictors of psychological distress. Two hundred individuals (95 unaffected and 105 affected with bipolar disorder, schizoaffective disorder manic type, or recurrent major disorder) were surveyed. Thirty-five percent of participants reported being "not at all willing to have children" or "less willing to have children" as a result of having a strong family history of bipolar disorder. Being not at all or less willing to have children was significantly associated with perceived stigma of bipolar disorder, endorsement of a genetic model, and being affected. Among unaffected participants only, endorsement of a genetic model was strongly positively correlated with perceived stigma. Among affected participants, perceived stigma was significantly correlated with psychological distress. Meiser and colleagues[62] concluded that having a genetic explanation for bipolar disorder may exacerbate associated stigma among unaffected members from families with multiple cases of bipolar disorder, whereas it does not impact on perceived stigma among affected family members. Meiser and colleagues recommended that affected family members may benefit from interventions to ameliorate the adverse effects of perceived stigma.

In another article from the same study, Meiser and colleagues[63] reported on interest in genetic testing for gene variations associated with bipolar disorder and associated information needs. The percentage of participants reporting interest in genetic testing was associated with the degree of certainty with which any test would indicate the development of bipolar disorder. Interest in genetic testing was lowest (with 77% of participants indicating interest) given a 25% lifetime risk scenario, and highest (92%) for the 100% lifetime risk scenario. Eighty percent of participants indicated interest in genetic testing of their own children; of these 30% reported wanting their children tested at birth, and 33% in early childhood. Forty-one percent of participants reported that they would be interested in preimplantation genetic diagnosis, and 54% in prenatal testing. These results indicated that uptake of genetic testing for genotyping for low-risk alleles related to bipolar disorder is likely to be lower than for testing for high-penetrance gene mutations that follow Mendelian inheritance.

In one of the few studies to examine attitudes toward genetic testing for families and clinicians of patients with schizophrenia, DeLisi and Bertisch[64] reported that the majority of family members who completed the survey (83%) indicated that they would want to be tested if a genetic test were to become available, and that more than half (56%) would want prenatal testing. Similarly, more than half of clinicians (56%) would recommend genetic testing, though intriguingly, only 25% of researchers reported that genetic testing would be a useful tool in the future. Austin and colleagues[65] used a Web-based survey of visitors to a psychosis information Web site to investigate perceptions of genetic risk, associated effects on reproductive decisions, and attitudes toward genetic testing among unaffected relatives of individuals with psychosis. This survey found that overestimating the risk of inheritance was associated with reproductive decisions favoring fewer children, and more positive attitudes toward genetic testing.

In a recent study, Laegsgaard and colleagues[66] surveyed 397 persons with major depression, bipolar disorder, schizophrenia, or anxiety disorder. A large proportion of patients expressed an interest in participating in genetic testing, though there was little support for prenatal testing. Interest in testing was associated with being a parent and a belief that test results would enable them to be better prepared for "fighting the disorder." A lack of interest was associated with concern about difficulty in coping with the results of genetic tests.

The authors' group has also been interested in attitudes and understanding of genetic risk testing for depression, arising largely out of a focus on gene-environment interactions in the origins of this condition. In 2006, the authors[67] replicated the gene-environment interaction between the serotonin transporter gene and stressful life events in depression that had been reported by Caspi and colleagues.[68,69] Although recent meta-analyses have failed to confirm such an interaction,[70,71] the authors' study of response of individuals to being informed of their "depression risk genotype,"[59] and that of Green[58] in individuals at risk of Alzheimer disease, nonetheless provide the only evidence hitherto of the response of individuals to an actual (ie, nonhypothetical) situation of receiving results from genetic testing. The authors[59] assessed predictors of the impact of receiving individual genotype data in 128 participants in a study of gene-environment interaction in depression onset. Two-thirds decided to learn their individual genotype results (receivers), and prior to disclosure this decision was associated with a perception of greater benefit from receipt of the information. Receivers completing the 2-week and 3-month follow-up generally reported feeling pleased with the information and having had a more positive experience than distress. However, distress was related to genotype, with those with the "high-risk" s/s allele being most affected. Those who elected not to learn their results generally did so because of feared repercussions of being compelled to provide insurance companies or workplaces with this information. Overall, there was high interest in, and satisfaction with, learning about this putative depression risk genotype. The recent report of Green and colleagues[58] in which children of patients with Alzheimer disease responded positively to receipt of their APOE genotype is in accordance with the authors' findings with risk of depression.

The authors have since gone on to examine attitudes in the general community to such potential genetic testing for depression risk, using serotonin transporter genotyping as an example. This series of studies has involved both qualitative and quantitative investigations. An overview of the qualitative research that is now in press is presented here. Quantitative findings from a national survey of more than 1000 respondents from the general population will be reported elsewhere. Wilde and colleagues[72] examined this issue with 4 structured focus groups comprising a total of 36 participants. The majority of participants indicated interest in having a genetic test for susceptibility to major depression, if it were available. Having a family history of mental illness was cited as a major reason. After discussion of perceived positive and negative implications of predictive genetic testing, one-quarter changed their mind about having such a test. Fear of genetic discrimination and privacy issues predominantly influenced change of attitude. All participants still interested in having a predictive genetic test for risk of depression reported they would only do so through trusted medical professionals. Participants were unanimously against DTC genetic testing marketed via the Internet, although some would consider it if there was suitable protection against discrimination. The study highlighted the importance of general practitioner and public education about psychiatric genetics, and the availability of appropriate treatment and support services before implementation of future predictive genetic testing services.

In a second report from this qualitative investigation, Wilde and colleagues[73] evaluated the preparedness of individuals identified with a hypothetical genetic risk for a depressive disorder to ameliorate risk through cognitive or behavioral intervention. Participants predominantly viewed genetic risk factors for depression as predisposing rather than causal, with environmental risk factors acting as triggers. Hypothetical identification with a genetic variant suggesting predisposition to depression prompted strong interest in seeking further information about predictive genetic testing from medical professionals; willingness to reduce life stress, drugs, and alcohol intake; willingness to increase exercise; and willingness to undertake cognitive and behavioral interventions at a presymptomatic stage. Mixed views prevailed about the potential for individuals to modify stress. Preventive intervention at a presymptomatic stage of depression was viewed negatively by a minority of participants, due to a fatalistic attitude toward a genetic predisposition and attitudes that intervention was futile in the absence of symptoms.

There have also been a few studies on the attitudes of psychiatrists to the future possibility of genetic testing for mental disorders. In one of the first reports, Finn and colleagues[74] surveyed psychiatrists attending a continuing medical education course. These investigators found that whereas a majority (83%) considered it their role to discuss genetic information with patients and families, less than a quarter felt prepared or competent to do so. A substantial proportion indicated willingness to use hypothetical genetic tests for diagnostic clarification, as well as presymptomatic and prenatal risk prediction. Hoop and colleagues[75,76] have surveyed a random national sample of United States psychiatrists to assess attitudes, knowledge, and clinical experience regarding genetics. The psychiatrists surveyed reported positive attitudes toward incorporating genetics into psychiatric practice, but indicated insufficient training in genetics. Furthermore, they believed that genetic testing would benefit many patients and would dramatically change the way that psychiatry is practiced. A large majority supported laws to prevent discrimination based on genetic tests, and endorsed restrictions on the sale of genetic tests direct to consumers.

GENETIC TESTING IN PSYCHIATRY AND STIGMA

There has been a long-standing belief in psychiatry that delineation of the underpinning biological dysfunction, and genetic abnormalities in particular, will end the stigma associated with mental illnesses and resulting discrimination. This belief is consistent with the so-called attribution theory, that is, a genetic explanation (an uncontrollable biological cause) will decrease stigma by alleviating self-blame and increasing sympathy.[77] The alternative hypothesis is related to the idea of "genetic essentialism," that is, the belief that genes form the basis of our human identity and that a genetic explanation could increase stigma by increasing perceptions of "differentness" and seriousness, thereby increasing "social distance."[78] Phelan[79] has expanded on this alternative hypothesis, suggesting that proven genetic origins and genetic testing could in fact make the ill person seem "defective" or "physically distinct," "almost a different species." Certainly the response of unaffected family members in the authors' own study of bipolar disorder pedigrees has been consistent with genetic essentialism,[62] indicating that this will be a critical area for community education about psychiatric genetic testing in the future. Spriggs and colleagues[80] have argued that such a possible response to future genetic testing emphasizes the need for genetic research to be accompanied by social science research on the ways that genetic findings influence the lives of those who are tested.

SUMMARY: CURRENT AND FUTURE DIAGNOSTIC AND PREDICTIVE GENETIC TESTS FOR MENTAL ILLNESSES

Given the development of clear definitional criteria for genetic testing as detailed in this article, and the experience now gained in the identification of susceptibility genes for the major psychiatric disorders, an analysis of how these 2 dimensions intersect is warranted.

Assays to deliver genetic tests results for mental illness have extremely high reliability and accuracy, resulting in excellent analytical validity. In contrast, as discussed earlier, the clinical validity for genetic tests for mental illness is much less robust. The strength of evidence for the link between genotype and disease is, at best, weak for risk factor alleles. This limitation results in poor test performance characteristics, including low sensitivity and specificity and low positive and negative predictive values. Measures of clinical utility are also correspondingly low. The question of test legitimacy is an area in which there is considerable opinion, although to date there is a paucity of empirical data. The ability of the genetic test to achieve its intended purpose is limited due to a low measure of clinical validity, thus leading to low efficacy and a low effectiveness. Because of these low measures, the appropriateness of the clinical utility is also argued to be low, because the expected benefit will be small and the expected negative consequences may be significant.

For example, with respect to APOE testing as a predictor of the development of Alzheimer disease in subjects with mild cognitive impairment (MCI), one study[81] found that the PPV of APOE ε-4 for predicting conversion from MCI to Alzheimer disease was 0.48, and the negative predictive value was 0.65. These predictive values were at a level that did not support their utility as a diagnostic test for predicting such progression. Examples of clinically available genetic tests in general medicine with accepted clinical utility are detailed in **Box 2**.

Given the early stage of development of genetic tests for mental illness, the feasibility of test delivery may be difficult to determine until empirical data on acceptability to meet the desires and expectations of patients and their families become available. A genetic test, or set of tests, with a high clinical validity and utility would presumably

---

Box 2
Examples of adult-onset disorders for which genetic testing is clinically available in many developed countries

Cancer syndromes

Hereditary breast/ovarian cancer syndromes, hereditary nonpolyposis colorectal cancer, familial adenomatous polyposis, Li-Fraumeni syndrome, ataxia telangiectasia, multiple endocrine neoplasia type 2

Neurodegenerative disorders

Huntington disease, hereditary cerebral hemorrhages with amyloidosis, familial early-onset Alzheimer disease, hereditary Pick disease

Progressive muscle disorders

Myotonic muscular dystrophy, Duchenne muscular dystrophy

Cardiovascular disorders

Hereditary hemorrhagic telangiectasia, hereditary hypertrophic cardiomyopathy

Genitourinary disorders

Polycystic kidney disease

Metabolic disorders

Familial hypercholesterolemia, hereditary hemochromatosis, diabetes mellitus type 1

Data from Meiser B, Gleeson MA, Tucker KM. Psychological impact of genetic testing for adult-onset disorders. An update for clinicians. Med J Aust 2000;172(3):126–9.

---

have a strong economic efficiency and optimality. However, as argued earlier, the authors' current assessment is that genetic tests for mental illness are of relatively low clinical validity and utility, and thus would have a low economic efficiency and optimality. Equity is unlikely to be a significant issue for a test of low clinical validity and utility.

Review of each of these criteria suggests that there are currently very limited reasons to advocate for the widespread introduction of genetic tests for diagnostic and predictive use in mental illnesses, and the same is true for other complex disorders. However, given the ability to market a new technology without the need to provide a clear evidentiary base, it may be that such tests find relatively widespread interest in the general population, perhaps as an example of individual empowerment that the Internet has provided in a range of health care behaviors.

In conclusion, it is the authors' opinion that there is currently no evidence justifying the marketing of predictive or diagnostic genetic tests for any mental illness. Growing evidence emanating from GWAS suggests that these conditions are caused by multiple common allele variants, and an uncertain number of rare allelic variants (both SNPs and CNVs). Future genetic testing is therefore likely to comprise algorithms involving both multiple low penetrant common and rare gene variants, and screening for rare highly penetrant de novo CNVs (although the lack of disease specificity for the latter is of concern).[82] Even if a firm evidence base for the clinical validity of such testing is achieved, widespread availability should not occur until clinical utility is confirmed. Furthermore, before such tests are marketed, specialized psychiatric genetic counseling programs will need to be developed[83] in conjunction with clinical and community education programs to minimize the possibility that such testing might increase stigma.

REFERENCES

1. Couzin J. Science and commerce. Gene tests for psychiatric risk polarize researchers. Science 2008;319(5861):274–7.
2. Barrett TB, Hauger RL, Kennedy JL, et al. Evidence that a single nucleotide polymorphism in the promoter of the G protein receptor kinase 3 gene is associated with bipolar disorder. Mol Psychiatry 2003;8(5):546–57.
3. Barrett TB, Emberto JE, Nievergelt CM, et al. Further evidence for association of GRK3 to bipolar disorder suggests a second disease mutation. Psychiatr Genet 2007;17(6):315–22.
4. Zhou X, Barrett TB, Kelsoe JR. Promoter variant in the GRK3 gene associated with bipolar disorder alters gene expression. Biol Psychiatry 2008;64(2):104–10.
5. Prata DP, Breen G, Munro J, et al. Bipolar 1 disorder is not associated with the RGS4, PRODH, COMT and GRK3 genes. Psychiatr Genet 2006;16(6):229–30.
6. Braff DL, Freedman R. Clinically responsible genetic testing in neuropsychiatric patients: a bridge too far and too soon. Am J Psychiatry 2008;165(8):952–5.
7. Burmeister M, McInnis MG, Zöllner S. Psychiatric genetics: progress amid controversy. Nat Rev Genet 2008;9:527–40.
8. Psychiatric GWAS, Consortium Coordinating Committee. Genomewide association studies: history, rationale, and prospects for psychiatric disorders. Am J Psychiatry 2009;166(5):540–56.
9. International Schizophrenia Consortium. Common polygenic variation contributes to risk of schizophrenia and bipolar disorder. Nature 2009;460(7256):748–52.
10. Shi J, Levinson DF, Duan J, et al. Common variants on chromosome 6p22.1 are associated with schizophrenia. Nature 2009;460(7256):753–7.
11. Stefansson H, Rujescu D, Cichon S, et al. Large recurrent microdeletions associated with schizophrenia. Nature 2008;455(7210):232–6.
12. International Schizophrenia Consortium. Rare chromosomal deletions and duplications increase risk of schizophrenia. Nature 2008;455(7210):237–41.
13. Bassett AS, Marshall CR, Lionel AC, et al. Copy number variations and risk for schizophrenia in 22q11.2 deletion syndrome. Hum Mol Genet 2008;17(24):4045–53.
14. Sebat J, Lakshmi B, Malhotra D, et al. Strong association of de novo copy number mutations with autism. Science 2007;316(5823):445–9.
15. Ferreira MA, O'Donovan MC, Meng YA, et al. Collaborative genome-wide association analysis supports a role for ANK3 and CACNA1C in bipolar disorder. Nat Genet 2008;40(9):1056–8.
16. Holmans P, Green EK, Pahwa JS, et al. Gene ontology analysis of GWA study data sets provides insights into the biology of bipolar disorder. Am J Hum Genet 2009;85(1):13–24.
17. Burke W, Zimmern R. Moving beyond ACCE: an expanded framework for genetic test evaluation. Cambridge (UK): PHG Foundation; 2007.
18. Melzer D, Hogarth S, Liddell K, et al. Genetic tests for common diseases: new insights, old concerns. BMJ 2008;336(7644):590–3.
19. Wellcome Trust Case Control Consortium. Genome-wide association study of 14,000 cases of seven common diseases and 3,000 shared controls. Nature 2007;447(7145):661–78.
20. Scott LJ, Muglia P, Kong XQ, et al. Genome-wide association and meta-analysis of bipolar disorder in individuals of European ancestry. Proc Natl Acad Sci U S A 2009;106(18):7501–6.

21. Stefansson H, Ophoff RA, Steinberg S, et al. Common variants conferring risk of schizophrenia. Nature 2009;460(7256):744–7.
22. Hardy J, Singleton A. Genomewide association studies and human disease. N Engl J Med 2009;360(17):1759–68.
23. Goldstein DB. Common genetic variation and human traits. N Engl J Med 2009; 360(17):1696–8.
24. Hirschhorn JN. Genomewide association studies—illuminating biologic pathways. N Engl J Med 2009;360(17):1699–701.
25. Kraft P, Hunter DJ. Genetic risk prediction—are we there yet? N Engl J Med 2009; 360(17):1701–3.
26. Weedon MN, Lango H, Lindgren CM, et al. Genome-wide association analysis identifies 20 loci that influence adult height. Nat Genet 2008;40(5):575–83.
27. Janssens AC, van Duijn CM. Genome-based prediction of common diseases: advances and prospects. Hum Mol Genet 2008;17(R2):R166–73.
28. Wray NR, Goddard ME, Visscher PM. Prediction of individual genetic risk to disease from genome-wide association studies. Genome Res 2007;17(10): 1520–8.
29. Hudson K, Javitt G, Burke W, et al. ASHG Statement* on direct-to-consumer genetic testing in the United States. Obstet Gynecol 2007;110(6):1392–5.
30. Hogarth S, Javitt G, Melzer D. The current landscape for direct-to-consumer genetic testing: legal, ethical, and policy issues. Annu Rev Genomics Hum Genet 2008;9:161–82.
31. Shetty P. Home DNA test kits cause controversy. Lancet 2008;371(9626): 1739–40.
32. Schmidt C. Regulators weigh risks of consumer genetic tests. Nat Biotechnol 2008;26(2):145–6.
33. Hudson KJG, Burke W, Byres P, et al. ASHG Statement on direct-to-consumer genetic testing in the United States. Am J Hum Genet 2007;81:635–7.
34. Human Genetics Commission. More genes direct: a report on developments in the availability, marketing and regulation of genetic tests supplied directly to the public. London (UK): Human Genetics Commission; 2007.
35. Abbing HD. Genetic testing for health care purposes, a Council of Europe Protocol. Eur J Health Law 2008;15(4):353–9.
36. Patch C, Sequeros J, Cornel MC. Genetic horoscopes: is it all in the genes? Points for regulatory control of direct-to-consumer genetic testing. Eur J Hum Genet 2009;17:857–9.
37. Janssens AC, Gwinn M, Bradley LA, et al. A critical appraisal of the scientific basis of commercial genomic profiles used to assess health risks and personalize health interventions. Am J Hum Genet 2008;82(3):593–9.
38. Zonno KD, Terry SF. Registry of genetic tests: a critical stepping stone to improving the genetic testing system. Genet Test Mol Biomarkers 2009;13(2): 153–4.
39. Hudson KL. Prohibiting genetic discrimination. N Engl J Med 2007;356(20): 2021–3.
40. Hudson KL, Holohan MK, Collins FS. Keeping pace with the times—the Genetic Information Nondiscrimination Act of 2008. N Engl J Med 2008;358(25):2661–3.
41. Arribas-Ayllon M, Sarangi S, Clarke A. The micropolitics of responsibility vis-a-vis autonomy: parental accounts of childhood genetic testing and (non)disclosure. Sociol Health Illn 2008;30(2):255–71.
42. Borry P, Evers-Kiebooms G, Cornel MC, et al. Genetic testing in asymptomatic minors. Eur J Hum Genet 2009;17:711–9.

43. Hathaway F, Burns E, Ostrer H. Consumers' desire towards current and prospective reproductive genetic testing. J Genet Couns 2009;18(2):137–46.
44. Rose S. The rise of neurogenetic determinism. Nature 1995;373(6513):380–2.
45. Rose SP. Neurogenetic determinism and the new euphenics. BMJ 1998; 317(7174):1707–8.
46. Craddock N, Jones IR, Kent L. Neurogenetic determinism and the new euphenics. Psychosocial and ethical issues in psychiatric genetics require constructive debate. BMJ 1999;318(7196):1488 [author reply: 1489].
47. Huntingtons Disease Collaborative Research Group. A novel gene containing a trinucleotide repeat that is expanded and unstable on Huntington's disease chromosomes. Cell 1993;72:971–83.
48. Meiser B, Dunn S. Psychological impact of genetic testing for Huntington's disease: an update of the literature. J Neurol Neurosurg Psychiatr 2000;69(5):574–8.
49. Klitzman R, Thorne D, Williamson J, et al. The roles of family members, health care workers, and others in decision-making processes about genetic testing among individuals at risk for Huntington disease. Genet Med 2007;9(6):358–71.
50. Klitzman R, Thorne D, Williamson J, et al. Disclosures of Huntington disease risk within families: patterns of decision-making and implications. Am J Med Genet A 2007;143A(16):1835–49.
51. Moeschler JB. Medical genetics diagnostic evaluation of the child with global developmental delay or intellectual disability. Curr Opin Neurol 2008;21(2):117–22.
52. Moeschler JB. Genetic evaluation of intellectual disabilities. Semin Pediatr Neurol 2008;15(1):2–9.
53. Lintas C, Persico AM. Autistic phenotypes and genetic testing: state-of-the-art for the clinical geneticist. J Med Genet 2009;46(1):1–8.
54. Munger KM, Gill CJ, Ormond KE, et al. The next exclusion debate: assessing technology, ethics, and intellectual disability after the Human Genome Project. Ment Retard Dev Disabil Res Rev 2007;13(2):121–8.
55. Farrer LA, Cupples LA, Haines JL, et al. Effects of age, sex, and ethnicity on the association between apolipoprotein E genotype and Alzheimer disease. A meta-analysis. APOE and Alzheimer Disease Meta Analysis Consortium. JAMA 1997; 278(16):1349–56.
56. Roberts JS, LaRusse SA, Katzen H, et al. Reasons for seeking genetic susceptibility testing among first-degree relatives of people with Alzheimer disease. Alzheimer Dis Assoc Disord 2003;17(2):86–93.
57. Roberts JS, Barber M, Brown TM, et al. Who seeks genetic susceptibility testing for Alzheimer's disease? Findings from a multisite, randomized clinical trial. Genet Med 2004;6(4):197–203.
58. Green RC, Roberts JS, Cupples LA, et al. Disclosure of APOE genotype for risk of Alzheimer's disease. N Engl J Med 2009;361(3):245–54.
59. Wilhelm K, Meiser B, Mitchell PB, et al. Issues concerning feedback about genetic testing and risk of depression. Br J Psychiatry 2009;194(5):404–10.
60. Trippitelli CL, Jamison KR, Folstein MF, et al. Pilot study on patients' and spouses' attitudes toward potential genetic testing for bipolar disorder. Am J Psychiatry 1998;155(7):899–904.
61. Meiser B, Mitchell PB, McGirr H, et al. Implications of genetic risk information in families with a high density of bipolar disorder: an exploratory study. Soc Sci Med 2005;60(1):109–18.
62. Meiser B, Mitchell PB, Kasparian NA, et al. Attitudes towards childbearing, causal attributions for bipolar disorder and psychological distress: a study of families with multiple cases of bipolar disorder. Psychol Med 2007;37(11):1601–11.

63. Meiser B, Kasparian NA, Mitchell PB, et al. Attitudes to genetic testing in families with multiple cases of bipolar disorder. Genet Test 2008;12(2): 233–43.
64. DeLisi LE, Bertisch H. A preliminary comparison of the hopes of researchers, clinicians, and families for the future ethical use of genetic findings on schizophrenia. Am J Med Genet B Neuropsychiatr Genet 2006;141B(1):110–5.
65. Austin JC, Smith GN, Honer WG. The genomic era and perceptions of psychotic disorders: genetic risk estimation, associations with reproductive decisions and views about predictive testing. Am J Med Genet B Neuropsychiatr Genet 2006; 141B(8):926–8.
66. Laegsgaard MM, Kristensen AS, Mors O. Potential consumers' attitudes toward psychiatric genetic research and testing and factors influencing their intentions to test. Genet Test Mol Biomarkers 2009;13(1):57–65.
67. Wilhelm K, Mitchell PB, Niven H, et al. Life events, first depression onset and the serotonin transporter gene. Br J Psychiatry 2006;188:210–5.
68. Caspi A, Moffitt TE. Gene-environment interactions in psychiatry: joining forces with neuroscience. Nat Rev Neurosci 2006;7(7):583–90.
69. Caspi A, Sugden K, Moffitt TE, et al. Influence of life stress on depression: moderation by a polymorphism in the 5-HTT gene. Science 2003;301(5631): 386–9.
70. Munafo MR, Durrant C, Lewis G, et al. Gene X environment interactions at the serotonin transporter locus. Biol Psychiatry 2009;65(3):211–9.
71. Risch N, Herrell R, Lehner T, et al. Interaction between the serotonin transporter gene (5-HTTLPR), stressful life events, and risk of depression: a meta-analysis. JAMA 2009;301(23):2462–71.
72. Wilde A, Meiser, B, Mitchell, PB. Public interest in predictive genetic testing for susceptibility to major depression. European Journal of Human Genetics 2009 [Epub ahead of print].
73. Wilde A, Meiser, B, Mitchell, PB, et al. Public attitudes towards mental health intervention for healthy people on the basis of genetic susceptibility. Australian and New Zealand Journal of Psychiatry, in press.
74. Finn CT, Wilcox MA, Korf BR, et al. Psychiatric genetics: a survey of psychiatrists' knowledge, opinions, and practice patterns. J Clin Psychiatry 2005; 66(7):821–30.
75. Hoop JG, Roberts LW, Green Hammond KA, et al. Psychiatrists' attitudes regarding genetic testing and patient safeguards: a preliminary study. Genet Test 2008;12(2):245–52.
76. Hoop JG, Roberts LW, Green Hammond KA, et al. Psychiatrists' attitudes, knowledge, and experience regarding genetics: a preliminary study. Genet Med 2008; 10(6):439–49.
77. Phelan JC. Geneticization of deviant behavior and consequences for stigma: the case of mental illness. J Health Soc Behav 2005;46(4):307–22.
78. Nelkin D, Lindee MS. "Genes made me do it": the appeal of biological explanations. Politics Life Sciences 1996;15(1):95–7.
79. Phelan JC. Genetic bases of mental illness—a cure for stigma? Trends Neurosci 2002;25(8):430–1.
80. Spriggs M, Olsson CA, Hall W. How will information about the genetic risk of mental disorders impact on stigma? Aust N Z J Psychiatry 2008;42(3):214–20.
81. Hsiung GY, Sadovnick AD, Feldman H. Apolipoprotein E epsilon4 genotype as a risk factor for cognitive decline and dementia: data from the Canadian Study of Health and Aging. CMAJ 2004;171(8):863–7.

82. Collier D, Vassos E, Holden S. Advances in the genetics of schizophrenia: will high risk copy number variants be useful in clinical genetics or diagnosis? F1000 Medicine Reports 2009;1:61.

83. Austin JC, Honer WG. The potential impact of genetic counseling for mental illness. Clin Genet 2005;67(2):134–42.

Index

NOTE: Page numbers of article titles are in **boldface** type.

A

Acetylcholine receptor (CHRNA4), in ADHD, 169
Addiction(s), alcohol, 108–113
    cocaine, 118–119
    genetics of, **107–124**
    nicotine, 108, 113–118
    substance use disorders and, 107–108
Age, as confounding bias, 25
Alcohol dependence, acetaldehyde in, 109
    ADH1B*2 in, 109
    ADH variants in, protective effects of, 111, 113
    alcohol metabolizing enzymes in, 109–110
    aldehyde dehydrogenase deficiency in, 108–109
    ALDH2*2 allele in, environment effect on, 109
        on *ADH1B* gene, 109
    ALDH2 gene in, 109
    chromosome 4 and, GABA receptor gene cluster in, 111–112
    chromosome 4 in, ADH genes on, 109–110
    environmental component in, 108
    gamma-aminobutyric acid receptors genes in, 111–112
    genetics of, 108–113
    heritable component in, 108
Antidepressants, candidate gene studies of, 183–184
    GWAS of, 183–184, 186
    history of, 182–183
    pharmacodynamic studies of, *BDNF* in, 185–186
        5HTT variants in, 185
        TPH in, 185–186
    pharmacogenetic studies of response to, 183–184
    pharmacokinetic studies of, 183, 185
        CYP2C19 in, 183–185
        CYP2D6 in, 183–185
Antipsychotics, candidate gene studies of response to, 188–189
    GWAS of, 191–192
        ANKS1B in, 191
        CERKL in, 192
        CNTNAP5 in, 191
        for response to, 189
        NPAS3 in, 192
        SLCO3A1 in, 192
    history of, 188

Psychiatr Clin N Am 33 (2010) 245–255
doi:10.1016/S0193-953X(10)00009-2
0193-953X/10/$ – see front matter © 2010 Elsevier Inc. All rights reserved.

psych.theclinics.com

Moving?

Make sure your subscription moves with you!

To notify us of your new address, find your **Clinics Account Number** (located on your mailing label above your name), and contact customer service at:

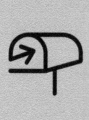

Email: journalscustomerservice-usa@elsevier.com

800-654-2452 (subscribers in the U.S. & Canada)
314-447-8871 (subscribers outside of the U.S. & Canada)

Fax number: 314-447-8029

Elsevier Health Sciences Division
Subscription Customer Service
3251 Riverport Lane
Maryland Heights, MO 63043

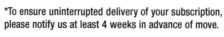

Printed and bound by CPI Group (UK) Ltd, Croydon, CR0 4YY

03/10/2024

01040450-0007